Editors:

CECILIA M. PEMBERTON, R.D.
CLIFFORD F. GASTINEAU, M.D., Ph.D.

Editorial Committee:

CARL F. ANDERSON, M.D.
JEANNE L. GILDEA, M.A., R.D.
KAREN E. MOXNESS, M.S., R.D.
JAMES C. ROSE, M.S., R.D.
SISTER MOIRA TIGHE, M.S., R.D.
JULIETTE VERNET, R.D.

Fifth Edition

MAYO CLINIC DIET MANUAL

A Handbook of Dietary Practices

PREPARED BY THE DIETETIC STAFFS OF
THE MAYO CLINIC
ROCHESTER METHODIST HOSPITAL
AND
ST. MARYS HOSPITAL OF
ROCHESTER, MINNESOTA

1981   W. B. SAUNDERS COMPANY
PHILADELPHIA · LONDON · TORONTO · SYDNEY

W. B. Saunders Company: West Washington Square
Philadelphia, Pa. 19105

1 St. Anne's Road
Eastbourne, East Sussex BN21 3UN, England

1 Goldthorne Avenue
Toronto, Ontario M8Z 5T9, Canada

Library of Congress Cataloging in Publication Data
Main entry under title:

Mayo Clinic diet manual.

Previous eds. by Mayo Clinic, Committee on Dietetics.
1. Diet therapy. 2. Diet in disease. 3. Mayo Clinic, Rochester, Minn. I. Pemberton, Cecilia M.
II. Gastineau, Clifford F. III. Mayo Clinic, Rochester, Minn. IV. Rochester, Minn. Methodist
Hospital. V. Saint Marys Hospital, Rochester, Minn. VI. Mayo Clinic, Rochester, Minn. Committee
on Dietetics. Mayo Clinic diet manual. [DNLM: 1. Diet therapy. WB 400 M473m]
RM219.M29 1981   615.8'54   77-88298

ISBN 0-7216-6212-9

Cover illustration by John W. Desley, Medical Illustrator

Mayo Clinic Diet Manual   ISBN 0-7216-6212-9

Last digit is the print number: 9 8 7 6 5 4 3 2 1

PREFACE

This edition of the Mayo Clinic Diet Manual reflects changes in the practice of dietetics and the greater awareness of nutritional principles by both physicians and dietitians. Diets are less likely to be regarded as specific treatment for a disease, and the dietitian's task is no longer solely a translation of diet orders into the serving of a predetermined pattern of foods. Physicians have become more aware of the influence of nutritional status on the disease process and are less rigid in prescribing specific diets. Consultations between physicians and dietitians are more common and more effective. These trends are desirable and should be cultivated.

In this edition of the Mayo Clinic Diet Manual, the rationale for each of the diets is provided. The discussion of the nature of the disorders and the dietary treatments is addressed equally to the physician and to the dietitian. By providing a rationale for the use of a diet, we hope that diet therapy can be carried out with more appropriate choices of kinds and degrees of control of dietary components. Some diet regimens are based on traditional dietary practices rather than on documented evidence. For this reason, the discussion of some diets does not provide a clear justification for them. We hope that when the next edition is prepared, investigators and practitioners will have recognized and remedied some of these deficiences.

Weight reduction diets variously called "Mayo Diet," "Mayo Clinic Two-Week Diet," or "Mayo Clinic Egg Diet" have been circulated widely throughout the United States. THESE DIETS DID NOT ORIGINATE AT THE MAYO CLINIC AND HAVE NEVER BEEN USED OR SANCTIONED BY THE CLINIC OR ANY OF ITS ASSOCIATED HOSPITALS. The recommended dietary programs for obesity are outlined on page 48.

The collaborative effort and counsel of all dietitians of the Mayo Clinic, Rochester Methodist Hospital, and St. Marys Hospital of Rochester have made this edition possible. The following dietitians have made major contributions in particular areas: Bill Badgley, vegetarian diets; Joan Gartner, lactose and gluten control; Janice Graner, protein control in renal disease; Patricia Hodgson, hyperlipoproteinemia; Diane Huse, pediatrics, anorexia nervosa, nutritional needs of the athlete, and dietary management of the patient with cancer; Ann Klause, pregnancy and lactation; LaVonne

Oenning, geriatrics and postgastrectomy dumping syndrome; and Joan Vogel, sodium control. We wish to thank all the physicians who reviewed material for this manual, particularly C. R. Fleming, L. K. Kvols, A. R. Lucas, L. H. Smith, and R. M. Tucker. We are indebted to Jane Haeflinger for typing copies that were circulated to physicians, dietitians, and committee members.

Cecilia Pemberton and Clifford F. Gastineau

Rochester, Minnesota

CONTENTS

SECTION 4   DIET DURING PREGNANCY AND LACTATION

SECTION 5   NORMAL NUTRITION AND THERAPEUTIC DIETS FOR INFANTS AND CHILDREN

SECTION 6 FORMULAS, FOOD SUPPLEMENTS, AND TOTAL PARENTERAL NUTRITION

SECTION 7 OTHER DIETARY PROGRAMS

APPENDIX

SECTION 1

GENERAL INFORMATION

NUTRITIONAL ADEQUACY

The Recommended Dietary Allowances (1974) of the National Research Council were used as a guide in assessing nutritional adequacy of the diets.

Nutrient composition for a 1-week cycle of menus was determined according to food composition values listed in United States Department of Agriculture Handbook No. 456 and data from food product manufacturers. Recommended Dietary Allowances for men and women from 23 to 50 years old were averaged and used as a reference point for assessing nutritional adequacy, except in the pregnancy and pediatric sections. Diets can be considered to provide at least 75% of the Recommended Dietary Allowances for nutrients analyzed, unless otherwise specified. A statement on nutritional content indicates a potential risk of inadequacy, especially if the diet is to be used for a prolonged period.

As proposed by the National Research Council, the Recommended Dietary Allowances should be used only as a guide for planning and evaluating diets. Recommended Dietary Allowances are intended to be used not as absolute requirements but rather as guidelines of acceptable nutrient intakes. Allowances (with the exception of calories) were estimated to "exceed the requirements of most individuals, and thereby ensure that the needs of nearly all are met."* The Recommended Dietary Allowances were not intended to cover the needs of those who are ill. However, for lack of more suitable guidelines, Recommended Dietary Allowances were used in evaluating the therapeutic diets presented in this manual.

Tables of approximate composition for specific nutrients are included with discussions of general hospital, clear liquid, full liquid, and soft diets. These values represent average composition of the diet from menu analysis for 1 week.

The 1979 Recommended Dietary Allowances became available during preparation of this manuscript and are given in the Appendix. Conclusions on nutritional adequacy are unchanged.

---

*National Research Council: Recommended Dietary Allowances. Eighth edition. Washington, D.C., National Academy of Sciences, 1974, p. 3.

SELECTED BIBLIOGRAPHY

Harper, A.E.: Recommended dietary allowances: Are they what we think they are? J. Am. Diet. Assoc., 64:151-156, 1974.
Hegsted, D.M.: Dietary standards. J. Am. Diet. Assoc., 66:13–21, 1975.
Hegsted, D.M.: Dietary standards (editorial). N. Engl. J. Med., 292:915–917, 1975.

PHYSICIAN'S GUIDELINES FOR ORDERING DIETS

The purpose of a diet order is to convey the intention of the physician to the dietitian. In formulating a diet order or diet prescription, one must consider the nature of the disease, what can be accomplished by the diet, and whether the diet will be accepted by the patient. Characteristics of a good diet order are as follows:

1. A diet order should be brief and specific. It should be concise enough to be conveyed by a few words or sentences.

2. A diet order should be clear and unambiguous. If the order can be interpreted to have a meaning other than that intended, it has been poorly written.

3. A diet order should be complete. All dietary modifications or restrictions must be repeated each time a diet order is altered. When changes are made in one portion of the diet order, it should not be assumed that the dietitian will automatically maintain the other modifications.

4. A diet order should be internally consistent. One dietary modification should not conflict with another.

5. If the diet order includes several modifications, the most important one should be listed first to give it priority.

6. A diet order should not be unnecessarily restrictive or complex. Although some disease states require very restrictive dietary measures, less stringent restrictions often accomplish what in intended.

7. Frequent changes in diet orders should be avoided. Although changing circumstances in the hospital may require dietary modifications, early in the hospital stay one should attempt to formulate the diet that will be used on dismissal. Early formulation gives the dietetic staff time to carry out instructions and gives the patient a better understanding of personal long-term dietary needs.

The degree of dietary control should be specified as clearly as possible. The term "minimum" indicates that the diet provides as small an amount of the substance as possible without making the diet distinctly inconvenient or unpalatable. "Low," "limited," and "restricted" are used to indicate an intermediate reduction in the amount of the substance in the diet. The terms "generous" and "high" indicate an increase of the substance in the diet that can be achieved with reasonable convenience. A range for the quantity implied by these general terms is specified, when practical, with the diet.

It should be the responsibility of the physician to inform the patient of the diet restrictions. If aware of the importance with which the physician regards the dietary modifications, the patient is more likely to accept this change in manner of living.

SECTION 2

NORMAL NUTRITION

GENERAL HOSPITAL DIET

The general hospital diet is intended for the adult patient who does not need specific dietary modifications. Menus are either selected by or planned for the patient according to food preferences. In either situation, the diet is aimed at supplying appropriate amounts of protein, calories, and other nutrients.

There are two general philosophies on the composition of a general hospital diet. One focuses on educating the patient in the principles of nutrition by example, and the other focuses on providing food the patient is willing and able to eat. Usually, a compromise is reached between these philosophies, with the emphasis adjusted to best meet the needs of a particular patient.

Some consider implementation of a diet based on control of sodium, cholesterol, and fat intake to foster advantageous health practices. If the patient is able to eat adequately, hospitalization may provide an opportune time to teach these principles to the patient. Either the American Heart Association General Dietary Recommendations or the Dietary Goals for the United States, U.S. Senate Select Committee on Nutrition and Human Needs (see Appendix, page 301) may be used as a guide. If such modifications are considered desirable, the physician should notify the dietitian, who will discuss them with the patient. The Mayo Clinic does not specifically endorse either of these formulations. Dietary restrictions are best adapted to the needs of the individual.

In many instances, hospitalization is not an appropriate time to impose undue dietary restrictions, especially if the modifications keep the patient from consuming enough protein and calories to meet the nutritional needs of convalescence from illness, injury, or surgery. The importance of adequate and appropriate food intake during these situations may warrant compromise in traditional meal-planning practices.

PHYSICIANS: HOW TO ORDER DIETS

The diet order should indicate general diet.

APPROXIMATE COMPOSITION*

Calories	Protein g	Fat g	Carbohydrate g	Sodium† meq	Potassium meq
2,030	80	80	250	125	85

*Amounts represent the diet as planned for or selected by most patients. There will be some variation according to individual food choices and preferences.
†Value is for the amount of sodium in food and for salt added in preparation; salt added at the table is not included.

SUGGESTED DAILY FOOD EXCHANGES*

Milk	Vegetables	Fruit	Starch	Meat	Fat	Dessert	Sweets
2	3–4	2–3	6	5	9	1	2–4

*Amounts represent the diet as planned for or selected by most patients. There will be some variation according to individual food choices and preferences.

GENERAL DIET WITH CONSISTENCY MODIFICATIONS

In this category of diets, the general hospital diet is modified in consistency or texture, or both, to accommodate acceptance and tolerance by the patient.

CLEAR LIQUID DIET

GENERAL DESCRIPTION

The diet consists of clear fluids and juices that provide little residue and are easily absorbed.

INDICATIONS AND RATIONALE

The diet is of use when one must severely restrict undigested material in the gastrointestinal tract because of temporarily decreased function. It is most often used as the first phase of postoperative dietary progressions and as dietary preparation for colon surgery.

NUTRITIONAL ADEQUACY

In comparison with the Recommended Dietary Allowances, this diet is very low in all nutrients, although it does provide some calories and vitamin C. Low residue or chemically defined formula diets (see page 143) are desirable if prolonged use of clear liquid feedings is indicated.

PHYSICIANS: HOW TO ORDER DIETS

The diet order should indicate **clear liquid diet**. The clear liquid diet may be ordered with other diet modifications, such as "clear liquid, no gastric stimulants."

*APPROXIMATE COMPOSITION**

Calories	Protein *g*	Fat *g*	Carbohydrate *g*	Sodium† *meq*	Potassium *meq*
400	5	trace	95	65	20

*Composition will vary, depending on the quantity of liquids actually served to and consumed by the patient.

†Value is for amount of salt used in preparation of food; salt added at the table is not included.

FOODS TO ALLOW AND FOODS TO AVOID

Food Groups	Allow	Avoid
Beverage	Coffee; tea; decaffeinated coffee; cereal beverage; carbonated beverage; artificially flavored fruit drink	All others
Meat	None	All
Fat	None	All
Milk	None	All
Starch	None	All
Vegetable	Tomato juice	All others
Fruit	All fruit juices	All others
Soup	Clear fat-free broth; bouillon	All others
Dessert	Gelatin; fruit ice; Popsicle	All others
Sweets	Sugar; hard candy; honey	All others
Miscellaneous	Salt	All others

SAMPLE MENU PATTERN

Breakfast*	Noon Meal*	OR	Evening Meal*
Juice†	Broth		Broth
Beverage	Juice†		Juice†
	Gelatin		Fruit ice
	Beverage		Beverage
Between-meal Feedings: Available if requested.			

*The size of the meal is usually kept small, since most postoperative patients accept only a small volume of liquids at first.

†Some postoperative patients are nauseated at first and do not tolerate juices. It may be advisable to avoid citrus juice and tomato juice at the first feeding. If nausea continues, the physician may want to request a clear liquid diet without juice.

FULL LIQUID DIET

GENERAL DESCRIPTION

This diet includes liquids and semisolid foods.

INDICATIONS AND RATIONALE

The diet is frequently used as an intermediate step in postoperative dietary regimens or other situations in which gastrointestinal function is moderately reduced. The diet may also be indicated for the individual who has difficulty chewing and swallowing solid foods.

NUTRITIONAL ADEQUACY

In comparison with the Recommended Dietary Allowances, this diet is very low in all nutrients, with the exception of calcium and ascorbic acid. The nutritional adequacy can easily be improved through the use of dietary supplements (see page 246).

PHYSICIANS: HOW TO ORDER DIETS

The diet order should indicate **full liquid diet**. The full liquid diet may be ordered with other diet modifications, such as "full liquid, no gastric stimulants."

APPROXIMATE COMPOSITION*

Calories	Protein g	Fat g	Carbohydrate g	Sodium† meq	Potassium meq
1,500	50	55	205	110	65

*Composition will vary, depending on the quantity of liquids actually served to and consumed by the patient.

†Value is for amount of salt used in preparation of food; salt added at the table is not included.

FOODS TO ALLOW AND FOODS TO AVOID

Food Groups	Allow	Avoid
Beverage	Coffee; tea; decaffeinated coffee; cereal beverage; carbonated beverage; artificially flavored fruit drink	None
Meat	Dried egg powder in milk drinks; pureed meat in soup	All others
Fat	Butter; margarine; cream	All others
Milk	Milk and milk beverages; yogurt without seeds or whole fruit	All others
Starch	Cooked cereal	Dry cereal; all others
Vegetable	All juices; pureed vegetables in soup	All others
Fruit	All juices	All others
Soup	Broth; bouillon; strained cream soup	All others
Dessert	Gelatin; sherbet; ice cream; custard; pudding	All others; any with coconut, nuts, or whole fruit
Sweets	Sugar; honey; candy	All others; any with coconut, nuts, or whole fruit
Miscellaneous	Salt; pepper; mild spices*; cocoa; chocolate syrup	All others

*Inclusion of spices and seasonings may be modified according to the tolerance and usual food preferences of the patient.

SAMPLE MENU PATTERN

Breakfast		Noon Meal		OR	Evening Meal	
Juice	1 serving	Juice	1 serving		Juice	1 serving
Cooked cereal	1 serving	Strained			Strained	
Milk*	1 cup	cream soup	1 serving		cream soup	1 serving
Beverage		Gelatin	1 serving		Ice cream	1 serving
		Milk*	1 cup		Milk*	1 cup
		Beverage			Beverage	

Between-meal Feedings: Available if requested.

*Although milk is allowed as a beverage, many patients do not tolerate milk well after surgery.

SOFT DIET

GENERAL DESCRIPTION

This diet is similar to the general diet. It consists of foods that are tender but not ground or pureed. Whole meat, cooked vegetables, and fruits are allowed. There are some limitations in seasoning.

INDICATIONS AND RATIONALE

The diet is frequently used as an intermediate step in postoperative dietary regimens. It may be of both psychologic and physiologic advantage when used as a transition diet for the postoperative patient or other individual whose diet has previously been restricted in amount and consistency of foods. The diet also may be useful for the debilitated patient to facilitate ease in eating.

PHYSICIANS: HOW TO ORDER DIETS

The diet order should indicate **soft diet.**

APPROXIMATE COMPOSITION

Calories	Protein g	Fat g	Carbohydrate g	Sodium* meq	Potassium meq
1,860	80	70	225	115	80

*Value is for amount of salt used in preparation of food; salt added at the table is not included.

FOODS TO ALLOW AND FOODS TO AVOID

Food Groups	Allow	Avoid
Beverage	Coffee; tea; decaffeinated coffee; cereal beverage; carbonated beverage	None
Meat	Any tender meat, fish, or fowl, all without tough connective tissue; eggs; cottage cheese; mild cheese; creamy-style peanut butter	Fried; highly seasoned (such as cold cuts); strong cheese*
Fat	Butter; margarine; cream; vegetable oil; crisp bacon; avocado; gravy; cream sauce; mildly seasoned salad dressing*	Olives; nuts; highly seasoned salad dressing*
Milk	Milk and milk beverages; yogurt with allowed fruits	All others
Starch	Any product made with white, refined wheat, light rye, or graham flours; refined cereals (cooked or ready-to-eat); potato and potato substitutes	Any product made with coarse, whole grains; any containing seeds, nuts, or dried fruits; any fried
Vegetable	Cooked mild-flavored vegetables: asparagus, green or wax beans, beets, carrots, mushrooms, peas, pumpkin, spinach, squash, tomato juice	All other cooked vegetables; all raw vegetables
Fruit	All juices; cooked or canned fruit: applesauce, apricots, cherries, peaches, pears, pineapple; raw fruit: banana and citrus fruit only without membrane	All other cooked fruits; all other fresh fruits; dried fruits
Soup	Broth; bouillon; cream or canned soups made with foods allowed	All others
Dessert	Gelatin; sherbet; ice cream; custard; pudding; cake; cookies; pastry	All others; any with coconut, nuts, or disallowed fruit
Sweets	Sugar; honey; jelly; candy	Any with coconut, nuts, or disallowed fruit
Miscellaneous	Salt; pepper; mild spices* and herbs*; catsup*; vinegar; chocolate	Strong spices*; mustard*; pickles; horseradish

*Inclusion of spices and seasonings may be modified according to the tolerance and usual food preferences of the patient.

SAMPLE MENU PATTERN

Breakfast*		Noon Meal		OR	Evening Meal	
Juice	1 serving	Meat	2 oz		Meat	2 oz
Cereal	1 serving	Potato	1 serving		Potato substitute	1 serving
Meat or egg	1 oz or 1 egg	Vegetable	1 serving		Vegetable	1 serving
Toast	1 serving	Bread	1 serving		Bread	1 serving
Fat	1 serving	Fat	1 serving		Fat	1 serving
Milk	1 cup	Fruit	1 serving		Dessert	1 serving
Beverage		Beverage			Beverage	
Sugar						

Between-meal Feedings: Available if requested.

*Breakfast is likely to be smaller when used as a transitional diet in the postoperative series.

MECHANICAL SOFT DIET

GENERAL DESCRIPTION

The mechanical soft diet differs from the general hospital diet in that modifications are made in texture. Initially, it includes ground meat and pureed vegetables and fruits. The dietitian later modifies the texture of the foods, according to acceptance and tolerance by the patient, to include soft, whole vegetables and fruit. Bread and other bakery products are permitted. The dietitian evaluates the patient's tolerance of bread products.* No restrictions in seasonings are made unless specified. If modification other than texture is necessary, it should be included in the diet order.

INDICATIONS AND RATIONALE

The mechanical soft diet is intended for the person who has difficulty in chewing or swallowing. It enables ingestion of foods with relative comfort and in sufficient amounts. The diet may be used as part of the postoperative series after plastic, laryngeal, and esophageal operations. Efforts should be made to adapt the diet to these special situations and to individual needs and capabilities.

PHYSICIANS: HOW TO ORDER DIETS

The diet order should indicate **mechanical soft diet**.

---

*Patients who have neurologic disorders and patients who are recovering from craniotomies are often unable to chew bread products. Patients who have had esophageal operations or radiation to the oral region (followed by decreased salivation) are likely to have difficulty swallowing bread products.

PREOPERATIVE DIETS

A general diet may be ordered the night before general surgery. Usually nothing is permitted by mouth after this evening meal.

If it is necessary to limit foods that produce residue in the gastrointestinal tract, a diet controlled in residue (see page 143) may be used before the operation. A clear liquid diet (which is low in residue) is generally preferred in preparing patients for colon operations.

GENERAL POSTOPERATIVE DIETS

GENERAL DESCRIPTION

Diets included in the standard postoperative regimens are clear liquid, full liquid, and soft diets. The rate of progression depends on the type of surgery and the subsequent response of the patient.

RATIONALE

Although glucose and electrolyte solutions given intravenously are sufficient to sustain most patients for a short part of the postoperative period without serious depletion of body protein and other stored nutrients, oral intake of food should be resumed as soon as possible. Enteral feeding of a liquid diet can begin when, in the judgment of the surgeon, the gastrointestinal tract can tolerate the feeding. Commonly, feedings are not begun until peristaltic sounds are heard and there is passage of flatus, but under special circumstances, liquid elemental diets that require little or no digestion and have negligible residue may be given cautiously before there is evidence of peristaltic activity. In all instances, one should be ready to discontinue feeding or to revert to an earlier stage in the dietary progression if there is abdominal distention, cramping, or other evidence of intolerance to the feeding. Alternate methods of feeding—such as dietary supplements, tube feedings, supplementary and peripherally administered amino acid, and total parenteral nutrition—should be considered for patients who are severely debilitated and malnourished or who for prolonged periods are unwilling or unable to eat adequately. See pages 237 and 246 for a discussion of dietary supplements and tube feedings.

GENERAL POSTOPERATIVE DIETARY PROGRESSIONS

The following diet progressions permit the surgeon to designate how rapidly the feeding is to be resumed after surgery. The dietitian and surgeon evaluate each patient's acceptance and tolerance of the diet and may adjust the rate of progression.

Start clear liquid diet (first meal) and advance to general diet by meal indicated for rate of progression desired.

Progression	Meal
Rapid	Third
Regular	Sixth
Slow	Ninth

PHYSICIANS: HOW TO ORDER DIETS

The diet order may indicate either the rate of progression (**rapid, regular,** or **slow progression**) *or* the specific diet (**clear liquid, full liquid,** or **soft diet**) at each stage in the patient's convalescence.

OTHER NORMAL DIETS

The following information on vegetarian diets, geriatric nutrition, Jewish dietary practices, and nutritional needs of the athlete is presented to promote understanding and consideration of unusual nutritional needs in meal planning. A special or unique diet is not offered in these areas.

VEGETARIAN DIETS

The three main categories of vegetarianism are *lacto-ovovegetarian*, the most popular type, in which plant foods are supplemented with dairy products and eggs; *lactovegetarian*, the same diet without eggs*; and *"pure" vegetarian*,* also referred to as *vegan*, the less common diet of purely plant origin.

Any detrimental effects of these dietary practices on the optimal nutritional status of the individual depend on the particular diet, the volume and variety of foods included, and the length of time practiced. The dietitian should first find out whether the practice is beneficial, neutral, or harmful. It should be noted that similar nutritional risks apply to other diet regimens.

Several factors that can increase the risk of nutritional deficiencies are history of weight loss, use of laxatives or enemas, restriction of fluids, and periods of fasting. Pregnant women, lactating women, and infants are especially vulnerable to nutritional inadequacies. Low rates of growth in vegetarian children are more apparent before 2 years of age, possibly because of inadequate supplemental feeding of breast-fed infants after 6 months of age (Shull et al., 1977). The diets of persons at high risk of nutritional deficiencies should be evaluated carefully.

Nutrients that may be limited or lacking in vegetarian diets are high-quality protein, vitamin B_{12}, riboflavin, calcium, and iron. Discussion of these nutrients follows.

PROTEIN

Plant proteins have a lower biologic value than proteins of animal origin. The biologic value of a protein is its ability to support growth and maintenance of body structure, and this ability depends on the number and proportion of the amino acids it contains. The proteins of legumes, whole grains, nuts, and vegetables contain all the essential amino acids but yield them at generally lower levels than do proteins of animal origin. The lower biologic value of plant proteins is the result of low levels of one or more of the essential amino acids. However, when a mixture of plant proteins is consumed, supplementation occurs and results in a mixture of all essential amino acids in proportions analogous to the proteins of animal origin. Vegetable mixtures supplying the essential amino acids in appropriate proportions are as efficient as proteins of animal origin in meeting protein needs at minimal levels of intake. In fact, when different proteins are combined in appropriate ways, vegetable proteins cannot be distinguished nutritionally from those of animal origin. Therefore, the derived amino acid profile and not the origin or "value" of a single protein should be considered as the nutritional criterion for meeting protein needs in vegetarian diets.

The sources of protein must be combined in such a way that the amount and proportion of amino acids that result will support normal growth and maintenance. To supply enough derived protein of high biologic value containing all the essential amino acids in desirable proportions, meals should consist of a combination of grains and legumes, grains and nuts or seeds, or grains and vegetables. The following chart simplifies the planning of vegetarian diets.

---

*When eggs or dairy products, or both, are excluded, items of food derived from them are also excluded.

AD-BAC PROTEIN SUPPLEMENTATION BALANCE

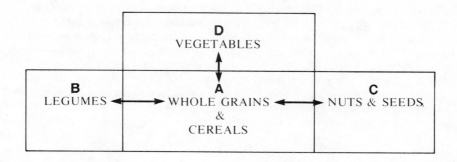

"A" Box — Whole Grains and Cereals

Wheat
Rye
Barley
Corn ⎬ and their products
Millet
Oats
Rice

"B" Box — Legumes

Peanuts	Lima beans
Peas	Soybeans
Mung beans	Black beans
Broad beans	Kidney beans
Black-eyed peas	Garbanzos
Lentils	Other beans

"C" Box — Nuts and Seeds

Cashews	Pumpkin seeds
Pistachios	Squash seeds
Walnuts	Sunflower seeds
Brazil nuts	Sesame seeds
Other nuts	

"D" Box — Vegetables

Potato
Dark green vegetables
Other vegetables

Whole grains and their products ("A" box) should be used in generous amounts in any vegetarian diet. They are sources of protein, iron, and riboflavin in addition to being the supplementing protein to the legumes ("B" box), the nuts and seeds ("C" box), and the vegetables ("D" box). In order to yield a balance of amino acids, a meal pattern should include food from the "A" box and a supplementing protein from the "B," "C," or "D" box. If a particular meal in a day's pattern does not include the selection of food from the "A" box, the resulting amino acid mixture will not be in balance, and the diet should be supplemented *either* by eggs or dairy products *or* by food from the appropriate protein box.

VITAMIN B_{12}

The lacto-ovovegetarian and lactovegetarian categories in general have adequate intake of vitamin B_{12}. Vitamin B_{12} is not present in plant foods in significant enough amounts to be considered a dietary source. However, some persons eating "pure" vegetarian, or vegan, diets appear to remain in good health for many years, or nearly a lifetime, without symptoms of deficiency developing. Others are forced to use supplementary vitamin B_{12} or to adopt a lactovegetarian or lacto-ovovegetarian diet after a few months or a few years. The reason for this variation is not clear, and results of nutritional studies are not uniform. Supplementary vitamin B_{12} for the "pure" vegetarian can be obtained from soybean milk (fortified with vitamin B_{12}) or commercial meat analogues (fortified with vitamin B_{12}).

RIBOFLAVIN, CALCIUM, AND IRON

If milk and milk products are not included in the diet, other sources of calcium (some dark green vegetables and some nuts) and riboflavin (most whole grain, enriched grain, and cereal products) can be included. Iron intake can be increased by using enriched grain and cereal products. The proportion of iron that is available for absorption can be increased by including a source of ascorbic acid in the meal.

GENERAL DIETARY RECOMMENDATIONS

Lacto-ovovegetarian and lactovegetarian diets are nutritionally sound, but a conscious effort must be made to select carefully the proper foods in sufficient amounts to maintain optimal weight and health. If selected appropriately, these diets are also adequate in meeting needs induced by stress during growth, pregnancy, and lactation. The modified basic four food guide on page 19 will facilitate proper selection for vegetarian diets.

Care must be taken in planning the "pure" vegetarian diet, since it lacks concentrated sources of a single protein with adequate proportions of essential amino acids and also is limited in calcium, iron, riboflavin, and vitamin B_{12}.

MODIFIED BASIC FOUR FOOD GUIDE FOR VEGETARIAN DIETS*

Food Group	Number of Servings	
	Adult	Pregnancy/Lactation
Milk and Milk Products	4	4+
Protein Foods		
Legumes	2	2
Nuts	1	1+
Whole Grain Products and Enriched Cereals	6	6
Vegetables and Fruits		
Rich in vitamin C	3	3
Dark green	1½	1½
Other	3	3

*Adapted from King, J. C., Cohenour, S. H., Corruccini, C. G., et al.: Evaluation and modification of the basic four food guide. J. Nutr. Educ., 10:27, 1978.

SELECTED BIBLIOGRAPHY

American Academy of Pediatrics, Committee on Nutrition: Nutritional aspects of vegetarianism, health foods, and fad diets, Pediatrics, 59:460-464, 1977.

Bressani, R., and Behar, M.: The use of plant protein foods in preventing malnutrition. *In* Proceedings of the 6th International Congress of Nutrition. Edinburgh, E. & S. Livingstone, 1964, p. 182.

Hardinge, M. G., and Crooks, H.: Non-flesh dietaries. II. Scientific literature. J. Am. Diet. Assoc., 43:550-558, 1963.

Lappé, F. M.: Diet for a Small Planet. New York, Ballantine Books, 1971.

Monsen, E. R., Hallberg, L., Layrisse, M., et al.: Estimation of available dietary iron. Am. J. Clin. Nutr., 31:134-141, 1978.

Raper, N. R., and Hill, M. M.: Vegetarian diets. Nutr. Rev., 32 (Suppl. 1):29-33, 1974.

Register, U. D., and Sonnenberg, L. M.: The vegetarian diet. J. Am. Diet. Assoc., 62:253-261, 1973.

Robertson, L., Flinders, C., and Godfrey, B.: Laurel's Kitchen: A Handbook for Vegetarian Cookery and Nutrition. Berkeley, California, Nilgiri Press, 1976.

Shull, M. W., Reed, R. B., Valadian, I., et al.: Velocities of growth in vegetarian preschool children. Pediatrics, 60:410-417, 1977.

Vyhmeister, I. B., Register, U. D., and Sonnenberg, L. M.: Safe vegetarian diets for children. Pediatr. Clin. North Am., 24:203-210, 1977.

Williams, E. R.: Making vegetarian diets nutritious. Am. J. Nurs., 75:2168-2173, 1975.

GERIATRIC NUTRITION

The dietary requirements of the older person may be influenced by general health, nutritional stresses of any disease present, the amount of physical activity, and other factors. The functional capacity of nearly every organ system decreases with age, but no clear inferences can be drawn about how such changes may influence nutritional needs. Ingrained food habits and preferences, psychiatric disorders such as depression and loneliness, altered taste or appetite from use of drugs, difficulties with chewing, less money, and difficulties in preparing food for a person living alone all may interfere with the elderly person's obtaining an adequate diet.

Aging results in a decrease in the rate of metabolism, and physical activity usually decreases as well. Thus, one must gradually lower calorie intake as one grows older to prevent weight gain and obesity.

Protein requirements of the elderly have not been proved to be different from those of younger adults. However, because the elderly are more frequently ill and illness commonly causes significant loss of protein from the body, diets planned for the elderly should provide a somewhat greater margin of safety.

The elderly are particularly vulnerable to various nutritional anemias. Reduced gastric acidity adversely affects the absorption of iron and vitamin B_{12}. Anemia due to folic acid deficiency may occur in conjunction with vitamin C deficiency when fresh fruits and vegetables are absent from the diet.

Calcium absorption is also reported to decrease with age, but the osteoporosis commonly seen in old age is apparently the consequence of many years of several factors, one of which may be poor intake of calcium. Whether increased intake of calcium by the elderly slows the progression of osteoporosis is problematic.

Because intestinal muscle tone diminishes with age, abdominal distension from certain foods and constipation are common. Therefore, it is good to encourage the use of tender vegetables, fruits, and whole grain cereals for their fiber content to promote normal peristalsis. Six to eight glasses of water daily also help control constipation. Inappropriate use of laxatives may be avoided by such dietary measures.

Mechanical soft or liquid diets may be prescribed for the elderly who have difficulty chewing regular foods.

SELECTED BIBLIOGRAPHY

Mitchell, H. S., Rynbergen, H. J., Anderson, L., and Dibble, M. V.: Nutrition in Health and Disease. Sixteenth edition. Philadelphia, J. B. Lippincott Company, 1976, pp. 277-283.
National Dairy Council: Nutrition of the elderly. Dairy Council Digest, 48:1-5, Jan.-Feb. 1977.
Robinson, C. H.: Normal and Therapeutic Nutrition. Fourteenth edition. New York, Macmillan, 1972, pp. 337-345.

JEWISH DIETARY PRACTICES

The following discussion of Jewish dietary habits is presented to promote better understanding and to facilitate service to the patient who follows kosher practices. The Mayo Clinic and associated hospitals do not have a kosher food service. Commercially prepared kosher dinners (regular and salt-free) are available.

"Kosher" means "fit." The term refers to foods that can be eaten in accordance with Jewish dietary laws, including specific foods and food combinations that are allowed or prohibited. The stringency with which these practices are followed varies among communities and individuals.

1. Meat and poultry must be slaughtered and processed in a specified manner to be kosher. Proper kosher procedure involves soaking the meat in water for at least 30 minutes and then salting with kosher salt; an alternative method is to broil meat until well done. Kosher meat may come only from cloven-hooved animals (such as cows, sheep, and goats) that graze and chew their cud. Pork is not allowed.

2. Only fish with fins and scales are permitted; shellfish and eels are not allowed.

3. Dairy and meat products may not be eaten at the same meal. Dairy products may be eaten just before a meal containing meat; there should be an interval of 3 to 6 hours after a meal containing meat before dairy products may be consumed again.

4. Separate facilities for food preparation and separate dishes and utensils for food service should be used for meat and dairy foods. In a nonkosher food service, food may be served in disposable dishes and utensils; disposable foil containers may be used for heating foods.

5. Leavened bread products are not allowed for 8 days during Passover. Foods leavened with eggs or steam may be used. During Passover, bread products are made from specially approved flour.

6. Most fruits, vegetables, fish, eggs, grains, coffees, and teas are "pareve," meaning "inherently kosher." They may be eaten in any combination with other foods. Therefore, nondairy creamers, margarine, and soy products may be included in meals containing either meat or milk products. (Grape juice and any jams or jellies containing grapes are kosher only if preparation is supervised.)

7. Symbols are used on processed foods to certify that the food is kosher. These include the emblem (U), copyrighted by the Union of Orthodox Jewish Congregations; the letter K, indicating rabbinical supervision by the individual company (not always approved by Orthodox rabbis; each item should be cleared with a local rabbi for suitability); the emblem (K), copyrighted by the Organized Kasrus Laboratories; (VH), the emblem used by Vaad-Harobonim of Massachusetts; (MK), the emblem used by Montreal Vaad-Hair; (C.O.R.), copyrighted emblem of the Council of Orthodox Rabbis of Toronto; and C.R.C., emblem of the Chicago Rabbinical Council.

8. Some therapeutic food products and dietary supplements are permissible for those following kosher practices (Natow et al., 1975). For information on the acceptability of a particular product, ask a rabbi or the Union of Orthodox Jewish Congregations of America, 84 Fifth Avenue, New York, New York.

9. Nonkosher food products may be used if considered essential to the treatment of an extremely ill person. A rabbi should be consulted on this or any similar matter.

SELECTED BIBLIOGRAPHY

Kaufman, M.: Adapting therapeutic diets to Jewish food customs. Am. J. Clin. Nutr., 5:676-681, 1957.
Natow, A. B., Heslin, J., and Raven, B. C.: Integrating the Jewish dietary laws into a dietetics program. J. Am. Diet. Assoc., 67:13-16, 1975.

NUTRITIONAL NEEDS OF THE ATHLETE

Both the nonathlete and the athlete need optimal nutrition to maintain top physical performance. Although little investigation has been done into the special nutritional needs that athletic performance may impose, evidence to date suggests that the optimal diet for the athlete meets calorie, protein, vitamin, and mineral needs; it is similar to the diet recommended for the general population.

The athlete's calorie needs are determined by the basal energy requirement, which is based on height, weight, age, and sex (see nomogram, page 282), and the energy needed for activity (work). To cover daily activities, the nonathlete or athlete who is not in training or competition needs additional calories equal to 20 to 30% of the basal energy requirements. The athlete, however, should add to this caloric requirement for basal needs and activity the calories required to participate in the athletic event.* The additional calories needed to participate in an athletic event depend on the intensity and duration of the event. A daily calorie intake appropriate for body size and activity is important. If the athlete's caloric intake exceeds needs, body fat will increase. This increase impairs the quality of performance in athletic competition and fosters eating habits and attitudes toward food that may promote obesity later in life. This problem is especially important to consider when dealing with the young athlete.

Combustion of protein is no higher during heavy exercise than during rest (Mayer and Bullen, 1960). Therefore, the daily adult protein requirement of 0.8 g/kg of body weight is adequate for the athlete and can easily be met in the diet without protein supplements. This amount also meets the requirements for muscle hypertrophy. Exercise, not increased protein intake, builds muscle mass.

Although frank vitamin deficiencies are known to impair the ability to perform efficiently, there are no data to support the common belief that vitamin and mineral supplementation enhances athletic performance.

The role of water in regulating body temperature is of particular importance to the athlete. The excessive heat generated by exercise is dissipated through the evaporation of sweat. Although salt as well as water is lost during sweating, the reduction in athletic performance that occurs with dehydration from exercise is not caused primarily by a decrease in extracellular water. Salt replacement is rarely needed during athletic activity; athletes eating a varied diet generally get enough sodium to meet the needs of vigorous athletic activity. Water lost during exercise should be replaced by small amounts of fluid taken at intervals, however.

----

*The approximate caloric cost of a variety of activities has been determined and reported (Consolazio et al., 1963).

An athlete's diet can be designed, after the calorie and protein requirements have been determined, in the same manner as that for other normal diets. A food exchange list or similar listing of food groups may be useful in formulating guidelines. Concentrated calories in the form of desserts and sugars and sweets may be included to achieve diets very high in calories. It is important for the athlete to understand that no single food or category of foods contains all the nutrients in amounts sufficient to maintain life and that a varied diet must be eaten if all the required nutrients are to be consumed.

The effect on performance of pregame or game-time eating (Nutrition for Athletes, 1971), although difficult to evaluate, is of questionable significance, because combined with, and probably more important than, the foods consumed is the psychologic significance ascribed to foods or combinations of foods by the athlete and the coach.

The optimal diet for an athlete is not essentially different from that of the nonathlete. If a varied diet is eaten—one that meets calorie, protein, vitamin, and mineral requirements—the athlete need not take supplements; all nutrient needs for growth, maintenance, and activity will be met by food.

SELECTED BIBLIOGRAPHY

Consolazio, C. F., Johnson, R. E., and Pecora, L. J.: Physiological Measurements of Metabolic Functions in Man. New York, McGraw-Hill Book Company, 1963.

Huse, D. M., and Nelson, R. A.: Basic, balanced diet meets requirements of athletes. Physician Sportsmed., 5:52-56, Jan. 1977.

Mayer, J., and Bullen, B.: Nutrition and athletic performance. Physiol. Rev., 40:369-397, 1960.

Nutrition for Athletes: A Handbook for Coaches. Washington, D.C., American Association for Health, Physical Education, and Recreation, 1971.

NOTES

SECTION 3

THERAPEUTIC DIET MODIFICATIONS

DIETARY MANAGEMENT OF DIABETES

GENERAL DESCRIPTION

Diets used in the management of diabetes mellitus are controlled in energy (calories) and macronutrients (protein, fat, and carbohydrates). Large amounts of simple, rapidly absorbed carbohydrates are to be avoided. Moderate restriction of cholesterol, saturated fats, and, to some extent, salt is usually advised.

NUTRITIONAL ADEQUACY

A multivitamin and mineral supplement may be appropriate for persons following diets that provide fewer than 1,000 to 1,200 calories.

INDICATIONS AND RATIONALE

A primary goal of management of diabetes is to achieve as nearly normal a state of metabolism as possible without undue inconvenience or risk of serious insulin reaction. With current techniques, however, it is not possible to keep plasma glucose levels within physiologic limits at all times. Dietary control is an important part of the management of diabetes and will do much to return plasma glucose levels toward normal and to minimize fluctuations in plasma glucose levels after meals. Dietary management is also directed at reducing the risk of premature or accelerated atherosclerosis, to which the person with diabetes is particularly vulnerable.

CATEGORIES OF DIABETES

There are currently two recognized descriptive categories of diabetes mellitus:

1. "Maturity-onset," "ketosis-resistant," or "insulin-independent" diabetes occurs in 80 to 90% of persons with diabetes. Persons having maturity-onset diabetes do not require injected insulin to prevent ketosis, since in these individuals the pancreas is capable of producing some insulin. In some, injection of insulin is needed in addition to dietary control to prevent undesirable elevations of plasma and urine glucose levels. If the impairment of insulin secretion is less severe, an oral hypoglycemic agent may lower plasma glucose. This type of diabetes usually appears in middle-aged persons, most of whom are overweight. Control of calorie intake is the most important dietary measure for the maturity-onset diabetic. Often, results of plasma and urine glucose tests improve remarkably within days after a low-calorie diet is begun, and further improvement often results from correction of obesity.

2. "Growth-onset," "juvenile-onset," "ketosis-prone," or "insulin-dependent" diabetes occurs in 10 to 20% of persons with diabetes. Persons having growth-onset diabetes require one or more injections of insulin daily to control plasma and urine glucose levels and to prevent ketosis. This type of diabetes usually appears early in life but may occur at any age. Consistency in composition and timing of meals and between-meal or bedtime snacks is important for control in this category of diabetes.

GENERAL DIETARY RECOMMENDATIONS

The diets for diabetes described in this manual utilize the 1976 "Exchange Lists for Meal Planning."*

Proportion of Calories from Protein, Fat, and Carbohydrate. The usual distribution of calories in weight maintenance diets is approximately 20% protein, 35% fat, and 45% carbohydrate. The proportions are slightly different for very low calorie diets, since it is necessary to maintain an adequate intake of protein.

Most patients find that the limitation in the amount of meat required to meet the recommended level of fat (35% of calories) is acceptable, although in many instances the amount of meat allowed is substantially less than the patient has been accustomed to consuming. Adherence to a diet restricted in fat much below 35% of calories, even a decrease to 30%, entails a sufficiently great change in the patient's usual choice of foods that only the well-motivated patient is likely to modify eating habits to this extent. Although diets containing a higher proportion of carbohydrate and lower proportion of fat have been found to be compatible with good clinical control of both juvenile-onset and adult-onset diabetes, evidence is lacking that these diets provide advantages that would justify recommending a major change in habitual choices of foods. There is probably no single ideal ratio of fat, carbohydrate, and protein for the diabetic person; a rather wide range of proportions appears to be compatible with good diabetic care.

Protein requirements of adult-onset diabetics are not different from those of nondiabetic individuals. In juvenile-onset diabetes, there are inevitable periods of suboptimal levels of circulating insulin and, hence, of accelerated protein catabolism. The juvenile-onset diabetic should receive the full quota of protein, particularly during the years of growth. Additional amounts of protein likely would yield no benefit.

Meal Plan. The total day's caloric intake should be distributed into meals and snacks according to the preferences, physical activity, and insulin requirement of the patient. Between-meal and bedtime snacks are ordinarily not necessary unless insulin is being used. A bedtime snack is routinely planned for the patient taking insulin injections and should provide one-fourth to one-half the calories of a meal. Midmorning and midafternoon snacks may be helpful to the unstable or juvenile-onset diabetic. The distribution of calories, protein, and carbohydrate among the three meals and bedtime snacks as given in the sample menu patterns on page 34 is satisfactory for most diabetics, but reapportionment according to the patient's preferences is often needed.

---

*American Diabetes Association, Inc., and The American Dietetic Association, 1976, 24 pp. Some modifications have been made in the original exchange list; these are noted.

Timing and Consistency of Meals. If insulin is being used, meals and snacks should be calculated in composition to distribute calories, carbohydrate, and protein in a consistent manner. The timing of meals and snacks should be consistent from day to day and be designed to be compatible with the usual pattern of physical activity and with the nature of insulin injected. If there is a consistent tendency toward glycosuria or hypoglycemia at a given time of day, shifting portions of food from one time of day to another may correct the problem. Adjustments in timing and size of meals and snacks sometimes achieve good control of glycemia and thus avoid the need for changing from simple to more complex insulin regimens.

If insulin is not used, timing and composition of meals are less crucial.

Simple Carbohydrates. Simple carbohydrates—particularly sucrose, and, therefore, sugar, jellies, and canned fruit packed in syrup—are generally restricted on the presumption that the rapidly absorbed sugar will cause a greater postprandial rise in plasma glucose. The amount of simple carbohydrates (for example, glucose, fructose, and sucrose) occurring naturally in fruits does not seem to be sufficient to disturb diabetic control when fruits are part of a meal.

The person who takes insulin should always have available a quickly absorbable source of carbohydrate, such as candy or sugar cubes, to counteract hypoglycemia if it occurs.

Adjustments for Increased Exercise. Exercise increases the utilization of glucose by muscles and may increase the rate of release of insulin from injection sites into the blood. Whenever the person who takes insulin indulges in vigorous and unscheduled physical activity, extra carbohydrate should be consumed before or during the exercise to avoid hypoglycemia. An extra feeding equivalent to a bread exchange may be appropriate for a person with unstable or juvenile-onset diabetes who is about to drive a car, unless a regular meal was eaten within the last two hours.

Other Dietary Modifications. Persons with diabetes are more vulnerable to the development of atherosclerosis at an earlier age and in a more severe degree than are nondiabetics. The American Heart Association has made general dietary recommendations as a means of lowering serum lipids of most people and thus possibly retarding atherosclerosis. The diets described herein are generally compatible with the recommendations of the American Heart Association (see page 300).

Moderate control of cholesterol (300 to 500 mg/day) is accomplished by limiting eggs to three a week and only occasionally allowing other high-cholesterol foods. Using fat exchanges as polyunsaturated fats and consuming skim milk are preferred.

Persons with diabetes are subject to the complications of diabetic nephropathy and the hypertension that results from these renal changes 10 to 20 years after the onset of diabetes. Essential hypertension is as likely to develop in diabetics as it is in the general population at any age. Therefore, advising the normotensive diabetic to avoid excessive use of salt and high-sodium foods is reasonable, but routinely recommending stringent sodium restriction is not justified.

Increased amounts of dietary fiber have been said to confer some amelioration of diabetes, but this has not been established. The conventional diet for diabetes, consisting as it does of a generous proportion of vegetables, is intrinsically somewhat higher in naturally occurring fiber than the usual American diet.

PRIORITIES FOR PLANNING DIETS

Maturity-onset	Juvenile- or growth-onset
High Priority	
If patient is obese, plan diet to reduce weight and then to maintain weight.	Keep timing and composition of meals regular from day to day; avoid large amounts of simple carbohydrates.
Stress nutritious, well-balanced meals and avoidance of large amounts of simple carbohydrates.	Add between-meal and bedtime snacks; shorten intervals between feedings insofar as convenience permits.
If hypertension or serum lipid abnormalities are present, modify diet.	Plan for food to be taken to correct hypoglycemic episodes resulting from exercise; plan for food to be taken during illness.
	In children, plan for enough calories and protein to permit growth.
Lower Priority	
Keep meal times and composition regular (more important if patient takes insulin).	Correct mild obesity (juvenile-onset diabetic patients are rarely obese) only if it is accompanied by hypertension or serum lipid disturbances.
Add snacks and bedtime feeding (not necessary unless patient takes insulin).	

DETERMINATION OF CALORIE LEVEL

The average calorie requirement of persons of the same age, sex, and body size under basal conditions can be determined from the food nomogram (see page 282). Ordinarily, "ideal" or "desirable" weight is used in nomogram calculations. More accurate determination of calorie requirements can be made through measurement of oxygen consumption or basal metabolic rate.*

For weight maintenance, the calorie level can be calculated by a diet history and verified with the nomogram. Basal calories are determined from the nomogram, and an increment of 10 to 50% is added—10% for the inactive person and up to 50% or more for the very active person. For hospitalized patients, "basal calories" are usually adequate. Adjustments should be made in the calorie level if the patient gains or loses weight on the diet. If weight gain is desirable, the increment above basal calories should include an allowance for activity and an additional 10 to 30%. In some juvenile-onset diabetics, an additional allowance must be made for calories lost as glycosuria.† See page 234 for guidelines for estimating caloric needs of children.

---

*Milliliters of oxygen used per minute multiplied by the factor 7 (0.0048 kcal/ml O_2 × 1,440 min/24 hr = 6.912) yields an estimate for calories expended in 24 hours under resting conditions.

†Multiply grams of glucose excreted in 24 hours by the factor 3.8 to obtain calories lost. This quantity commonly varies considerably from day to day. Some juvenile-onset diabetics, even with best efforts at control, may lose several hundred calories daily by this route.

The question of establishing a "goal weight" or "ideal weight" is important in diabetes because of the insulin resistance associated with obesity. In general, the patient with diabetes should be somewhat lean or toward the lower side of average weight ranges. For weight to be lost at a perceptible rate, the diet should provide a daily calorie deficit of at least 500 calories. See page 50 for prediction of weight loss.

PHYSICIANS: HOW TO ORDER DIETS

The diet order should indicate that the patient has diabetes and may (1) specify the patient's height and weight and indicate a calorie level that is equal to **basal calories** or **an increment above basal calories** (for example, B + 20%) *or* (2) indicate whether **weight reduction** or **weight maintenance** is necessary (the dietitian will determine the appropriate calorie level) *or* (3) specify the **calorie level** (for example, 1,800 calories).

When the diabetic patient undergoes surgery, the custom at the Mayo institutions is for the physician responsible for care of diabetes to order **"usual diabetic diet is _____ ; diet progression according to surgeon's orders."** The surgeon orders the usual diet progression according to his judgment of the patient's progress, as though the patient were not diabetic. The dietitian then incorporates modifications for diabetes into the surgeon's orders.

DIABETES AND PREGNANCY

The diet during pregnancy follows the same basic principles outlined previously. The calorie level should be adjusted periodically for appropriate weight gain. Between-meal feedings may be desirable. For further information, see page 173.

DIABETES AND HYPERLIPIDEMIA

Moderate restriction of cholesterol and substitution of polyunsaturated fats for saturated fats are generally encouraged in diabetic diets. If the patient has hypercholesterolemia, more strict dietary control may be needed. See page 52 for additional modifications.

DIABETIC DIET WITH SODIUM CONTROL

If control of sodium is necessary, considerations for determining the calorie level and meal plan remain the same, but the sodium exchange lists (see page 67) should be used. These exchange lists, based on the food lists used for diabetes, are subdivided according to sodium content.

DIABETIC DIET WITH PROTEIN CONTROL

When protein intake is limited because of renal failure, some compromises may have to be made in the principles of the diabetic diet. The exchange list for control of protein, sodium, and potassium should be used. The principles of a diet controlled in protein (see page 80) generally take priority, especially at the very low levels of protein intake.

DIET DURING ILLNESS

No precise rules can be laid down for eating during an illness, particularly if there is nausea or vomiting. Adult-onset diabetics are vulnerable to dehydration and "nonketotic hyperosmolar coma" during an illness if there is persistent glycosuria. Generous consumption of water is an important precaution. In juvenile-onset or ketosis-prone diabetes, adequate amounts of both insulin and carbohydrate are needed to prevent the development of ketoacidosis during illness. Sugar or carbohydrate of any sort should be taken at frequent intervals and in whatever amounts can be tolerated when nausea is present. When illness prevents taking the usual diet but nausea is not a problem, systematic replacement of carbohydrate is appropriate.

REPLACEMENT OF AVAILABLE CARBOHYDRATE

If the insulin-taking diabetic misses a meal in preparation for diagnostic tests or during illness, the amount of available carbohydrate in the meal plan should be replaced with other sources of carbohydrate. Available carbohydrate is the proportion of macronutrients that can be converted into glucose by the body (100% of carbohydrate, 60% of protein, and 10% of fat). Substitutions can be made by use of sweetened carbonated beverages, sweetened gelatin, sugar, and fruit juice.

Food Groups	Grams of Available Carbohydrates in 1 Exchange
Meat	5.0
Fat	0.5
Nonfat milk	17.0
Bread	16.0
Fruit	10.0
Vegetable	6.0

For hospital patients on clear liquid diets, precise calculation of available carbohydrate is not necessary. Stress and trauma are likely to alter insulin requirements, and glucose is often given intravenously to supplement oral feeding.

APPROXIMATE COMPOSITION

Calorie Level	Protein g	Fat g	Carbohydrate g
800	55	25	80
1,000	60	35	110
1,200	70	45	125
1,400	80	55	155
1,600	85	60	180
1,800	95	70	210
2,000	100	75	220
2,200	120	80	260
2,400	120	95	275
2,600	125	100	300
2,800	130	110	325
3,000	140	115	345

SUGGESTED DAILY FOOD EXCHANGES

| Exchange Group | \
Calorie Level | | | | | | | | | | | |
|---|---|---|---|---|---|---|---|---|---|---|---|---|
| | 800 | 1,000 | 1,200 | 1,400 | 1,600 | 1,800 | 2,000 | 2,200 | 2,400 | 2,600 | 2,800 | 3,000 |
| Meat* | 5 | 5 | 6 | 7 | 7 | 8 | 8 | 9 | 9 | 9 | 10 | 10 |
| Fat | 0 | 2 | 3 | 4 | 5 | 6 | 7 | 7 | 10 | 11 | 12 | 13 |
| Milk, nonfat† | 2 | 2 | 2 | 2 | 2 | 2 | 3 | 4 | 4 | 4 | 4 | 5 |
| Starch | 1 | 3 | 4 | 6 | 7 | 9 | 9 | 10 | 11 | 12 | 13 | 13 |
| Vegetable | 2 | 2 | 2 | 2 | 2 | 2 | 2 | 2 | 2 | 2 | 2 | 2 |
| Fruit | 3 | 3 | 3 | 3 | 4 | 4 | 4 | 5 | 5 | 6 | 7 | 8 |

*Calculations are based on values for medium-fat meats.
†If low-fat or whole milk is used, there should be an appropriate decrease in fat exchanges.

SAMPLE MENU PATTERNS

Examples of distribution of total daily food exchanges are shown below. They are intended only as a guide. Meal plans should be based as much as possible on individual needs and preferences.

Exchange List	Calorie Level											
	800	1,000	1,200	1,400	1,600	1,800	2,000	2,200	2,400	2,600	2,800	3,000
Breakfast												
Meat	1	1	1	1	1	1	1	1	1	1	1	1
Fat	...	1	1	1	1	1	1	1	2	2	2	2
Nonfat milk	...	...	...	...	...	...	1	1	1	1	1	1
Starch	1	1	1	2	2	2	2	2	3	3	3	3
Fruit	1	1	1	1	1	1	1	1	1	2	2	2
Noon Meal												
Meat	2	2	2	3	3	3	3	3	3	3	3	3
Fat	...	...	1	1	2	2	2	2	3	4	4	5
Nonfat milk	1	1	1	1	1	1	1	1	1	1	1	2
Starch	...	...	1	1	2	2	2	3	3	4	4	4
Vegetable	1	1	1	1	1	1	1	1	1	1	1	1
Fruit	1	1	1	1	2	2	2	2	2	2	2	2
Evening Meal												
Meat	2	2	3	3	3	3	3	4	4	4	4	4
Fat	...	1	1	2	2	2	3	3	4	4	5	5
Nonfat milk	...	...	...	...	...	...	...	1	1	1	1	1
Starch	...	1	1	2	2	3	3	3	3	3	4	4
Vegetable	1	1	1	1	1	1	1	1	1	1	1	1
Fruit	1	1	1	1	1	1	1	2	2	2	2	2
Bedtime Snack												
Meat	...	...	...	...	...	1	1	1	1	1	2	2
Fat	...	...	...	...	...	1	1	1	1	1	1	1
Nonfat milk	1	1	1	1	1	1	1	1	1	1	1	1
Starch	...	1	1	1	1	2	2	2	2	2	2	2
Fruit	...	...	...	...	...	...	...	...	...	...	1	2

FOODS TO AVOID

All foods containing large amounts of added sugar should be avoided, except in special circumstances, since they cause a relatively rapid increase in blood glucose. The following foods should be avoided.

Candy	Pudding	Marmalade
Cake	Sweet rolls	Molasses
Cookies	Sugar	Syrup
Pastries	Honey	Sweetened condensed milk
Pies	Jam	Sweetened soft drinks
	Jelly	Chewing gum

FOODS AS DESIRED

The following foods contain negligible amounts of protein, fat, or carbohydrate and may be used as desired without calculation into the meal plan.

Beverages
  Coffee
  Tea
  Decaffeinated coffee
Condiments
  Catsup (limit to 1 tbsp)
  Barbecue sauce (limit to 1 tbsp)
  Horseradish
  Mustard
  Meat sauces (prepared without sugar)
  Pickles (prepared without sugar)
Flavoring extracts
Cocoa powder (limit to 1 tbsp)

Seasonings
  Salt
  Pepper
  Herbs
  Spices
Lemon
Lime
Gelatin, plain, unflavored
Salad dressings
  Low-calorie (limit to 1 tbsp)
  Lemon juice
  Lime juice
  Vinegar
Bouillon or broth (fat-free)

FOOD EXCHANGE LIST*

This food exchange list is intended to be used as a reference tool. For this reason, a more comprehensive list of foods is given than may actually be used for instruction of individuals.

LIST 1: MEAT EXCHANGES†

Measure or wt	Gram wt	Lean meat—protein, 7 g; fat, 3 g; 55 kcal
1 oz	30	Beef: baby beef (very lean), chipped beef, chuck, flank steak, tenderloin, plate ribs, plate skirt steak, round (bottom, top), all rump cuts, spareribs, tripe, ground (preceding meats trimmed of fat and ground)
1 oz	30	Lamb: leg, rib, sirloin, loin (roast and chops), shank, shoulder
1 oz	30	Pork: leg (whole rump, center shank), smoked ham (center slices)
1 oz	30	Veal: leg, loin, rib, shank, shoulder, cutlets
1 oz	30	Poultry (meat without skin): chicken, turkey, cornish hen, guinea hen, pheasant
1 oz	30	Fish, any fresh or frozen
1/4 cup	30	Canned salmon, tuna, mackerel, crab, lobster
1 oz (about 5)	30	Clams, oysters, scallops, shrimp
3	30	Sardines, drained
1/4 cup	60	Egg substitutes, fat-free
1 oz	30	Cheeses containing less than 5% butterfat (specialty cheese products)
1/4 cup	45	Cottage cheese: dry, 1% butterfat, 2% butterfat
1/2 cup	100	Dried beans and peas, cooked (omit 1 starch exchange)

Measure or wt	Gram wt	Medium-fat meat—protein, 7 g; fat, 5 g; 73 kcal; OR 1 lean meat + 1/2 fat exchange
1 oz	30	Beef: ground (less than 20% fat), corned beef (canned), rib eye, round (ground commercial)
1 oz	30	Pork: loin (all tenderloin cuts), shoulder arm (picnic), shoulder blade, Boston butt, Canadian bacon, boiled ham
1 oz	30	Liver, heart, kidney, sweetbreads
1/4 cup	45	Cottage cheese, creamed
1 oz	30	Cheese: mozzarella, ricotta, Neufchatel, farmer cheese
3 tbsp	15	Cheese, Parmesan
1	50	Egg
1 oz	30	Roasted soybeans
1 oz	30	Peanuts, sunflower seeds, pumpkin seeds, squash seeds (omit 2 fat exchanges)
2 tbsp	30	Peanut butter (omit 2 fat exchanges)

LIST 1: MEAT EXCHANGES† (Continued)

Measure or wt	Gram wt	High-fat meat—protein, 7 g; fat, 8 g; 100 kcal; OR 1 lean meat + 1 fat exchange
1 oz	30	Beef: brisket, corned beef (brisket), ground (more than 20% fat), hamburger (commercial), chuck (ground commercial), roasts (rib), steaks (club and rib)
1 oz	30	Lamb, breast
1 oz	30	Pork: spareribs, loin (back ribs), ground, country-style ham, deviled ham
1 oz	30	Veal, breast
1 oz	30	Poultry: capon, duck (domestic), goose
1 oz	30	Cheese: all others, including cheddar types
2 tbsp	30	Cheese spreads
1 slice, 4 1/2 in. by 1/8 in.	45	Cold cuts
1 small	45	Frankfurter

*Based on "Exchange Lists for Meal Planning," American Diabetes Association, Inc., and The American Dietetic Association, 1976, 24 pp. Variations from the original list are given on page 45.

†Nutrient values for three meat groups (lean, medium-fat, and high-fat) are given to encourage use of lower-fat meats. However, basing calculations on medium-fat meats is generally acceptable unless precise control of fat is necessary.

LIST 2: FAT EXCHANGES—fat, 5 g; 45 kcal

Measure	Gram wt	Predominantly polyunsaturated or monounsaturated fats
1 tsp	5	Margarine: soft, tub, stick*
1/8	30	Avocado, 4 in. in diameter†
1 tsp	5	Oil: corn, cottonseed, safflower, soy, sunflower
1 tsp	5	Olive oil†
1 tsp	5	Peanut oil†
2 tbsp	30	Nondairy cream substitute*
1 tbsp	15	French or Italian salad dressing*
1 tsp	5	Mayonnaise*
2 tsp	10	Mayonnaise-type salad dressing*
5 small	50	Olives†
10 whole	10	Almonds†
2 large whole	5	Pecans†
6 small	8	Walnuts
6 small	8	Nuts, other†
		Predominantly saturated fats
1 tsp	5	Butter
1 tsp	5	Bacon fat
1 strip	10	Bacon, crisp
2 tbsp	30	Cream: light, sour
1 tbsp	15	Cream, heavy
2 tbsp	30	Other nondairy cream substitutes
1 tbsp	15	Cream cheese
2 tbsp	30	Gravy
1 tsp	5	Lard
3/4-in. cube	5	Salt pork

*Made with corn, cottonseed, safflower, soy, or sunflower oil only.
†Fat content is primarily monounsaturated.

LIST 3: MILK EXCHANGES

Measure	Gram wt	Nonfat fortified milk—protein, 8 g; carbohydrate, 12 g; fat, trace; 80 kcal
1 cup	240	Skim or nonfat milk
1/3 cup	25	Powdered milk (nonfat dry, before adding liquid)
1/2 cup	120	Canned, evaporated skim milk
1 cup	240	Buttermilk made from skim milk
1 cup	240	Yogurt made from skim milk (plain, unflavored)
		1% fat fortified milk (1 nonfat milk + 1/2 fat exchange)— protein, 8 g; carbohydrate, 12 g; fat, 2.5 g; 102 kcal
1 cup	240	1% milk
1 cup	240	Low-fat buttermilk
		2% fat fortified milk (1 nonfat milk + 1 fat exchange)— protein, 8 g; carbohydrate, 12 g; fat, 5 g; 125 kcal
1 cup	240	2% milk
1 cup	240	Yogurt made from 2% milk (plain, unflavored)
		Whole milk (1 nonfat milk + 2 fat exchanges)— protein, 8 g; carbohydrate, 12 g; fat, 10 g; 160 kcal
1 cup	240	Whole milk
1/2 cup	120	Canned, evaporated whole milk
1 cup	240	Buttermilk made from whole milk
1 cup	240	Yogurt made from whole milk (plain, unflavored)

LIST 4: STARCH EXCHANGES–protein, 2 g; carbohydrate, 15 g; 68 kcal

Measure	Gram wt	Bread
1 slice	25	White, including French and Italian
1 slice	25	Whole wheat
1 slice	25	Rye or pumpernickel
1 slice	25	Raisin
1/2	30	Bagel, small
1/2	30	English muffin, small
1	35	Plain roll, bread
1/2	35	Frankfurter roll
1/2	35	Hamburger bun
3 tbsp	20	Dried bread crumbs
1	30	Tortilla, 6 in.
4	20	Breadsticks, 3 1/2 in. long

Measure	Gram wt	Cereal
1/2 cup	20	Bran flakes
3/4 cup	20	Other ready-to-eat, unsweetened cereal
1 cup	15	Puffed cereal, unfrosted
1/4 cup	30	Grape-Nuts
1/2 cup	30	100% bran cereals
1/2 cup	100	Cooked cereal
1/2 cup	100	Grits, cooked
1/2 cup	100	Rice or barley, cooked
1/2 cup	100	Pasta, spaghetti, noodles, macaroni (cooked)
		Popcorn (popped, no fat added)
3 cups	45	Large kernel
1 1/2 cups	20	Small kernel
2 tbsp	15	Cornmeal, dry
2 1/2 tbsp	20	Flour
2 tbsp	25	Tapioca
1/4 cup	25	Wheat germ

LIST 4: STARCH EXCHANGES—protein, 2 g; carbohydrate, 15 g; 68 kcal *(Continued)*

Measure	Gram wt	Crackers
3	20	Arrowroot
2	20	Graham, 2 1/2 in. sq
1/2	20	Matzoth, 4 in. by 6 in.
4	20	Melba toast, 3 3/4 in. by 2 in.
20	20	Oyster
25	20	Pretzels, 3 1/8 in. long by 1/8 in. in diameter
3	20	Rye wafers, 2 in. by 3 1/2 in.
6	20	Saltines
4	20	Soda, 2 1/2 in. sq

		Dried beans, peas, and lentils (omit 1 meat exchange)
1/2 cup	100	Beans, peas, lentils (dried, cooked)
1/4 cup	50	Baked beans (canned, no pork)

		Starchy vegetables
1/3 cup	80	Corn
1 small	100	Corn on the cob
1/2 cup	100	Green peas, canned or frozen
1/2 cup	100	Lima beans
2/3 cup	125	Parsnips
1 small	100	Potato, baked or boiled
1/2 cup	100	Potato, mashed
3/4 cup	150	Pumpkin
1/2 cup	100	Winter squash: acorn, butternut
1/4 cup	60	Yam or sweet potato

LIST 4: STARCH EXCHANGES– protein, 2 g; carbohydrate, 15 g; 68 kcal *(Continued)*

Measure	Gram wt	Prepared foods (omit 1 fat exchange)
1	35	Biscuit, 2 in. in diameter
1	45	Corn bread, 2 in. by 2 in. by 1 in.
1	40	Corn muffin, 2 in. in diameter
5	20	Crackers, round butter type
1	40	Plain muffin, small
1	60	Pancake, 5 in. by 1/2 in.
15	30	Potato or corn chips (omit 2 fat exchanges)
8	40	Potatoes, French fried, 2 in. to 3 1/2 in. long
1	35	Waffle, 5 in. by 1/2 in.

		Additional starch exchanges (Many of the following foods contain added sugar. They should be used only occasionally, in limited amounts, and with other foods.)
1/16 of 10-in. cake (1½ in.)	25	Angel food cake, plain
8	15	Animal crackers
1/2 cup	100	Commercial flavored gelatin
5	20	Gingersnaps, 1 in.
1/2 cup	70	Ice cream (omit 2 fat exchanges)
1/2 cup	60	Ice milk (omit 1 fat exchange)
1/4 cup	50	Sherbet
1/16 of 10-in. cake (1½ in.)	25	Sponge cake
5	20	Vanilla wafers, 1 in.

LIST 5: VEGETABLE EXCHANGES— protein, 2 g; carbohydrate, 5 g; 25 kcal;
1 exchange is 1/2 cup (100 g)

Asparagus	Greens	Onions
Bean sprouts	Chards	Rutabaga
Beets	Collards	Sauerkraut
Broccoli	Dandelion	String beans, green or yellow
Brussels sprouts	Kale	Tomatoes
Carrots	Spinach	Tomato juice
Eggplant	Okra	Turnips
		Vegetable juice cocktail

The following vegetables have little protein, fat, or carbohydrate. They may be used as desired.

Cabbage	Escarole	Mushrooms
Cauliflower	Green pepper	Parsley
Celery	Greens	Radishes
Chicory	Beet	Rhubarb
Chinese cabbage	Mustard	Summer squash
Cucumber	Turnip	Watercress
Endive	Lettuce	Zucchini

LIST 6: FRUIT EXCHANGES—carbohydrate, 10 g; 40 kcal
(all fruits are unsweetened)

Measure	Gram wt		Measure	Gram wt	
1 small	80	Apple			Melon
1/3 cup	80	Apple juice	1/4 small	200	Cantaloupe
1/2 cup	100	Applesauce	1/8 medium	150	Honeydew
2 medium	100	Apricots, fresh	1 cup	175	Watermelon
4 halves	20	Apricots, dried	1 small	80	Nectarine
1/3 cup	80	Apricot nectar	1 small	100	Orange
1/2 small	50	Banana	1/2 cup	120	Orange juice
		Berries	1/2 cup	100	Orange sections
1/2 cup	70	Blackberries	3/4 cup	100	Papaya
1/2 cup	70	Blueberries	1 medium	100	Peach
1/2 cup	70	Raspberries	2 halves	20	Peach, dried
3/4 cup	110	Strawberries	1/2 cup	100	Peaches, canned
10 large	100	Cherries	1/3 cup	80	Peach nectar
1/2 cup	100	Cherries, canned	1 small	100	Pear
1/3 cup	80	Cider	2 halves	20	Pear, dried
1/3 cup	80	Cranberry juice cocktail	1/2 cup	100	Pears, canned
2	15	Dates	1/3 cup	80	Pear nectar
1	50	Figs, fresh	1 medium	30	Persimmon, native
1	15	Figs, dried	1/2 cup	100	Pineapple
1/2 cup	100	Figs, canned	1/3 cup	80	Pineapple juice
1/2 cup	100	Fruit cocktail	2 medium	100	Plums
1/2	100	Grapefruit	1/2 cup	100	Plums, canned
1/2 cup	120	Grapefruit juice	2 medium	25	Prunes
1/2 cup	100	Grapefruit sections	1/4 cup	60	Prune juice
12	75	Grapes	2 tbsp	15	Raisins
1/4 cup	60	Grape juice	1 medium	100	Tangerine
1/2 cup	100	Grapes, canned	1/2 cup	100	Tangerine juice
1/2 small	70	Mango	1/2 cup	100	Tangerine sections

MISCELLANEOUS EXCHANGES

The following substitutions may be made occasionally to allow flexibility and variation in diet.
    1 medium-fat meat exchange = 1 nonfat milk exchange*
    1 fruit exchange = 1 vegetable exchange = 1/2 starch exchange

CHANGES IN FOOD EXCHANGE LIST

The food exchange list in this chapter is based on the list published by the American Diabetes Association and The American Dietetic Association but differs from it in the following ways:
    1. Seasonings and Free Foods. — Cocoa powder is added.
    2. Meat Exchanges. — Lean ground meat is added. Egg substitutes are included in the lean category because of the greater availability of fat-free products. The percentage of fat designated for medium-fat ground meat has been changed from "15%" to "less than 20%." Peanuts and some other seeds and nuts are included in the meat group to permit greater use of plant protein sources. Cheese spreads are added to the high-fat meat group.
    As the fat content of meat increases, the protein content decreases for portions of equal weight. Usually of little concern, this circumstance may be of importance in diets in which protein is closely controlled.
    3. Fat Exchanges. — Salad dressings are included in the first group, since they are generally made with polyunsaturated or monounsaturated oils. Nondairy cream substitutes are also included in the first group because some made with polyunsaturated fats are available on the market. Gravy is included in the saturated fat category.
    One teaspoon (approximately 5 g) of butter or margarine provides 4 g of fat and 36 calories. Use of these values may be justified if a more nearly precise determination of calories from fat is needed or if the patient intends to use only butter or margarine in preference to other fat exchanges.
    4. Starch Exchanges. — Exchange values for bran cereals, Grape-Nuts, tapioca, small-kernel popcorn, breadsticks, and melba toast are added.
    If more nearly precise control of calories is needed, the following exchanges are suggested: wheat germ, 3 tbsp; dried beans, peas, and lentils, 1 starch exchange plus 1 meat exchange.
    Some sugar-sweetened foods are included. Guidelines for their use are given.
    5. Vegetable Exchanges. — The following vegetables provide less than 2.5 g of carbohydrate per 1/2 cup: cabbage, cauliflower, celery, cucumber, green pepper, beet greens, mustard greens, turnip greens, mushrooms, rhubarb, summer squash, and zucchini. These are included in the category of vegetables that may be used as desired.
    6. Fruit Exchanges. — The list has been expanded to include more canned fruits, fruit nectars, and cranberry juice cocktail.

---

*The carbohydrate content is not equal.

ARTIFICIAL SWEETENERS AND DIETETIC FOODS

The use of commercial food products labeled "dietetic," "sugar-free," "diet," or "low-calorie" should be discussed thoroughly with the patient. The nutritive value of these foods is often misinterpreted.

If foods or beverages containing non-nutritive sweeteners (for example, saccharin) are permitted, they should be used in limited amounts.

Sorbitol may not be completely absorbed in the small intestine. Therefore, when taken in large amounts, it may cause diarrhea. That which is absorbed contributes calories. Sorbitol is not ordinarily permitted because of its caloric value and because the sorbitol content of processed foods is generally not specified.

Fructose has been proposed as a substitute for table sugar. Fructose does not cause as rapid a rise in plasma glucose as sucrose does, but fructose is a source of calories from carbohydrate. Use of fructose is generally not encouraged, but if fructose is permitted, it should be used in limited amounts and be included in the meal plan as a substitute for a fruit exchange.

A summary of the 1978 Food and Drug Administration labeling regulations for foods making weight-control claims is given to help clarify questions and concerns about food labeling.

1. Foods making weight-control claims must be accompanied by nutrition labeling (unless otherwise exempt) and a statement describing the purpose of the food (that is, "low-calorie," "reduced-calorie," or "for calorie-restricted diet").

2. Terms such as "diet," "dietetic," and "artificially sweetened" may be used only if the food qualifies for labeling as low-calorie or reduced-calorie.

3. Terms such as "sugar-free," "sugarless," and "no sugar" may be used only if the food is also labeled as low-calorie or reduced-calorie, with one exception. If the term is used in reference to a purpose other than weight control (for example, sugarless gum), the term must be accompanied by an explanatory statement (for example, "not for weight control" or "does not promote tooth decay").

4. Presence of non-nutritive sweeteners must be indicated on the label. If a food contains both non-nutritive and nutritive sweeteners, the presence of both must be indicated. Other non-nutritive ingredients that help a food achieve its weight-control claims must be identified, and the percentage by weight must be declared.

5. A "low-calorie" food is defined as one containing no more than 40 calories per serving and having a caloric density of no more than 0.4 kcal/g as consumed. Foods that are naturally low in calories must be labeled so that this fact is clear (for example, "celery, a low-calorie food" rather than "low-calorie celery").

6. A "reduced-calorie" food is defined as one having a caloric reduction of at least one-third from the compared food. The label must describe the comparison on which the reduced-calorie claim is based.

7. Any other food may be labeled as "useful for weight control" or for use in "calorie-restricted" diets if the basis for this claim is also declared on the label.

8. Foods represented as being useful in the diet of diabetics must be accompanied by nutrition labeling and the statement "Diabetics: This product may be useful in your diet on the advice of a physician. This food is not a reduced-calorie food." This last sentence may be deleted if the food is otherwise labeled for reducing or maintaining caloric intake or body weight.

ALCOHOLIC BEVERAGES

Alcohol tends to be both ketogenic and hypoglycemic, but in the well-nourished diabetic who is eating regularly and taking appropriate amounts of insulin, alcohol often has little effect on the state of diabetes. Alcohol, if allowed, should be taken with food. Alcohol is high in calories and should therefore be used infrequently, if at all, by the patient consuming a low-calorie reduction diet.

The lean diabetic may be permitted to use alcohol occasionally, in moderation, without isocaloric substitution for other foods. Isocaloric substitution of alcohol for fat is also acceptable, although the metabolism of alcohol does not permit its classification as protein, fat, or carbohydrate. Substitution for fat is based on the reasoning that fat, like alcohol, has a less immediate effect on blood glucose than does either carbohydrate or protein. Unfortunately, designation of alcohol as a fat exchange implies a greater degree of nutritional identity than is justified. Distilled spirits (gin, rum, Scotch, vodka, and whiskey) may be traded as 1/2 oz for one fat exchange (1 jigger equals 3 fat exchanges). Fermented spirits (beer, wine, and ale) contain a substantial amount of carbohydrate in addition to alcohol, both of which should be considered in the exchange (12 oz of beer equals 1 bread exchange and 2 fat exchanges; 3 1/2 oz of dry wine equals 1/4 bread exchange and 1 1/2 fat exchanges).

SELECTED BIBLIOGRAPHY

A Guide for Professionals: The Effective Application of "Exchange Lists for Meal Planning." American Diabetes Association, Inc., American Dietetic Association, 1977.

American Heart Association, Committee on Nutrition: Diet and Coronary Heart Disease, pamphlet EM 379, New York, 1973.

Bierman, E. L., Albrink, M. J., Arky, R. A., et al.: Principles of nutrition and dietary recommendations for patients with diabetes mellitus: 1971. Diabetes, 20:633-634, 1971.

Labeling of foods for special dietary use. Federal Register, 43:43248-43262, 1978.

Lenner, R. A.: Studies of glycemia and glucosuria in diabetics after breakfast meals of different composition. Am. J. Clin. Nutr., 29:716-725, 1976.

Miranda, P. M., and Horwitz, D. L.: High-fiber diets in the treatment of diabetes mellitus. Ann. Intern. Med., 88:482-486, 1978.

Nuttall, F. Q., and Brunzell, J. D.: Principles of nutrition and dietary recommendations for individuals with diabetes mellitus: 1979. Diabetes, 28:1027-1030, 1979.

West, K. M.: Diet therapy of diabetes: An analysis of failure. Ann. Intern. Med., 79:425-434, 1973.

DIETARY MANAGEMENT OF OBESITY

GENERAL DESCRIPTION

The diets recommended for weight reduction are low-calorie modifications of the general diet. Intake of calories from all sources is limited. Simple carbohydrates, such as those in sweets and other foods with added sugar, are usually not planned in the diets, and alcohol is inadvisable because of its high caloric value.

NUTRITIONAL ADEQUACY

A multivitamin and mineral supplement may be appropriate for persons following diets that provide fewer than 1,000 to 1,200 calories.

INDICATIONS AND RATIONALE

Obesity seems to be associated with and complicates a number of diseases, including diabetes mellitus, hyperlipidemia, coronary heart disease, hypertension, and degenerative arthritis. Complications during some acute illnesses and after accidents, general anesthesia, and surgery are more common among obese than among nonobese patients.

There is no absolute definition of obesity. Body composition can be measured by several techniques, and skin fold measurements give a reasonable approximation (see page 279). These techniques yield estimates of body fat expressed as percentages of body weight. The generally accepted normal proportions of body fat are 15 to 20% of body weight for men and 20 to 25% for women. In extremely obese persons, 50 to 60% of body weight may be fat, whereas in marathon runners or gymnasts, fat may contribute less than 5% of body weight. Whether there is a particular percentage of weight as fat that provides optimal health has not been established. Persons having one of the disorders aggravated by obesity may profit by reducing weight to a distinct degree of leanness. For practical purposes, weight remains the most frequently used indicator of obesity.

Accumulation of adipose tissue is the consequence of consumption of calories in excess of expenditure. For obese persons, the basal metabolic rate expressed as a percentage above or below normal and corrected for age, surface area, and sex is similar in average and distribution to that of the reference population (Nelson et al., 1973). This finding implies that under basal conditions, the calorie expenditure of obese persons is greater than that of their normal-weight counterparts of the same age, height, and sex by the ratio of their surface areas.

Obesity may be treated by several methods, including prescribed diet, behavioral modification, anorectic drugs, and surgery. The success of anorectic drugs has been variable and generally temporary; some risks are associated with their use. Gastroplasty and jejunoileal bypass have substantial risks and have not been used at the Mayo Clinic. Behavioral modification, which aims to revise eating habits, has had excellent results in some circumstances. Some of the principles and techniques of behavioral modification can be used in conjunction with conventional low-calorie diets. Low-calorie diets adapted to the patient's preferred meal times and foods constitute the basic approach to obesity. The goals of low-calorie weight reduction diets are to provide essential nutrients while causing loss of weight and to help establish permanent and more desirable eating habits. Ideally, a diet similar to the low-calorie diet in selection of foods and in meal pattern and controlled in calories for weight maintenance should be provided when the goal weight has been achieved.

Proportions of protein, fat, and carbohydrate used in weight reduction diets can vary widely, and no particular proportion seems to have a clear advantage. Diets very low in carbohydrate, or ketogenic diets, may promote a more rapid loss of weight initially through diuresis, but loss of body fat is not significantly different from that achieved by isocaloric diets containing conventional proportions of carbohydrate. The diet should provide 0.8 to 1 g of protein* per kilogram of ideal body weight. Protein intake above this range does not seem to confer any benefit.

Exercise promotes calorie expenditure and, therefore, weight loss. Planned exercise is particularly important if the obese person is otherwise inactive. There is a dual benefit, since exercise utilizes excess calories and generally is associated with decreased appetite and food intake. The dietitian should evaluate the patient's activity patterns and suggest ways of utilizing them to increase regular activity. If there are any constraints on activity for medical reasons, the physician should tell the patient what kinds and amounts of activity are appropriate.

There should be some type of follow-up after the initial diet instruction to encourage the patient to adhere to the diet and to allow the dietitian to answer any questions. Follow-up may take the form of either regular visits to the dietitian for brief discussions and weighings or a weight loss record (see page 283) that is returned to the dietitian periodically. After the patient reaches the weight goal, a weight maintenance diet should be planned to help the patient continue to control weight.

DETERMINATION OF IDEAL WEIGHT

The height-weight table (see page 278) can be used as a guide for determining "ideal" or "desirable" weight. If the patient considers this weight to be inappropriate or unattainable, a "goal" or "preferred" weight should be established with the patient's agreement. The goal should be realistic. It may be helpful to set intermediate goal weights. When an intermediate weight is reached, the need for further reduction can be assessed by clinical means, which may include skin fold measurements. The patient would have the option of following a weight maintenance diet before resuming efforts to lose weight.

In determining the ideal weight, coexisting diseases that may be aggravated by obesity, such as diabetes mellitus, hypertension, and hyperlipidemia, should be taken into consideration. If such a disease is present, leanness or a weight at a lower end of the range of acceptable weight for height is often desirable.

DETERMINATION OF CALORIE LEVEL

The diet selected should be low enough in calories to cause a perceptible loss in weight. An average loss of 1 to 2 lb a week is a reasonable goal. If the diet selected causes a weight loss of less than, perhaps, 1/2 lb a week, the patient may become discouraged by the slow results.

Body size, age, and activity determine calorie expenditure and should be considered in arriving at the calorie level of the diet. A daily calorie deficit (calorie expenditure minus the calorie content of the diet) of at least 500 calories is usually appropriate. If the planned daily deficit is fewer than 500 calories, small errors in preparation of the diet may increase calorie intake to the point that weight loss is negligible. If the person is short and inactive, a diet of 800 or 1,000 calories may be necessary to achieve a perceptible loss (1 to 2 lb a week). Larger, more active persons may lose satisfactorily with a diet providing 1,400 or 1,600 calories.

---

*Recommended dietary allowance for protein is 0.8 g/kg of body weight.

USE OF THE NOMOGRAM TO PREDICT WEIGHT LOSS

The nomogram (see page 282) can be used to obtain the average basal calorie requirements according to the person's age, sex, and body size. The weight used to predict loss is from 10 to 20 lb less than actual weight.* To allow for calories expended through activity, one must add to basal calories an increment of 10 to 50%—10% for the inactive person and up to 50% or more for the very active person. The resulting figure is an estimation of average daily calorie expenditure. The calorie deficit is the difference between calories expended and calories consumed. Multiplied by 0.002, this figure gives an estimate in pounds of projected loss of weight a week. A deficit of 500 calories a day results in a deficit of 3,500 calories a week, which is equivalent to 1 lb of fat.

The nomogram indicates average basal caloric requirements. Caloric requirements can be determined more accurately by measuring oxygen consumption or the basal metabolic rate. Milliliters of oxygen used per minute multiplied by 7† yields an estimate of calories expended in 24 hours under resting conditions.

The patient should be told that the projected weight loss is an average figure and that the rate of weight loss varies considerably from person to person. Also, a steady rate of weight loss from week to week is unlikely. Decrease in weight tends to be greater in the first week or two weeks than later, especially if the carbohydrate and sodium content of the diet is substantially less than that of the previous diet. Several pounds of the first weight lost are likely to be from excretion of water and electrolytes. There may also be "plateaus"—periods of several weeks or more when the patient's weight remains the same despite close dietary adherence. The usual cause is temporary variation in the amount of body water. The patient should be told that the purpose of the diet is to lose fat tissue and that total weight does not always accurately reflect recent changes in the amount of body fat.

PHYSICIANS: HOW TO ORDER DIETS

The diet order may (1) indicate **weight reduction diet** (the dietitian will determine an appropriate calorie level) *or* (2) specify the daily **calorie deficit** desired (for example, 500- or 1,000-calorie daily deficit) *or* (3) specify the **calorie level** (for example, 1,000-, 1,200-, or 1,400-caloric diet).

GENERAL DIETARY RECOMMENDATIONS

1. A diet history is taken to assess the patient's weight, physical activity, and eating habits.
2. Ideal weight (see height-weight table, page 278) or a realistic weight goal is determined with the help of the patient. The patient's weight history and associated medical problems are considered.
3. A calorie level that will promote a reasonable and perceptible loss of weight is determined.
4. The food exchange list beginning on page 36 and the suggested daily food exchanges on page 51 may be used as a guide. Simple carbohydrates and alcohol should be avoided or allowed in only small amounts.
5. The diet should be adapted as closely as possible to the patient's preferences.
6. The diet should be directed at changing the patient's eating habits. If necessary, guidelines should be given to increase the patient's activity.
7. The diet should be flexible enough to allow the patient some variety in food choices, and it should be adaptable to restaurant dining or bag lunches.
8. The dietitian should evaluate the patient's progress, provide encouragement, and adjust the diet as needed.
9. A weight maintenance diet should be planned for the patient when the goal weight is reached.

---

*The lower weight is used in calculations because it reflects more accurately the weight of the patient during the period of loss than does the initial weight.

†0.0048 kcal/ml O_2 × 1,440 min/24 hr = 6.912.

APPROXIMATE COMPOSITION

	Protein	Fat	Carbohydrate
Calorie Level	g	g	g
800	55	25	80
1,000	60	35	110
1,200	70	45	125
1,400	80	55	155
1,600	85	60	180

SUGGESTED DAILY FOOD EXCHANGES*

	Calorie Level†				
Exchange Group	800	1,000	1,200	1,400	1,600
Meat‡	5	5	6	7	7
Fat	0	2	3	4	5
Milk, nonfat§	2	2	2	2	2
Starch	1	3	4	6	7
Vegetable	2	2	2	2	2
Fruit	3	3	3	3	4

*Use the food exchange list, page 36.

†These are the most frequently used levels. Intermediate levels may also be used.

‡Calculations are based on values for medium-fat meats. Use of lean and medium-fat meats rather than high-fat meats is encouraged.

§Use of nonfat milk is suggested; if low-fat or whole milk is used, the number of fat exchanges should be decreased.

SELECTED BIBLIOGRAPHY

Bray, G. A. (ed.): Obesity in Perspective (DHEW Publication No. [NIH] 75-708). Washington D.C., Government Printing Office, 1975.

Bray, G. A.: The obese patient. Major Probl. Intern. Med., 9:1-445, 1976.

Gastineau, C. F.: The prediction of weight loss on a reducing diet (editorial). Minn. Med., 43:255-257, 1960.

Nelson, R. A., Anderson, L. F., Gastineau, C. F., et al.: Physiology and natural history of obesity. J.A.M.A., 223:627-630, 1973.

Yang, M.-U., and Van Itallie, T. B.: Composition of weight lost during short-term weight reduction: Metabolic responses of obese subjects to starvation and low-calorie ketogenic and nonketogenic diets. J. Clin. Invest., 58:722-730, 1976.

DIETARY MANAGEMENT OF HYPERLIPIDEMIA (TYPES I-V)

GENERAL DESCRIPTION

Dietary treatment for the hyperlipidemias emphasizes control of weight. Management of dietary constituents—fat (amount and kind), cholesterol, carbohydrate, and alcohol—is determined by which lipids are elevated in the blood. Also, the particular abnormal pattern of lipoproteins should be considered if one is to achieve the greatest effect with diet.

INDICATIONS AND RATIONALE

Elevation of cholesterol or triglycerides is of medical concern because of its association with the development of atherosclerosis. Treatment is based on the assumption that normalization of values reduces the rate of atherogenesis. Normal values, however, do not necessarily indicate an absence of risk for atherosclerosis.

"Hyperlipidemia" is a general term that refers to increased levels of cholesterol and triglycerides. "Hyperlipoproteinemia" refers to abnormal levels of any one of the lipoprotein fractions that carry lipids in the blood. Six abnormal types of hyperlipoproteinemia have been identified; classification of each is determined by which lipoproteins are increased. The diagnosis of hyperlipidemia is based on the laboratory determination of cholesterol and triglyceride values. When the laboratory diagnosis is unclear, lipoprotein analysis may be done to determine whether abnormal lipoprotein values are present and the type of hyperlipoproteinemia.

The chart below illustrates the different amounts of protein, cholesterol, triglycerides, and phospholipids in each lipoprotein fraction. An increase in any of the fractions causes a proportionate increase in the associated lipids in the blood.

Lipoprotein Fractions	Protein %	Cholesterol %	Triglyceride %	Phospholipid %
Chylomicrons	2	5	90	3
Very Low-density Lipoproteins (VLDL)	10	12	60	18
Intermediate-density Lipoproteins (IDL)	10	30	40	20
Low-density Lipoproteins (LDL)	25	50	10	15
High-density Lipoproteins (HDL)	50	20	5	25

Hyperlipoproteinemias can occur with other disease states. Treatment of the underlying disease usually corrects these secondary forms of hyperlipoproteinemia.

Primary hyperlipoproteinemias are a result of either genetic abnormalities or environmental factors. Severe forms often are inheritable; a modified diet and, often, drugs are necessary for treatment. Milder forms may be associated with dietary indiscretions. Modifying the diet produces a small to moderate reduction in serum cholesterol concentration or, less frequently, normalizes the serum cholesterol value.

The dietary-related hyperlipidemias found most often in medical practice are elevated serum cholesterol values due to abnormal concentrations of LDL and elevated serum triglyceride values due to abnormal concentrations of VLDL. Diets high in fat, saturated fat, and cholesterol increase levels of LDL; consuming less of these constituents and isocalorically substituting polyunsaturated fats reduce LDL levels. Diets high in calories, carbohydrates, or alcohol increase levels of VLDL; reducing weight and consuming less carbohydrate and alcohol normalize VLDL levels. It is also generally recommended that very large meals and high-fat meals be avoided.

Lipid disorders are first treated by modifying the diet. Drugs may be prescribed if dietary regulations are unsuccessful. Because the effects of diet and drugs are additive, dietary modification should be continued during drug therapy. Continuation of the diet is advised even with normalization of blood lipids and lipoprotein pattern.

TYPES OF HYPERLIPOPROTEINEMIAS

Lipid abnormalities are classified by types I, IIa, IIb, III, IV, and V. The specific lipid disorders of these types are as follows:

Type	Lipid Abnormality	Elevated Lipoprotein
I	Hyperchylomicronemia	Chylomicrons
IIa	Hypercholesterolemia	LDL
IIb	Combined hypercholesterolemia and endogenous hypertriglyceridemia	LDL and VLDL
III	Dysbetalipoproteinemia (broad beta pattern)	IDL
IV	Hypertriglyceridemia	Chylomicrons and VLDL
V	Hypertriglyceridemia	VLDL and chylomicrons

Hyperchylomicronemia (Type I). Rare; detected in early childhood.

Abnormal blood lipids: Severe elevation of triglycerides (more than 1,000 mg/dl) due to a deficiency of lipoprotein lipase, an enzyme thought to be responsible for the clearning of chylomicrons.

Major Dietary Emphasis.—Preventing chylomicron formation by severely restricting dietary fat.

Dietary fat	25 to 35 g/day; see page 145 for fat-restricted diets
Medium-chain triglycerides (do not cause chylomicron formation)	20 to 40 g/day; see page 147
Alcohol	None

Hypercholesterolemia (Type IIa). Common; may be familial (detected in early childhood or adulthood) or environmental (detected in adulthood).

Abnormal blood lipids: Elevated LDL cholesterol. Familial forms—cholesterol elevations are often in the range of 700 to 1,000 mg/dl; drugs usually are needed in addition to dietary modifications. Environmental forms—cholesterol elevations are generally less (300 to 500 mg/dl); modifying dietary composition alone may suffice for normalizing cholesterol levels.

Major Dietary Emphasis.—Reduction of dietary intake of cholesterol and saturated fat as one means of decreasing excess LDL; substitution of polyunsaturated fats for saturated fats.

Cholesterol	≤200 mg/day
Total fat	≤35% of calories
Saturated fat	≤10% of calories
Polyunsaturated fats	Isocaloric substitution for saturated fats

Caloric restriction may have minimal effect on lowering lipids. See page 58 for foods allowed.

Hypercholesterolemia with Endogenous Hypertriglyceridemia (Type IIb). Similar to type IIa.

Abnormal blood lipids: Elevated LDL cholesterol (genetic and environmental forms same as type IIa) and elevated triglycerides (less than 400 mg/dl) generally due to increased VLDL production from intake of excess calories, carbohydrates, or alcohol.

Major Dietary Emphasis.—Same as type IIa; restriction of calories until ideal body weight is achieved and limitation of carbohydrate intake* to control excess production of VLDL.

Weight reduction	See page 49 for information on ideal weight
Cholesterol	⩽200 mg/day
Total fat	⩽35% of calories
Saturated fat	⩽10% of calories
Polyunsaturated fats	Isocaloric substitution for saturated fats
Carbohydrate*	⩽45% of calories

See page 58 for foods allowed.

Dysbetalipoproteinemia (Type III). Relatively uncommon; detected from early adulthood.
Abnormal blood lipids: Elevated LDL cholesterol and VLDL triglycerides due to accumulation of intermediate forms of lipoproteins (IDL) as a result of a block in normal conversion of VLDL to LDL.

Major Dietary Emphasis.—Dietary modifications similar to those for type IIb, except that cholesterol restriction is less severe.

Weight reduction†	See page 49 for information on ideal weight
Cholesterol	⩽300 mg/day
Total fat	⩽35% of calories
Saturated fat	⩽10% of calories
Polyunsaturated fats	Isocaloric substitution for saturated fats
Carbohydrate	⩽45% of calories (see type IIb for use of complex and refined carbohydrates and alcohol)

See page 58 for foods allowed.

---

*Complex carbohydrates are emphasized. Simple carbohydrates and alcohol are generally not included in weight reduction diets. They may be allowed in weight maintenance diets if the calorie level is sufficiently high and the physician approves. If simple carbohydrates or alcohol is allowed, substitutions can be made from the starch group (page 61). The physician should discuss use of alcohol with the patient and also inform the dietitian.

†Achievement of ideal body weight and controlled carbohydrate intake usually is effective in normalizing blood lipids.

Hypertriglyceridemia (Type IV). Common; detected in adulthood, generally during the middle years.

Abnormal blood lipids: Elevated triglycerides (usually less than 1,000 mg/dl), generally due to increased VLDL production from intake of excess calories, carbohydrates, or alcohol.

Major Dietary Emphasis.—Reduction of glucose intolerance by restricting calories until ideal body weight is achieved and by controlling carbohydrate intake.* Some physicians also may specify lowering of cholesterol intake and modifying of fat content; guidelines for type II should be followed.

Weight reduction	See page 49 for information on ideal weight
Carbohydrate*	≤45% of calories

See page 48 for weight reduction diets.

Mixed Hyperlipidemia (Type V). Relatively uncommon; detected from early adulthood.

Abnormal blood lipids: Elevated triglycerides (more than 10,000 mg/dl) due to accumulation of both VLDL and chylomicrons caused by a defect in the metabolism of endogenous and exogenous triglycerides (reduced lipoprotein lipase activity).

Major Dietary Emphasis.—Reduction of fat and carbohydrate intolerance by restricting calories and achieving ideal body weight, by severely limiting total fat intake, by controlling carbohydrate intake,* and by avoiding alcohol. Moderate cholesterol and modified fat measures also are included.

Weight reduction	See page 49 for information on ideal weight
Carbohydrate*	≤50% of calories
Total fat	≤30% of calories
Alcohol	None
Cholesterol	≤500 mg/day
Polyunsaturated fats	Isocaloric substitution for saturated fats within 30% fat allowance

See page 58 for foods allowed.

---

*Complex carbohydrates are emphasized. Simple carbohydrates and alcohol are generally not included in weight reduction diets. They may be allowed in weight maintenance diets if the calorie level is sufficiently high and the physician approves. If simple carbohydrates or alcohol is allowed, substitutions can be made from the starch group (page 61). The physician should discuss use of alcohol with the patient and also inform the dietitian.

DIETARY PRESCRIPTION FOR THE HYPERLIPIDEMIAS

	Type of Hyperlipoproteinemia					
	I	IIa	IIb	III	IV	V
Calories	Weight maintenance	Weight control	Weight control	Weight control	Weight control	Weight control
Fat	25–35 g (any type); MCT, 20–40 g	35% kcal; 10% SF; use PUSF	35% kcal; 10% SF; use PUSF	35% kcal; 10% SF; use PUSF	Not restricted unless physician requests	<30% kcal; use PUSF
Carbohydrate	Not restricted	Not restricted	≤45% kcal*	≤45% kcal*	≤45% kcal*	≤50% kcal*
Alcohol	Avoid	Not restricted	Restricted	Restricted	Restricted	Avoid
Cholesterol	Not restricted	≤200 mg†	≤200 mg†	≤300 mg	Not restricted unless physician requests	≤500 mg

MCT = medium-chain triglycerides; SF = saturated fat (percentage of fat from saturated fat is based on meat sources); PUSF = polyunsaturated fats.
*Emphasize complex carbohydrate.
†Meat is major source.

PHYSICIANS: HOW TO ORDER DIETS

The diet order should either indicate the **type of hyperlipoproteinemia** (for example, type II) *or* specify the **diet modification** (for example, low cholesterol and saturated fats).

FOODS TO ALLOW AND FOODS TO AVOID

The items listed apply only to control of *cholesterol* and *saturated fat* for weight maintenance diets. To determine the appropriate portion to serve, see the food exchange list, page 36. The cholesterol and fatty acid contents of selected foods are listed in the Appendix, page 284.

Food Groups	Allow	Avoid
Beverage	Coffee; tea; decaffeinated coffee; cereal beverage; carbonated beverage	Beverage mixes containing whole milk solids, cocoa butter, hydrogenated vegetable fats, coconut oil, or palm oil
Meat	Lean meats (no more than 15% fat) trimmed of visible fat and prepared without added fat; low-fat cold cuts and frankfurters	High-fat meats (more than 15% fat): cold cuts, frankfurters, sausage, canned meats, corned beef, spareribs, ground beef with more than 15% fat; fried meats; meat with added fat; organ meats: brains, heart, liver, kidney, sweetbreads, tongue
	Fish; shellfish (except shrimp)	Shrimp; fish canned in oil; caviar
	Chicken and turkey (without skin)	Duck; goose; capon
	Peanut butter*; vegetable protein meat substitutes*	
	Egg whites; low-cholesterol egg substitutes	Egg yolks†
	Cheese low in butterfat (no more than 15% fat) Natural—mozzarella, part skim; ricotta, whole milk; cream cheese, part skim; sapsago; cottage cheese, creamed (4% fat) and low-fat (2% or less fat); dried curd cheese, such as farmer, pot, hoop, and baker's cheeses	Cheese high in fat (more than 15% fat) Natural—all except those in "Allow" column
	Processed—low-fat cheese food made primarily from skim milk; filled skim milk cheese made with corn, cottonseed, safflower, or sunflower seed oil*	Processed—high-fat cheese food made primarily from whole milk or cream; filled cheese made with coconut or palm oil

Food Groups	Allow	Avoid
Fat	Vegetable oils with a ratio of poly-unsaturated fat to saturated fat of 2 or more (listed in order of preference): safflower, corn, sunflower, walnut, wheat germ, sesame, soybean, cottonseed	Coconut oil; palm oil; cocoa butter; avocado; butter; lard; salt pork; meat fat; poultry skin; bacon; suet; cream; sour cream; other cream products; fish liver oil‡
	Peanut oil§; olive oil§	
	Margarines (preferably soft) and shortenings listing liquid vegetable oil as the first ingredient and having a ratio of polyunsaturated fat to saturated fat of 2 or more**; diet margarine††	Margarine and shortening containing animal fat; completely hydrogenated vegetable oil
	Margarines and shortenings listing partially hydrogenated vegetable oil as the first ingredient§	
	Mayonnaise; mayonnaise-type salad dressing; salad dressing prepared with recommended vegetable oils without cream or cheese	Salad dressing containing cream, cheese, hydrogenated vegetable oil, coconut oil, or palm oil
	Imitation cream products made with polyunsaturated fats	Cream; half-and-half; other cream products; nondairy coffee lighteners and imitation cream products made with coconut, palm, or hydrogenated vegetable oil
	Almonds; pecans; walnuts; other nuts,§ except those in "Avoid" column	Cashews; macadamia nuts
Milk	Milk and milk products containing less than 1% butterfat: skim milk, nonfat dry milk, buttermilk made from skim milk, yogurt made from skim milk	Milk and milk products containing 1% or more butterfat: whole milk, 2% milk, 1% milk, evaporated milk, sweetened condensed milk, buttermilk made from whole or low-fat milk, yogurt made from whole or low-fat milk, any milk beverage containing whole milk solids or cocoa butter, chocolate milk
	Imitation dairy products made with allowed fats*	Imitation dairy products made with coconut, palm, or hydrogenated vegetable oil

Food Groups	Allow	Avoid
Starch	Any product containing less than 1 g of fat per serving: white or whole grain breads, rolls, cereals; plain crackers; starchy vegetables; wheat germ*; popcorn; pasta (except egg noodles)	Any product containing 1 g or more of fat per serving (unless prepared with allowed fats*): pancakes, waffles, biscuits, muffins; variety or butter-type snack crackers; French fries; potato or corn chips; egg noodles
	Any homemade or commercially prepared baked goods containing skim milk, low-cholesterol egg substitutes, and allowed fats*	Any homemade or commercially prepared baked goods or mixes containing whole milk, butterfat, other animal fats, hydrogenated shortening, or egg yolks†
Vegetable	Any prepared without fat or with allowed fats*	None
Fruit	Any	None
Soup	Any fat-free soup or any containing less than 1 g of fat per serving: bouillon, fat-free broth, soups with base of skim milk, packaged dehydrated soups	Any with added fat or containing 1 g or more of fat per serving: commercial canned soups, cream soups, soups containing whole milk products
Dessert	Angel food cake; gelatin; fruit ice; meringues; sherbet, ice milk, and puddings made with skim milk; vanilla wafers; gingersnaps; commercial fig bars; any homemade or commercially prepared dessert containing allowed ingredients, skim milk, egg whites, egg substitutes, allowed fats and margarines,* cocoa powder, or carob powder	Any homemade or commercially prepared desserts or mixes containing whole milk, cream, butterfat, other animal fats, hydrogenated fats, egg yolks,† chocolate, cocoa butter, coconut, cashews, or macadamia nuts
Sweets	Sugar; honey; jam; jelly; syrup; plain sugar candy (hard candy, gumdrops, jelly beans, marshmallows)	Any containing whole milk, cream, chocolate, cocoa butter, hydrogenated fats, coconut, cashews, or macadamia nuts
Miscellaneous	Salt; pepper; herbs; spices; pickles; relishes; catsup; mustard; meat sauces and extracts; vinegar; cocoa powder; fat-free butter flavoring; flavoring extracts	Any product containing ingredients that must be avoided

*Total fat allowance should be reduced proportionately.

†Three egg yolks are allowed each week for diets with moderate control of cholesterol—300 to 500 mg/day.

‡Cholesterol content varies but is generally high.

§These fats have a ratio of polyunsaturated fat to saturated fat of less than 2; they may be used as part of the fat allowance for diets with moderate cholesterol control.

**The content of polyunsaturates should be obtained periodically from the manufacturer. The amount may vary depending on the proportion of partially hydrogenated vegetable oils added.

††Diet margarines that are high in polyunsaturated fats are acceptable but are not recommended. Since the main ingredient is water, approximately twice as much margarine is needed to provide the same amount of polyunsaturated fat as regular margarine.

SIMPLE CARBOHYDRATES AND ALCOHOL

Diets high in calories, carbohydrate, or alcohol increase VLDL levels. Simple carbohydrates and alcohol are generally not included in weight reduction diets. However, they may be included in weight maintenance diets if the allowable calorie level is sufficiently high and the physician approves.

Alcohol-Carbohydrate Substitutions. Any of the following quantities of alcoholic beverages is 1 serving and may be used in place of 1 serving from the starch allowance in diets with carbohydrate restrictions (diets for types IIb, III, IV, and V).

1 oz	Gin, rum, whiskey, vodka
1 1/2 oz	Dessert or sweet wine
2 1/2 oz	Dry table wine
5 oz	Beer

Dessert-Carbohydrate Substitutions. Any of the following quantities of desserts is 1 serving and may be used in place of 1 serving from the starch allowance in diets with carbohydrate restrictions (diets for types IIb, III, IV, and V).

1/2 cup	Commercial flavored gelatin
1/4 cup	Sherbet or fruit ice
1/2 cup	Plain pudding
5	Vanilla wafers or gingersnaps
1 1/2 in. cube	Plain cake
1/10	16-in. angel food or sponge cake

SELECTED BIBLIOGRAPHY

Fredrickson, D. S., Levy, R. I., Bonnell, M., et al.: The Dietary Management of Hyperlipoproteinemia: A Handbook for Physicians and Dieticians (DHEW Publication No. [NIH] 75-110). Bethesda, Maryland, National Heart and Lung Institute, 1974.

Gotto, A. M., Jr., DeBakey, M. E., Foreyt, J. P., et al.: Dietary treatment of type IV hyperlipoproteinemia. J.A.M.A., 237:1212-1215, 1977.

Grundy, S. M.: Effects of polyunsaturated fats on lipid metabolism in patients with hypertriglyceridemia. J. Clin. Invest., 55: 269-282, 1975.

Grundy, S. M.: Treatment of hypercholesterolemia. Am. J. Clin. Nutr., 30:985-992, 1977.

Kummerow, F. A.: Nutrition imbalance and angiotoxins as dietary risk factors in coronary heart disease. Am. J. Clin. Nutr., 32:58-83, 1979.

Levy, R. I., Morganroth, J., and Rifkind, B. M.: Treatment of hyperlipidemia. N. Engl. J. Med., 290:1295-1301, 1974.

Murphy, B. F.: Management of hyperlipidemias. J.A.M.A., 230:1683-1691, 1974.

Olefsky, J., Reaven, G. M., and Farquhar, J. W.: Effects of weight reduction on obesity: Studies of lipid and carbohydrate metabolism in normal and hyperlipoproteinemic subjects. J. Clin. Invest., 53:64-76, 1974.

Palumbo, P. J., Briones, E. R., Nelson, R. A., et al.: Sucrose sensitivity of patients with coronary-artery disease. Am. J. Clin. Nutr., 30:394-401, 1977.

Roen, P. B.: The evening meal and atherosclerosis. J. Am. Geriatr. Soc., 26:284-285, 1978.

Stone, N. J.: When to worry about plasma lipids. Cardiovasc. Med., 1:143-158, 1976.

Taylor, C. B., Peng, S.-K., Werthessen, N. T., et al.: Spontaneously occurring angiotoxic derivatives of cholesterol. Am. J. Clin. Nutr., 32:40-57, 1979.

SODIUM CONTROL

GENERAL DESCRIPTION

Sources of dietary sodium are (1) table salt, or sodium chloride, (2) foods to which salt or sodium compounds have been added, (3) foods that inherently contain sodium, and (4) chemically softened water containing sodium salts. The level of sodium restriction—20 meq (500 mg), 40 meq (1,000 mg), 90 meq (2,000 mg), or no extra salt*: 90 to 150 meq (2,000 to 3,500 mg)—depends on the severity of the disorder.

In diets restricting sodium to 20, 40, or 90 meq, the calculated amount of sodium should be no greater than 10% above the prescribed level. It is acceptable for the calculated level of sodium to be more than 10% below the prescribed level. In most situations, special efforts (such as adding extra salt) need not be made to bring sodium intake up to the prescribed level. The level of sodium prescribed for the disorders discussed in this section is usually considered the maximal acceptable level.

INDICATIONS AND RATIONALE

Sodium-controlled diets are prescribed primarily for the prevention and control of edema and for the control of hypertension. The following chart summarizes disorders and the level of sodium restriction usually prescribed.

Sodium meq	Condition
20	Congestive heart failure; cirrhosis with massive ascites (occasionally)
20–90	Congestive heart failure
40–90	Hypertension; cirrhosis with ascites
90–150 (no extra salt)*	Mild hypertension; mild fluid retention

These sodium levels are only general guidelines, and the degree of restriction should be based on the severity of the disease. However, a restriction of less than 40 meq may be difficult to maintain for long periods outside a hospital setting.

Congestive Heart Failure. Congestive heart failure results when the heart is unable to pump enough blood to satisfy the body's metabolic requirements. Reduced blood flow, through a complex system of mechanical and hormonal processes, results in diminished renal function and retention of sodium and water. This results in an increase in extracellular fluid volume with congestion in the lungs (pulmonary edema) and edema in the extremities.

---

*The sodium content of a no-extra-salt diet varies according to calorie level. The diet allows only limited amounts of salt in cooking and does not allow additional salt (that is, the saltshaker) or foods excessively high in sodium. See page 66 for further explanation of the no-extra-salt diet.

Sodium restriction, by reducing extracellular fluid volume, decreases the work required of the heart, and this may promote diuresis. The level of restriction needed depends on the severity of the heart failure and the effectiveness of diuretics. A diet restricting sodium to 20 meq may be prescribed initially. When edema is controlled, the intake of sodium may be increased to 40 meq. A diet containing 90 meq of sodium is generally sufficient to control edema after the patient leaves the hospital. See page 253 for other dietary modifications that may be appropriate for congestive heart failure.

Cirrhosis with Ascites. Chronic disease of the liver may be accompanied by ascites, which is the accumulation of abnormal amounts of fluid in the abdomen. This may occur as a result of portal vein hypertension, reduced oncotic pressure, impaired water excretion, and increased sodium retention. Initially, a diet of 20 meq of sodium or 40 meq of sodium may be instituted. A diet containing 90 meq of sodium, when used in conjunction with diuretics, is often eventually sufficient to control fluid retention.

Hypertension. Sustained elevation of the blood pressure is known as hypertension. Most patients have essential hypertension—hypertension unrelated to any identifiable cause. Weight control, sodium restriction, and drug therapy are the major methods of treating these hypertensive patients.

Generally, dietary management is selected as the initial means of treatment for mild and, sometimes, for moderate hypertension. Usually, efforts to control moderate or severe hypertension require drug therapy in addition to dietary measures as the initial means of management. The effectiveness of medication may be enhanced by control of sodium intake.

Restriction of sodium decreases circulatory blood volume. Maximal intake of 90 meq of sodium is prescribed for most patients. In very mild cases, a no-extra-salt diet may be sufficient to control high blood pressure, especially if previous sodium intake has been excessive. In severe hypertension, greater restrictions may be necessary, for example, 40 meq.

Weight reduction is recommended for any hypertensive patient above ideal weight. If serum lipid levels are abnormal or even slightly elevated, modification of cholesterol and fat intake may be warranted (see page 58), since atherosclerosis may be aggravated by persistent elevation of blood pressure. If cholesterol intake is to be reduced and polyunsaturated fats are to be substituted, these modifications should be indicated on the diet request form.

Diuretic drugs may reduce the blood levels of potassium; reduced levels affect renal, muscle, and cardiac function. Levels may be increased to normal by use of a potassium-sparing diuretic, a potassium chloride supplement, or a salt substitute containing potassium chloride or by an increase in dietary potassium (foods high in potassium content are listed on page 109). These methods are directed at repletion of potassium loss; however, urinary loss of potassium can often be minimized by controlling the sodium intake of patients on diuretic therapy.

Since control of sodium and calories may potentiate the action of antihypertensive agents, consistent observation of dietary precautions is needed to properly adjust the dose of these agents.

Caffeine has been reported to increase blood pressure, perhaps through stimulation of secretion of renin and of catecholamines. For this reason, caffeine-containing beverages (and medications) should be used in moderation.

PHYSICIANS: HOW TO ORDER DIETS

The diet order should indicate a specific level of sodium (for example, **20 meq**, **40 meq**, or **90 meq of sodium**) *or* a **no-extra salt diet**. If a specific amount is ordered, the dietitian will plan a diet that does not exceed that amount by more than 10%. In some diets (for example, calorie-restricted, 90 meq of sodium), the amount of sodium provided by foods is often substantially less than 90 meq; a measured amount of salt will *not* be added unless specifically requested by the physician.

SOURCES OF SODIUM IN THE DIET

The sodium content of the American diet is estimated to be 110 to 260 meq (2,500 to 6,000 mg), which is equivalent to 6 to 15 g of salt. The inherent sodium content of foods and the sodium added by food manufacturers must be considered when a sodium-controlled diet is prescribed. The major source of sodium in the diet is table salt (40% sodium), commonly used in cooking, in food processing, and at the table.

Foods. Sodium inherent in some foods must be calculated as part of the sodium allowance. Animal foods such as meats, eggs, and dairy products and some vegetables contain sodium and should be used in controlled amounts. Sodium compounds are used in food processing for various reasons; for example, sodium benzoate is a preservative in relishes, sauces, and margarine, and sodium citrate enhances the flavor of gelatin desserts and beverages. It is important to read labels on foods purchased. There are many low-sodium products on the market. If such a product contains no more than 10 mg of sodium per serving, it may be used.

Medications. Antacids, laxatives, cough medicines, and other medications may contain significant amounts of sodium. One should check the label or ask a local pharmacist or the manufacturer for the sodium content.

Softened Water. Drinking water, either natural or softened, may be a significant source of sodium. Patients on diets of 20 meq are advised to ask the public health department about the sodium content of the local water supply. If the content exceeds 40 parts per million (2 meq, or 40 mg, of sodium per liter), distilled water should be used. Patients who are limited to 20 meq of sodium in the diet and whose water supply must be softened should have the softener attached only to the hot water line so that cold water used in cooking and for drinking will not contribute to sodium intake.

SODIUM DEPLETION

Symptoms of sodium depletion are weakness, lethargy, abdominal cramps, and oliguria. Other problems related to sodium depletion are azotemia and disturbances in the acid-base balance; severe sodium loss may precipitate peripheral circulatory failure (shock). The chance of sodium deficiency may be increased by profuse perspiration, vomiting, diarrhea, surgery, some renal disturbances and diuretics. Dietary sodium restriction alone should not cause sodium depletion but will contribute to the risk of sodium depletion resulting from the preceding factors.

SAMPLE DAILY FOOD EXCHANGES*

Food Groups	Sodium (meq) Exchange†	20 meq of Sodium		40 meq of Sodium		90 meq of Sodium	
		1,000-calorie	2,000-calorie	1,000-calorie	2,000-calorie	1,000-calorie	2,000-calorie
Meat‡							
Salted	3	...	...	5	...	5	5
Unsalted	1	5	5	...	5	...	...
Fat							
Salted	2	...	...	2	...	2	9
Unsalted	...	2	9	...	9	...	...
Milk							
Nonfat§	5	2	...	2	...	2	...
Low-fat or whole	5	...	2	...	2	...	2
Starch**							
Group 1	1	3	6	1	3	...	2
Group 2	5	...	...	2	2	...	2
Group 3	10	...	...	...	1	3	2
Vegetable							
Salted	12	...	...	...	...	2	...
Unsalted	0.5	2	2 or 3	2	2 or 3	...	2 or 3
Fruit	0	3	2 or 3	3	2 or 3	3	2 or 3
Sweets	0	...	2 to 4	...	2 to 4	...	2 to 4
Dessert							
Regular	5–10	...	...	...	...	...	1
Special, low-sodium	1	...	1	...	1	...	...
Beverages††							

*Sample exchanges for two calorie levels are given only for diets of 20, 40, and 90 meq of sodium. For no-extra-salt diets, the number of exchanges from particular food groups is not limited, unless there is need for weight reduction. See further explanation of the no-extra-salt diet on page 66.

†The list of food exchanges includes both salted and unsalted foods to improve acceptance by the patient and to allow greater flexibility in meal planning. In most cases, salted fats and breads are the regular commercial products to which salt is added in processing. Salted meats, vegetables, potatoes, and cereals are those that have a measured amount of salt added in preparation (1/8 tsp of salt per serving of vegetables, cooked cereal, potatoes, and potato substitutes; 1/4 tsp of salt per pound of meat). Unsalted products are those that do not have salt added in preparation or processing; in some cases, they are referred to as "low-sodium" or "salt-free."

‡Calculations are based on values for medium-fat meats. Use of lean and medium-fat meats rather than high-fat meats is encouraged in weight reduction and modified-fat diets.

§Nonfat milk is generally encouraged in weight reduction diets; however, low-fat or whole milk may be used with appropriate reduction of fat allowance.

**The starch group is subdivided into groups of 1, 5, and 10 meq of sodium. For diets allowing 90 meq of sodium that include foods from both the 5- and the 10-meq groups, basing calculations on an average of 8 meq of sodium per starch exchange may be sufficiently accurate.

††Sweetened carbonated beverages, low-calorie beverages, and alcoholic beverages may be included by adjusting the number of exchanges from other food groups.

NO-EXTRA-SALT DIET

The sodium content of the no-extra-salt diet varies according to the calorie level; the usual range is 90 to 150 meq. Guidelines for this diet are as follows:

1. Do not add salt to food at the table.
2. Use only limited amounts of salt in food preparation: 1/4 tsp of salt per pound of meat; 1/8 tsp of salt per serving of cooked cereal, potatoes, potato substitutes, and cooked vegetables.
3. Avoid the following foods:
   - Salt-cured meats; salted canned or processed meats, fish, and fowl; bacon; ham; dried beef; corned beef; frankfurters; processed cold cuts; sausages; sardines; salted cheese and cheese foods; salted peanuts; commercial casserole mixes; frozen dinners
   - Commercially prepared salted salad dressings (except mayonnaise and mayonnaise-type salad dressing); commercial gravy and gravy mixes; salt pork
   - Salted snack foods; salted crackers; salted popcorn; pretzels; potato chips; corn chips; salted nuts; canned soups; dried soup mixes; broth; bouillon (except salt-free)
   - Sauerkraut; pickled vegetables; commercially frozen vegetable mixes with sauces
   - Seasoning salt; seasoning mixes; meat tenderizer; monosodium glutamate; catsup; prepared mustard; prepared horseradish; soy sauce; bottled meat and barbecue sauce; olives; pickles
   - Cultured buttermilk; cocoa mixes; cocktail beverage mixes; club soda; Gatorade
4. Limit the following foods:
   - Organ meats (such as liver, heart, and kidney), shellfish (such as shrimp, clams, and lobster), or peanut butter to 2 servings per week. Additional servings of salt-free peanut butter may be used.
   - Tomato juice or vegetable juice cocktail to 1/2 cup per day. Additional servings of salt-free tomato juice or salt-free vegetable juice cocktail may be used.

(Foods not listed here are allowed on the no-extra-salt diet.)

FOOD EXCHANGE LIST FOR SODIUM CONTROL*

This food exchange list is intended to be used as a reference tool. For this reason, a more comprehensive list of foods is given than may actually be used for instruction of individuals.

LIST 1: MEAT EXCHANGES – Unsalted: **1 meq of sodium**
Salted with 1/4 tsp/lb: **3 meq of sodium**

Measure or wt	Gram wt	Lean meat—protein, 7 g; fat, 3 g; 55 kcal
1 oz	30	Beef: baby beef (very lean), chuck, flank steak, tenderloin, plate skirt steak, round (bottom, top), all rump cuts, spareribs, tripe,† ground (preceding meats trimmed of fat and ground)
1 oz	30	Lamb: leg, rib, sirloin, loin (roast and chops), shank, shoulder
1 oz	30	Pork: leg (whole rump, center shank)
1 oz	30	Veal: leg, loin, rib, shank, shoulder, cutlets
1 oz	30	Poultry (meat without skin): chicken, turkey, cornish hen, guinea hen, pheasant
1 oz	30	Fish: any fresh or frozen, unsalted
1/4 cup	30	Canned salmon, tuna
1 oz	30	Mackerel, crab,† lobster†
1 oz (about 5)	30	Clams,† oysters,† scallops,† shrimp†
1/2 cup	100	Dried beans and peas (omit 1 starch exchange)
1/4 cup	60	Egg substitutes, fat-free
		Medium-fat meat—protein, 7 g; fat, 5 g; 73 kcal; OR 1 lean meat + 1/2 fat exchange
1 oz	30	Beef: ground (less than 20% fat), rib eye, round (ground commercial)
1 oz	30	Pork: loin (all tenderloin cuts), shoulder arm (picnic), shoulder blade, Boston butt
1 oz	30	Liver,† heart,† kidney,† sweetbreads†
1	50	Egg‡
2 tbsp	30	Peanut butter, unsalted or fresh ground (omit 2 fat exchanges)
1 oz	30	Peanuts, unsalted (omit 2 fat exchanges)

LIST 1: MEAT EXCHANGES – Unsalted: **1 meq of sodium**
Salted with 1/4 tsp/lb: **3 meq of sodium** *(Continued)*

Measure or wt	Gram wt	High-fat meat—protein, 7 g; fat, 8 g; 100 kcal; OR 1 lean meat + 1 fat exchange
1 oz	30	Beef: brisket, ground (more than 20% fat), hamburger (commercial), chuck (ground commercial), roasts (rib), steaks (club and rib)
1 oz	30	Lamb, breast
1 oz	30	Pork: spareribs, loin (back ribs), ground
1 oz	30	Veal, breast
1 oz	30	Poultry: capon, duck (domestic),† goose†
1 oz	30	Cheese, unsalted cheddar types

Avoid: Salt-cured meats; salted canned or processed meats, fish, and fowl; bacon; ham; dried beef; corned beef; frankfurters; processed cold cuts; sausages; sardines; salted cheese and cheese foods; salted peanut butter; salted peanuts; commercial casserole mixes; frozen dinners

*The sodium exchange list is based on "Exchange Lists for Meal Planning" (American Diabetes Association, Inc., and the American Dietetic Association, 1976), with modifications for sodium control. See page 45 for changes made in the original list.

†Limit to 2 servings per week from this group because of higher natural sodium content. Values range from 1 to 5 meq per exchange.

‡Eggs must count as salted meat exchanges.

LIST 2: *FAT EXCHANGES* – fat, 5 g; 45 kcal

Measure	Gram wt	Trace of sodium
		Predominantly polyunsaturated or monounsaturated fats
1 tsp	5	Margarine,* unsalted
1/8	30	Avocado,† 4 in. in diameter
1 tsp	5	Mayonnaise, unsalted
2 tsp	10	Mayonnaise-type salad dressing,* unsalted
1 tsp	5	Oil: corn, cottonseed, safflower, soy, sunflower
1 tsp	5	Oil: olive,† peanut†
2 tbsp	30	Nondairy cream substitute*
10 whole	10	Almonds,† unsalted
2 large whole	5	Pecans,† unsalted
6 small	8	Walnuts, unsalted
6 small	8	Nuts, other† (unsalted)
		Predominantly saturated fats
1 tsp	5	Butter, unsalted
2 tbsp	30	Cream: light, sour
1 tbsp	15	Cream, heavy
1 tsp	5	Lard
2 tbsp	30	Other nondairy cream substitutes
		2 meq of sodium
		Predominantly polyunsaturated or monounsaturated fats
1 tsp	5	Margarine,* salted
1 tsp	5	Mayonnaise,* salted
2 tsp	10	Mayonnaise-type salad dressing,* salted
		Predominantly saturated fats
1 tsp	5	Butter, salted
1 tbsp	15	Cream cheese

Avoid: Salted nuts; commercially prepared salad dressing (other than those listed); bacon; salt pork; olives; commercial gravy and gravy mixes

*Made with corn, cottonseed, safflower, soy, or sunflower oil only.
†Fat content is primarily monounsaturated.

LIST 3: *MILK EXCHANGES* — 5 meq of sodium

Measure	Gram wt	Nonfat fortified milk—protein, 8 g; carbohydrate, 12 g; fat, trace; 80 kcal
1 cup	240	Skim or nonfat milk
1/3 cup	25	Powdered milk (nonfat dry, before adding liquid)
1/2 cup	120	Canned, evaporated skim milk
1 cup	240	Yogurt made from skim milk (plain, unflavored)
		1% fat fortified milk (1 nonfat milk + 1/2 fat exchange)— protein, 8 g; carbohydrate, 12 g; fat, 2.5 g; 102 kcal
1 cup	240	1% milk
		2% fat fortified milk (1 nonfat milk + 1 fat exchange)— protein, 8 g; carbohydrate, 12 g; fat, 5 g; 125 kcal
1 cup	240	2% milk
1/4 cup	45	Cottage cheese
3 tbsp	15	Parmesan cheese
1 cup	240	Yogurt made from 2% milk (plain, unflavored)
		Whole milk (1 nonfat milk + 2 fat exchanges) — protein, 8 g; carbohydrate, 12 g; fat, 10 g; 160 kcal
1 cup	240	Whole milk
1/2 cup	120	Canned, evaporated whole milk
1 cup	240	Chocolate milk
1 cup	240	Yogurt made from whole milk (plain, unflavored)
Avoid:		Cultured buttermilk; instant cocoa mixes

LIST 4: STARCH EXCHANGES* — protein, 2 g; carbohydrate, 15 g; 68 kcal

Measure	Gram wt	Group 1: 1 meq of sodium
		Bread
1 slice	25	Unsalted bread
1	30	Tortilla, 6 in.
		Cereal
3/4 cup	20	Corn flakes, unsalted
1 cup	15	Puffed wheat or rice, unsalted
1 biscuit	15	Shredded wheat, unsalted
1/2 cup	100	Cooked cereal, no salt
1/2 cup	100	Grits (cooked, no salt)
1/2 cup	100	Rice or barley (cooked, no salt)
1/2 cup	100	Pasta, spaghetti, noodles, macaroni (cooked, no salt)
		Popcorn (popped, no salt, no added fat)
3 cups	45	Large kernel
1 1/2 cups	20	Small kernel
2 tbsp	15	Cornmeal, dry
2 1/2 tbsp	20	Flour
1/4 cup	25	Wheat germ
2 tbsp	25	Tapioca
		Crackers
4	20	Salt-free soda crackers, 2 1/2 in. sq
		Dried beans, peas, and lentils (omit 1 meat exchange)
1/2 cup	100	Beans, peas, lentils (dried, cooked, no salt)
		Starchy vegetables
1/3 cup	80	Corn: fresh, frozen, or canned (low-sodium); cooked
1 small	100	Corn on the cob
1/2 cup	100	Lima beans: fresh, frozen, or canned (low-sodium); cooked
1/2 cup	100	Peas, fresh or canned (low-sodium); cooked
1/2 cup	100	Parsnips, cooked
1 small	100	Potato, baked or boiled
1/2 cup	100	Potato, mashed
3/4 cup	150	Pumpkin, canned
1/2 cup	100	Winter squash: acorn, butternut (baked)
1/4 cup	60	Yam or sweet potato, baked in skin

LIST 4: STARCH EXCHANGES* — protein, 2 g; carbohydrate, 15 g; 68 kcal *(Continued)*

Measure	Gram wt	Group 2: 5 meq of sodium
		Bread
1 slice	25	White, including French and Italian
1 slice	25	Whole wheat
1 slice	25	Rye or pumpernickel
1 slice	25	Raisin
1/2	30	Bagel, small
1/2	30	English muffin, small
1	40	Plain muffin, small
3 tbsp	20	Dried bread crumbs
		Cereal
1 cup	15	Puffed rice
		Crackers
2	20	Graham, 2 1/2 in. sq
1/2	20	Matzoth, 4 in. by 6 in.
4	20	Melba toast, 3 3/4 in. by 2 in.
3	20	Rye wafers, 2 in. by 3 1/2 in.
		Starchy vegetables
1/3 cup	80	Corn, regular
1/2 cup	100	Peas, frozen (cooked)
1/2 cup	100	Mixed vegetables, frozen (cooked)
1/4 cup	60	Sweet potato, canned

LIST 4: STARCH EXCHANGES* — protein, 2 g; carbohydrate, 15 g; 68 kcal *(Continued)*

Measure	Gram wt	Group 3: 10 meq of sodium
		Bread
1	35	Plain roll
1/2	35	Hamburger bun
1	45	Corn bread, 2 in. by 2 in. by 1 in.
1	60	Pancake, 5 in. by 1/2 in.
1	35	Waffle, 5 in. by 1/2 in.
		Cereal
3/4 cup	20	Corn, wheat, or wheat and malted barley flakes
1/2 cup	20	Bran or oat flakes
1 cup	25	Puffed oats†
1/2 cup	100	Cooked cereal (with 1/8 tsp of salt)
1/2 cup	100	Grits, cooked (with 1/8 tsp of salt)
1/2 cup	100	Rice or barley, cooked (with 1/8 tsp of salt)
1/2 cup	100	Pasta, spaghetti, noodles, macaroni (cooked; with 1/8 tsp of salt)
		Starchy vegetables
1/2 cup	100	Potatoes, cooked (with 1/8 tsp of salt)

Avoid: Salted snack foods; salted crackers; potato chips; corn chips; pretzels; salted popcorn; commercial mixes; commercially frozen convenience foods; commercial soups; dried soup mixes; broth; bouillon

*The starch group is subdivided into groups of 1, 5, and 10 meq of sodium. For diets allowing 90 meq of sodium that include foods from both the 5- and the 10-meq groups, basing calculations on an average of 8 meq of sodium per starch exchange may be sufficiently accurate.

†Contain 13 meq of sodium per cup.

LIST 5: VEGETABLE EXCHANGES – protein, 2 g; carbohydrate, 5 g; 25 kcal;
1 exchange is 1/2 cup (100 g)
Unsalted: **0.5 meq of sodium***
Salted with 1/8 tsp/1/2 cup: **12 meq of sodium***

Asparagus	Eggplant	Tomatoes
Bean sprouts	Okra	Tomato juice, unsalted
Broccoli	Onions	Turnips
Brussels sprouts	Rutabaga	Vegetable juice cocktail, unsalted
Collards	String beans, green or yellow	

The following vegetables, higher in natural sodium (2 to 4 meq) than the preceding, should be limited to 1/2 cup (100 g) per day for diets of 40 meq of sodium or less.

Artichoke	Greens
Beets	Beet
Carrots	Chards
Celery	Dandelion
Chinese cabbage	Kale
	Spinach
Watercress	Turnip

The following vegetables have little protein, fat, or carbohydrate and may be used as desired.

Cabbage	Escarole	Parsley
Cauliflower	Green pepper	Radishes
Chicory	Lettuce	Rhubarb
Cucumber	Mushrooms	Summer squash
Endive	Mustard greens	Zucchini

Avoid: Sauerkraut; pickled vegetables; salted tomato juice; salted vegetable juice cocktail; seasoned tomato sauces; commercially frozen vegetable mixes with sauces

---

*Unsalted vegetables are those that do not have salt added in preparation or processing, including fresh, frozen (no salt added), and canned (low-sodium) vegetables. Regular canned vegetables and frozen vegetables with salt added in processing are considered to be "salted" vegetables; salt should not be added in cooking.

LIST 6: *FRUIT EXCHANGES* – Unsweetened: carbohydrate, 10 g; 40 kcal
Sweetened: carbohydrate, 17 g; 68 kcal
Trace of sodium

Measure	Gram wt		Measure	Gram wt	
1 small	80	Apple			Melons
1/3 cup	80	Apple juice	1/4 small	200	Cantaloupe
1/2 cup	100	Applesauce	1/8 medium	150	Honeydew
2 medium	100	Apricots, fresh	1 cup	175	Watermelon
4 halves	20	Apricots, dried	1 small	80	Nectarine
1/3 cup	80	Apricot nectar	1 small	100	Orange
1/2 small	50	Banana	1/2 cup	120	Orange juice
		Berries	1/2 cup	100	Orange sections
1/2 cup	70	Blackberries	3/4 cup	100	Papaya
1/2 cup	70	Blueberries	1 medium	100	Peach
1/2 cup	70	Raspberries	2 halves	20	Peach, dried
3/4 cup	110	Strawberries	1/2 cup	100	Peaches, canned
10 large	100	Cherries	1/3 cup	80	Peach nectar
1/2 cup	100	Cherries, canned	1 small	100	Pear
1/3 cup	80	Cider	2 halves	20	Pear, dried
1/3 cup	80	Cranberry juice cocktail	1/2 cup	100	Pears, canned
2	15	Dates	1/3 cup	80	Pear nectar
1	50	Figs, fresh	1 medium	30	Persimmon, native
1	15	Figs, dried	1/2 cup	100	Pineapple
1/2 cup	100	Figs, canned	1/3 cup	80	Pineapple juice
1/2 cup	100	Fruit cocktail	2 medium	100	Plums
1/2	100	Grapefruit	1/2 cup	100	Plums, canned
1/2 cup	120	Grapefruit juice	2 medium	25	Prunes
1/2 cup	100	Grapefruit sections	1/4 cup	60	Prune juice
12	75	Grapes	2 tbsp	15	Raisins
1/4 cup	60	Grape juice	1 medium	100	Tangerine
1/2 cup	100	Grapes, canned	1/2 cup	120	Tangerine juice
1/2 small	70	Mango	1/2 cup	100	Tangerine sections

Avoid: Fruits that have been crystallized, glazed, or dried with a sodium compound

LIST 7: CANDY AND OTHER SWEETS

Sweets—carbohydrate, 13 g; 50 kcal; <1 meq of sodium

1 tbsp	Sugar
1 tbsp	Honey
1 tbsp	Maple syrup
1 tbsp	Jam, jellies

Candy—fat, 4 g; carbohydrate, 20 g; 120 kcal; <1 meq of sodium

1 oz	Butterscotch
1 oz	Plain milk chocolate
1 oz	Gumdrops
1 oz	Hard candies
1 oz	Jelly beans
1 oz	Marshmallows

Avoid: Candies containing salted nuts

LIST 8: **DESSERTS** – protein, 3 g; fat, 6 g; carbohydrate, 24 g; 175 kcal
Regular, containing salt: **5 to 10 meq of sodium**
Special, low-sodium: **1 meq of sodium***

1/10 of 10 in. cake	Angel food cake†
2 in. by 3 in. by 2 in.	Cake†
2	Cookies,† assorted (2 in. in diameter)
1 medium	Doughnut, cake or raised
1 cup	Gelatin, flavored
3/4 cup	Ice cream
1 cup	Ice milk
1/8 of 9 in. pie	Pie,† cream or fruit (unsalted crust)
1/2 cup	Pudding,† vanilla or chocolate
Avoid: Commercial mixes	

*Special low-sodium desserts are those that are prepared without salt and contain low-sodium baking powder rather than regular baking powder or baking soda.
†Use home recipes only. Do not use commercially prepared mixes.

LIST 9: BEVERAGES*

Coffee; decaffeinated coffee; tea

Sweetened, carbonated beverages† — 100 kcal

<1 meq of sodium

8 oz	Colas, ginger ale, tonic water

1 to 3 meq of sodium

8 oz	All others

Low-calorie beverages — less than 1 kcal/fl oz; 1 to 3 meq of sodium

8 oz	All sugar-free carbonated

Alcoholic beverages — 100 kcal; 1 meq of sodium

8 oz	Beer†
1 1/2 oz	Gin, rum, vodka, whiskey
3 1/2 oz	Wine
1 oz	Brandy

Avoid: Cocoa mixes; cocktail beverage mixes; Gatorade; club soda

---

*Caffeine-containing beverages should be used in moderation by persons following a low-sodium diet for control of hypertension.

†Sodium content of beer and carbonated beverages may vary owing to differences in sodium content of the water supply from which they are made.

LIST 10: MISCELLANEOUS

Allow: Spices and herbs; garlic and onion powder; dry mustard; fresh horseradish; flavoring extracts; vinegar; lemon juice; lime juice; unsalted bouillon

Avoid: Salt (except as allowed); seasoning salts; seasoning mixes; meat tenderizer; monosodium glutamate; catsup; prepared mustard and horseradish; soy sauce; bottled meat and barbecue sauce; olives; pickles

SELECTED BIBLIOGRAPHY

Iacono, J. M., Marshall, M. W., Dougherty, R. M., et al.: Reduction in blood pressure associated with high polyunsaturated fat diets that reduce blood cholesterol in man. Prev. Med., 4:426-443, 1975.

Margie, J. D., and Hunt, J. C.: Living With High Blood Pressure: The Hypertension Diet Cookbook. Bloomfield, New Jersey, HLS Press, 1978.

Moore, M. A.: Hypertension in the ambulatory patient. Am. Fam. Physician, 16:188-197, Nov. 1977.

Reisin, E., Abel, R., Modan, M., et al.: Effect of weight loss without salt restriction on the reduction of blood pressure in overweight hypertensive patients. N. Engl. J. Med., 298:1-6, 1978.

Robertson, D., and Frölich, J. C.: Coffee and hypertension (letter to the editor). N. Engl. J. Med., 298:1092, 1978.

Robertson, D., Frölich, J. C., Carr, R. K., et al.: Effects of caffeine on plasma renin activity, catecholamines and blood pressure. N. Engl. J. Med., 298:181-186, 1978.

Robinson, C. H., and Lawler, M. R.: Normal and Therapeutic Nutrition. Fifteenth edition. New York, Macmillan Publishing Company, 1977, pp. 541-551.

Thiele, V. F.: Clinical Nutrition. St. Louis, C. V. Mosby Company, 1976, pp. 138-140.

Vergroesen, A. J.: Physiological effects of dietary linoleic acid. Nutr. Rev., 35:1-5, 1977.

PROTEIN CONTROL

DIETARY MANAGEMENT OF RENAL FAILURE

GENERAL DESCRIPTION

The diet emphasizes controlled intake of protein and sodium and an adequate intake of essential amino acids and calories to meet the needs of the patient with a specific degree of renal failure.

NUTRITIONAL ADEQUACY

Diets containing 40 g of protein or less are inadequate in calcium and folic acid and low in phosphorus, thiamine, niacin, and riboflavin. Diets that contain 50 g of protein are inadequate in calcium and low in phosphorus, thiamine, riboflavin, niacin, and folic acid. Therefore, daily supplements of one multiple vitamin containing folic acid are recommended for patients following diets that provide 50 g of protein or less. Diets containing more than 50 g of protein are nutritionally adequate according to the Recommended Dietary Allowances.

INDICATIONS AND RATIONALE

The kidney functions as an excretory, regulatory, and endocrine organ. The kidney excretes the end products of protein metabolism and maintains both the electrolyte and the water balances of the body. Nephrons are the minute structural units of the kidney in which these functions are carried out. In the diseased kidney, the number of functioning nephrons is decreased. As the disease progresses, the waste products (urea, creatinine, uric acid, sulfate, and organic acids) increase in the blood, and the capacity of the kidney to excrete and conserve both water and electrolytes is impaired.

Fortunately, kidneys have a great reserve of capacity. Even if 60% of the nephrons have been destroyed, kidneys can maintain their functioning capacity without symptomatic complications to the individual. Usually, the patient does not become aware of symptoms until the residual kidney function is less than 30%, as reflected clinically by a creatinine clearance of 30 to 40 ml/minute per 1.73 m^2 or less. At this level of renal function, serum concentrations of urea and creatinine are elevated. It is important to recognize that normal limits of serum creatinine concentration are much lower for infants and small children than for adults. Accumulation of protein waste products may contribute to tiredness, nausea, vomiting, and anorexia. Excess dietary sodium increases the possibility of edema, weight gain, and hypertension, whereas insufficient dietary sodium may result in weight loss, depletion of extracellular fluid volume, orthostatic hypotension, and a further decrease in glomerular filtration rate.

The patient's symptoms, as well as the degree of impairment of renal function, should be considered when the amount of protein control is determined. The table that follows shows the initial suggested intake of protein per kilogram of body weight at the corresponding level of renal function in the adult patient.

| Creatinine Clearance ml/min/1.73 m^2 | Daily Protein Intake* | |
	Body Weight g/kg	Man g/70 kg
30 to 20	0.60	49 to 35
19 to 5	0.45	27
5	0.30	18

*Plus an amount of protein equal to the 24-hour urinary protein loss.

Close follow-up of patients is advised so that the amount of protein can be modified according to the patient's course. Although optimal protein intake has not been determined in children with renal insufficiency, their protein intake should not be reduced below 1 to 1.3 g/kg per day to assure that there is adequate protein for growth. This level of protein intake is a definite reduction from the usual child's intake of 2 to 4 g of protein per kilogram of body weight per day but generally allows for a satisfactory clinical response. If proteinuria is present, an amount of protein equal to that lost in the urine, as determined by a 24-hour urine collection, should be added to the calculated daily protein allowance (see "Dietary Management of Nephrotic Syndrome," page 84). At least 75% of the total protein should be of high biologic value (eggs, milk, and meat) to assure an adequate intake of essential amino acids.

The level of sodium intake should be specific to the patient's needs. Maximal renal function is achieved when sodium intake is increased to a level just below that which will cause edema or hypertension (or both). If edema or hypertension is present, a sodium intake of 60 to 90 meq per day is often indicated. In the extremely edematous patient, more strict control (less than 60 meq of sodium per day) and diuretics may be needed initially (see "Sodium Control," page 62). The diet should be planned to provide the prescribed level of sodium ±10%. For example, if a diet of 90 meq of sodium is requested, the diet should be calculated to provide between 81 and 99 meq of sodium. In some instances, a measured amount of added salt may be necessary.

Utilization of dietary protein is directly influenced by total caloric intake. Therefore, adequate caloric intake is of vital importance to the patient with renal disease to prevent catabolism of body protein, to ensure that dietary protein is not used as an energy source, and to maintain a constant body weight and energy level. In children with significant loss of renal function, adequate caloric intake becomes the single most important factor in the prevention of growth retardation. Patients need to be reminded continually to maintain an adequate caloric intake, since they often adhere more closely to protein control and neglect their caloric needs. Caloric intake of children should be no less than 80% of the recommended allowance for age (approximately 60 to 80 kcal/kg of ideal body weight). To maintain ideal weight, adults usually need at least 35 kcal/kg of ideal body weight per day. Fats and carbohydrates should be eaten along with the dietary protein or, if provided as a supplement, should be given within 4 hours of protein ingestion. Patients below ideal weight may need 35 to 50 kcal/kg of body weight to gain to ideal weight. For obese patients, moderate calorie control (daily deficit of 300 to 500 calories) is recommended. Obese patients should be carefully observed by the dietitian and the physician. Unless immediate weight loss is compelling, stringent calorie restriction is not recommended, since it may be hazardous, especially if renal function is less than 15% of normal. Attempts to achieve rapid loss of weight by drastic caloric restriction are not advisable, since body protein catabolism will result.

When urinary volume is normal, the serum potassium level usually remains within the normal range. Dietary potassium control becomes more important in end-stage renal failure, when urine volume decreases below normal. However, as a precaution, patients should be advised to avoid potassium chloride (salt substitutes) unless the physician prescribes it as a medication to correct hypokalemia. With normal urine output, hypokalemia does not usually occur unless excess sodium intake necessitates increased use of diuretics and a corresponding loss of potassium.

As the glomerular filtration rate declines to 30% of normal or less, the dietary phosphate load is greater than the kidney can excrete. Consequently, the serum phosphorus concentration rises and, in turn, causes the serum calcium level to decrease. The lowered serum calcium concentration stimulates increased secretion of parathyroid hormone. Renal osteodystrophy and metastatic calcification are two of the demonstrable complications that may result from the body's adjustments to normalize serum calcium and phosphorus levels. Unfortunately, dietary phosphorus and calcium are difficult to control. On a protein-controlled diet, the daily phosphorus intake is already well below the usual American intake (1,500 mg/day). The phosphorus intake can be decreased even more if dairy products and whole-grain breads and cereals are eliminated from the diet. However, the use of phosphate binders (aluminum hydroxide or aluminum carbonate) is usually necessary to lower serum phosphorus. Increased calcium needs are often best met by calcium supplements.

CHRONIC RENAL FAILURE AND DIABETES

When diabetes mellitus is complicated by renal failure, some compromises must be made in the usual diabetic diet. The requirements of the protein-controlled diet generally take priority, especially at very low levels of protein intake.

The decrease in protein intake requires a corresponding increase in intake of fat and carbohydrate. Low-protein bread products can be used as a source of calories. To assure adequate calories, one may also have to include simple carbohydrates, such as sugar, jellies, and sugar-sweetened fruit. If simple carbohydrates are consumed, they should be measured carefully and distributed evenly throughout the day to minimize fluctuation in blood sugar levels. Patients are often reluctant to eat simple sugars; thus, the rationale behind their incorporation must be clearly stated to ensure compliance.

The food exchange list for protein, sodium, and potassium control should be used rather than the diabetic food exchange list. Consistency in timing and composition of meals and the use of additional food for increased exercise to prevent hypoglycemic reactions are still appropriate.

PHYSICIANS: HOW TO ORDER DIETS

The diet order should indicate specific **levels of protein and sodium** and specify if **weight loss** is to be achieved. The dietitian will calculate caloric need for the nonobese patient. For nondialysis patients, the amounts of protein most commonly specified are **30, 40,** and **50 g.** The levels of sodium most commonly specified are **60** and **90 meq.**

DIETARY MANAGEMENT OF PATIENTS ON HEMODIALYSIS

GENERAL DESCRIPTION

The diet emphasizes controlled yet adequate amounts of protein, sodium, potassium, fluid, and calories according to the needs of the individual patient and to the frequency of dialysis.

NUTRITIONAL ADEQUACY

Amino acids and water-soluble vitamins lost in the dialysate should be replaced. A multivitamin containing ascorbic acid, pyridoxine, and folic acid and fortified with calcium and iron should be taken daily.

INDICATIONS AND RATIONALE

Nutritional management is extremely important for all hemodialysis patients. Although the dialysis machine is capable of duplicating much of the kidney's function, it does not have the flexibility of the normal kidney; if no nutritional controls are imposed, dangerous waste products will accumulate between dialyses. The diet should be correlated with the frequency of dialysis, the level of residual renal function, and the size of the patient.

Dialysis removes not only unwanted waste products but also some needed nutrients. Amino acids and water-soluble vitamins are two nutrients lost during dialysis. Because of this loss, the diet should be supplemented with folic acid, ascorbic acid, and pyridoxine (Kopple and Swendseid, 1975).

The protein intake of the patient must be sufficient to maintain nitrogen balance and to replace amino acids lost during dialysis and yet be low enough to prevent excessive interdialytic accumulation of waste products. The protein need for the average adult with minimal residual renal function who requires dialysis three times a week can usually be supplied by a diet that provides 1 g of protein per kilogram of ideal body weight. Seventy-five percent of the total protein intake should be of high biologic value. Children should not be restricted in protein below 1.5 to 2 g/kg per day (Spinozzi and Grupe, 1977). Adult patients who receive intermittent peritoneal dialyses should receive 1.5 g of protein per kilogram of body weight per day, since the amount of protein lost during peritoneal dialysis is greater than that lost during hemodialysis.

Adequate caloric intake is as important for dialysis patients as for nondialysis patients who are in the beginning stages of renal failure. The caloric need remains the same as it was before the need for dialysis (see page 81).

Sodium control (40 to 120 meq/day) is usually necessary to control hypertension and edema. Sodium control is extremely helpful in blunting thirst and thus in preventing excessive fluid intake. A high sodium intake during dialysis is not encouraged, as it contributes to excessive thirst that may persist beyond the dialysis.

Potassium control of the diet is essential. Hyperkalemia can result in cardiac dysrhythmia and even cardiac arrest. Generally, the potassium level of the diet is largely determined by the potassium concentration of the dialysate. With a dialysate concentration of 1 meq or more of potassium per liter, dietary potassium must be limited to 60 meq or less per day. With a dialysate concentration of less than 1 meq of potassium per liter, dietary potassium may be more liberal (about 100 meq or less).

Fluid control is often the most difficult part of the diet for the dialysis patient. Fluid sources are (1) beverages and foods that are liquid at room temperature, such as ice cream and gelatin, (2) water content of foods, and (3) the water formed from the oxidation of food (Vetter and Shapiro, 1975). The total fluid content of the diet is the sum of these three sources. In the stable dialysis patient, fluid is lost from the body by (1) urine excretion and (2) "insensible" routed (perspiration, respiration, and fecal losses). Insensible loss of water varies with body size and temperature but can be estimated as 750 to 1,000 ml/day for the adult patient, 30 ml/kg per day in infants up to 1 year of age, and 20 ml/kg per day to a maximum of 400 to 500 ml in older children. To achieve an interdialytic weight gain of 1 lb (0.45 kg) or less per day, one can calculate total dietary fluid allowed (from all three sources) by adding urine volume and insensible fluid loss and 1 lb (0.45 kg) of fluid (450 to 500 ml). In other words, total dietary fluid equals 1 lb of fluid plus insensible loss plus 24-hour urine volume. For practical purposes, the sum of the liquid content of foods and the water formed from the oxidation of foods can be considered equal to insensible water loss. Therefore, the usual practice is to estimate allowance of free dietary fluid (from beverages and foods that are liquid at room temperature) by adding the daily urine volume and 1 lb (0.45 kg) of fluid (450 to 500 ml). In other words, free dietary fluid equals 1 lb of fluid plus 24-hour urine volume.

Serum calcium and phosphorus levels are difficult to alter by dietary means. Limitations invoked by protein control generally also decrease calcium and phosphorus intake below usual levels. Phosphorus and calcium are best controlled by the use of phosphate binders and calcium supplements. However, it may be appropriate to further limit high-phosphorus foods. Calcium and phosphorus values of food may be found in the Appendix on page 292.

PHYSICIANS: HOW TO ORDER DIETS

The diet order should indicate the specific **levels of protein, sodium, potassium, and fluid** and specify if **weight loss** is to be achieved. The dietitian will calculate caloric need.

DIETARY MANAGEMENT OF NEPHROTIC SYNDROME

GENERAL DESCRIPTION

Dietary management of nephrotic syndrome emphasizes a high intake of protein, control of sodium, and adequate calories.

INDICATIONS AND RATIONALE

Nephrotic syndrome—or "massive proteinuria," as it is commonly called today—suggests a kidney malfunction. Massive proteinuria is defined as a 24-hour urine protein loss of 3.5 g or more. In most cases, some form of kidney disease is the cause of the massive proteinuria. Often, a kidney biopsy is necessary to determine the specific cause. In adults, some form of glomerulonephritis is usually found. In children, a common cause is lipoid nephrosis. In both adults and children, edema, hypertension, increased serum lipoprotein values, and decreased serum albumin concentration commonly accompany massive proteinuria. Some investigators still use the term "nephrotic syndrome" to describe this combination of findings.

Dietary treatment of nephrotic syndrome is directed toward control of edema, proteinuria, and hypoproteinemia. High dietary protein intake (to replace urinary protein loss), controlled sodium intake (to correct edema), and adequate calories (to prevent muscle catabolism and supply adequate energy) are the primary therapeutic measures. The patient's nutritional state and underlying renal condition must be taken into consideration when the diet is prescribed. Because many edematous nephrotic patients are also anorectic, particular attention and supervision should be given to their actual dietary intakes.

If the glomerular filtration rate is normal, 100 g or more of protein (1 1/2 to 2 g/kg of body weight for adults) per day and adequate calories are appropriate. Adult men may eat 100 to 140 g of protein for long periods, but women seldom eat more than 100 g.

The protein need for children with nephrotic syndrome is increased to 2 to 3 g/kg of body weight (Recommended Dietary Allowance: 1.2 to 1.5 g/kg of ideal body weight) to allow for positive nitrogen balance and growth. Commercial dietary supplements are available for patients who are unable to consume the recommended protein and calories. Dried milk can also be mixed with milk (to form double-strength milk) or other foods to increase the protein content. If the glomerular filtration rate is decreased, the amount of dietary protein allowed should be determined in the same way as it is for other patients with chronic renal failure, with an increment in dietary protein equivalent to the 24-hour urinary protein loss (see page 81). Protein of high biologic value should be used to supply at least 75% of the total protein in the diet.

After the initial diuresis, control of edema and hypertension can usually be maintained by a sodium allowance of 90 meq or less per day.

Caloric intake for patients who are not obese should be individualized according to height, weight, age, sex, and daily activity. Weight reduction for the obese patient should be approached cautiously. See page 50 for estimation of caloric deficits. Because of the patient's need for a high protein intake, weight reduction is best achieved at calorie levels of 1,600 to 1,800 calories. At this caloric level, commercial protein supplements are not necessary and the diet is more palatable.

The patient should be encouraged to record weight daily and to report any sudden gain or loss of more than 5 lb (2.27 kg) to the physician. Such sudden weight change may be a loss or gain of fluid rather than of fat tissue and is an important symptom that needs attention.

Hypercholesterolemia and hypertriglyceridemia frequently occur in patients with nephrotic syndrome. However, the impact of this form of hyperlipidemia on the potential development of atherosclerosis in the nephrotic patient is uncertain. Moderate control of cholesterol (300 to 500 mg/day) and reduction of free sugars can be achieved with good dietary planning. Such dietary modifications are desirable but of lower priority than maintenance of calorie and protein intake.

PHYSICIANS: HOW TO ORDER DIETS

The diet order should indicate the specific **level of sodium (60 or 90 meq)** and the **level of protein** according to the patient's needs. The dietitian will calculate caloric need. The dietitian will restrict cholesterol and free sugar only to the extent compatible with the patient's calorie and protein needs.

SELECTED BIBLIOGRAPHY

Anderson, C. F., Nelson, R. A., Margie, J. D., et al.: Nutritional therapy for adults with renal disease. J.A.M.A., 223:68-72, 1973.

Betts, P. R., and Magrath, G.: Growth pattern and dietary intake of children with chronic renal insufficiency. Br. Med. J., 2:189-193, 1974.

Goodhart, R. S., and Shils, M. E. (eds.): Modern Nutrition in Health and Disease: Dietotherapy. Fifth edition. Philadelphia, Lea & Febiger, 1973.

Kopple, J. D., and Swendseid, M. E.: Vitamin nutrition in patients undergoing maintenance hemodialysis. Kidney Int., 7 [Suppl.] 2:79-84, 1975.

Lewy, P. R., and Hurley, J. K.: Chronic renal insufficiency. Pediatr. Clin. North Am., 23:829-842, 1976.

Mitchell, H. S., Rynbergen, H. J., Anderson, L., et al.: Nutrition in Health and Disease. Sixteenth edition. Philadelphia, J. B. Lippincott Company, 1976.

Spinozzi, N. S., and Grupe, W. E.: Nutritional implications of renal disease. IV. Nutritional aspects of chronic renal insufficiency in childhood. J. Am. Diet. Assoc., 70:493-497, 1977.

Vetter, L., and Shapiro, R.: An approach to dietary management of the patient with renal disease. J. Am. Diet. Assoc., 66:158-162, 1975.

DIETARY MANAGEMENT OF HEPATIC COMA

GENERAL DESCRIPTION

The protein, sodium, and calorie contents of the diet are controlled according to individual needs.

NUTRITIONAL ADEQUACY

The nutritional adequacy of hepatic coma diets is similar to that of other protein-controlled diets. Since these diets are used for only a few days or weeks, vitamin and mineral supplements are generally not necessary unless the patient has previously been malnourished or has specific vitamin and mineral deficiencies.

INDICATIONS AND RATIONALE

Hepatic coma is a potential and serious complication of advanced liver disease. In many cases, hepatic coma is completely reversible or largely controllable. The early stages have been referred to as "precoma" or "impending hepatic coma." The characteristics of hepatic coma are broadly categorized as altered mental state (usually disorientation and confusion), tremor (may have asterixis, or flapping tremor), and electroencephalographic changes. Not all patients are comatose, and the degree to which the characteristics of hepatic coma are present varies somewhat.

Abnormalities in ammonia metabolism are involved in the pathogenesis of hepatic coma. Ammonia, a potentially toxic substance, is produced from dietary protein or other sources of nitrogen through the action of gastrointestinal bacteria. An important function of the liver is to remove ammonia from the blood by converting it to urea. Another source of ammonia is the enterohepatic circulation: ingested urea and urea that diffuses into the intestinal lumen from the blood are converted to ammonia, which enters the portal circulation and is delivered to the liver. Although the direct causes of hepatic coma have not been established, several predisposing or precipitating factors have been identified. Among these are gastrointestinal bleeding and excessive dietary protein intake (provide substrate for increased ammonia production), renal failure (increased availability of urea for enterohepatic circulation), infection (increased catabolism of body protein), and constipation (increased ammonia production and absorption). A number of other factors, such as overuse of diuretics and sedatives, anesthesia and surgery, and fluid and electrolyte imbalances, have been implicated in the development of hepatic coma.

The diet should be planned with use of the exchange list for protein, sodium, and potassium control* (see page 90). Although the diet should be individualized according to the needs of the patient, the following general guidelines may be helpful. Protein intake may be moderately restricted (40-, 50-, or 60-g protein diets) in the very early stages of impending hepatic coma or for patients having compensated, but advanced, liver disease. When the patient is in hepatic coma or impending hepatic coma, dietary protein may be restricted to 20 g or less, or perhaps to 0 to 5 g. As the condition of the patient improves, the protein level is increased gradually, and as tolerated, to 30, 40, or 50 g.

Calorie intake should be sufficient to prevent catabolism of body protein for energy. Caloric needs are generally not unusually high unless the patient is extremely restless or agitated. They can be estimated as basal plus 20% (from the nomogram) or 25 to 30 kcal/kg of ideal body weight. Many patients are anorexic and drowsy and may have difficulty consuming enough calories.

---

*This food exchange list is recommended in preference to other exchange lists because it permits more nearly precise control of protein. Since potassium is not limited in the treatment of hepatic coma, all restrictions based on potassium content can be disregarded.

Sodium intake may be restricted to 20 meq or less if ascites is present. A sodium intake of 90 meq or less is appropriate if ascites and edema are not present. However, a rapid gain in weight may indicate that some fluid is being retained, and the sodium level may need to be reduced to 40 meq or less.

Fluid intake is often restricted in the management of hepatic coma because of associated renal failure. When both fluid and protein are greatly restricted (for example, 600 ml of fluid and 0 to 5 g of protein), it is difficult to plan a diet adequate in calories.

PHYSICIANS: HOW TO ORDER DIETS

The diet order should specify the **levels of protein and sodium.** The dietitian will calculate calorie needs.

SELECTED BIBLIOGRAPHY

Breen, K. J., and Schenker, S.: Hepatic coma: Present concepts of pathogenesis and therapy. Prog. Liver Dis., 4:301-332, 1972.
Davidson, C. S., and Gabuzda, G. J.: Hepatic coma. *In* Schiff, L., ed.: Diseases of the Liver. Fourth edition. Philadelphia, J. B. Lippincott Company, 1975, pp. 466-499.

DIETARY CARE OF THE PATIENT WITH BURNS

GENERAL DESCRIPTION

Nutritional support of patients hospitalized because of severe trauma or extensive thermal injury emphasizes a high-protein, high-calorie diet. Dietary supplements are often necessary. Tube feedings and parenteral nutrition may be needed if intake of adequate calories and protein cannot be achieved through a normal diet.

NUTRITIONAL ADEQUACY

There is some evidence for increased needs of some vitamins, minerals, and trace elements. The optimal amounts are controversial. Generally, at least daily supplementation with a multivitamin is recommended.

INDICATIONS AND RATIONALE

Extensive burn injury is one of the most severe stresses known to man. It is characterized by increased metabolic rate and accelerated protein metabolism. The magnitude of response is directly related to the extent of injury, that is, the degree of burn (full-thickness or partial-thickness) and the total surface area affected.

The metabolic rate increases in proportion to the extent of burn and is up to two times greater than normal when there are burns over about 50% of the total body surface. By rule of thumb, caloric needs can be estimated as either (kilograms of body weight X 25) + (percentage of body burned X 40) or 40 to 60 kcal/kg of body weight.* Actual caloric expenditure can be estimated by measurement of oxygen consumption. Milliliters of oxygen consumed per minute multiplied by the factor 7 yields calories expended per 24 hours. Since change in the patient's weight can be used as an indicator of appropriateness of calorie intake, the patient should be weighed regularly.

---

*Usual caloric needs are approximately 25 kcal/kg of body weight.

Protein requirements have been estimated to be two to four times greater than normal.* A goal of 2 to 3 g of protein per kilogram of body weight can be used as an initial guide. Protein needs of individuals can be estimated through measurement of urinary nitrogen. Minimal protein losses can be calculated by multiplying the amount by which urinary nitrogen exceeds dietary nitrogen by the factor 6.25. The minimal loss of lean body tissue can be estimated by multiplying the amount by which urinary nitrogen exceeds dietary nitrogen by the factor 30. Some loss of protein occurs in the form of exudate from the burn.

The increase in metabolic rate is thought to be related primarily to increased secretion of catecholamines in response to stress. Evaporational water loss and surface cooling may also have some influence on the increased metabolic rate. Increased protein requirements are a result of mobilization of body protein for repair of body tissues, increased gluconeogenesis in response to increased levels of catabolic hormones, and exudation of protein from the wound.

During the period immediately after the burn, management of electrolyte and fluid needs is of primary importance. Ileus is common in the first week and often impedes oral intake. Calories from parenteral sources, such as intravenously administered glucose and amino acid solutions, have some protein-sparing effect, even though full calorie replacement may not be achieved. In some instances, total parenteral nutrition (see page 248) may be needed. During this period, which generally lasts several days to a week, the dietitian estimates nutritional needs and plans dietary strategy.

In the second phase, gastrointestinal function returns and electrolyte and fluid needs stabilize. Catabolism, which is the characteristic feature of this phase, continues until skin grafting is done or the surface barrier is reestablished.

The third phase of the period after the burn is the convalescent, or anabolic, phase. The metabolic rate returns to normal.

The objectives of dietary management are to minimize catabolism of body protein and to avoid the consequences of protein-calorie malnutrition, including impaired immune mechanisms with enhanced susceptibility to infection, retarded synthesis of blood proteins and hemoglobin, decreased vigor and muscular strength, and impaired wound healing. For a patient whose body weight was at or above ideal before the injury, a reasonable goal would be to avoid loss of more than 10% of that weight. Because of the risk of increased catabolism of body protein, efforts to reduce the weight of obese patients should not be undertaken during hospitalization.

---

*The Recommended Dietary Allowance (1980) for protein is 0.8 g/kg of body weight.

GENERAL DIETARY RECOMMENDATIONS

The following guidelines are given as a starting point; modifications should be made as needed.

1. Calculate the protein goal as 2 to 3 g/kg of body weight per 24 hours. The exchange list for protein control (see page 90) may be used as a guide.

2. Calculate calorie goals as (kilograms of body weight X 25) + (percentage of body burned X 40) or as 40 to 60 kcal/kg of body weight per 24 hours. Adequacy of caloric intake can be verified by periodic measurements of oxygen consumption or by frequent (preferably daily) weighings of the patient. The success of calorie and protein feeding can be assessed by urinary nitrogen measurements. Even with intensive feeding efforts, urinary nitrogen is likely to exceed intake in the early weeks after the burn, but one should try to approach nitrogen balance (urinary nitrogen equal to or less than intake) after this interval. Positive nitrogen balance (which indicates repair of protein deficits) may not be possible until the burn is healed or successfully covered with grafts.

3. Encourage the patient to achieve these goals by eating 5 or 6 small meals or regular meals with snacks. The calorie and protein contribution of foods may be increased by fortification with skim milk powder or use of dietary supplements (see page 247).

4. Monitor the patient's intake daily. Protein and calorie intake should be recorded. The diet should be planned to include tube feedings, oral dietary supplements, or parenteral nutrition as needed.

PHYSICIANS: HOW TO ORDER DIETS

The diet order should specify **high-calorie, high-protein diet.** The dietitian will estimate calorie and protein intake according to the guidelines given.

SELECTED BIBLIOGRAPHY

Bartlett, R. H., Allyn, P. A., Medley, T., et al.: Nutritional therapy based on positive caloric balance in burn patients. Arch. Surg., 112:974-980,1977.

Curreri, P. W., Richmond, D., Marvin, J., et al.: Dietary requirements of patients with major burns. J. Am. Diet. Assoc., 65:415-417, 1974.

Shuck, J. M., Eaton, R. P., Shuck, L. W., et al.: Dynamics of insulin and glucagon secretions in severely burned patients. J. Trauma, 17:706-712, 1977.

Wilmore, D. W., Long, J. M., Mason, A. D., Jr., et al.: Catecholamines: Mediator of the hypermetabolic response to thermal injury. Ann. Surg., 180:653-668, 1974.

FOOD EXCHANGE LIST FOR PROTEIN, SODIUM, AND POTASSIUM CONTROL

*COMPOSITION VALUES**

Food	Approximate Amount	Protein g	Fat g	Carbohydrate g	Calories	Sodium, meq Unsalted	Sodium, meq Salted	Potassium meq	Fluid† ml
Meat or meat substitute‡	1 oz	7	5	...	73	1	3§	2.5	20
Egg	1 medium	7	5	...	73	3	...	2	35
Milk or milk products	1/2 cup**	4	14	6	170	2.5	2.5	4	80
	(varies)		(varies)	(varies)	(varies)				varies
Starches (average)	1 serving	2	...	15	68	1	5-10	1.5	
Bread	1 slice	2	...	15	68	1	5	1	10
Cereal, dry	1 serving	2	...	15	68	1	10	1	1
Cereal, cooked	1/2 cup	2	...	15	68	1	10††	1.5	85
Vegetables	1 serving	2	...	15	68	0.5	10††	5	65
Vegetables (average)	1 serving	1	...	4	20	0.5	12	4	70
Group 1	1 serving	1	...	3	16	0.5	12	3	60
Group 2	1 serving	1	...	5	24	0.5	12	5	80
Fruits (average)	1 serving	0.5	...	17	70	...	...	3	85
Group 1	1 serving	0.5	...	17	70	...	...	2.5	85
Group 2	1 serving	0.5	...	17	70	...	...	5	85
Low-protein products	1 serving	0.2	1	27	120	0.5	varies	...	varies
Low-protein bread	1 slice (40 g)	0.2	3	22	115	0.5	varies	0.3	10
Low-protein hot cereal	4 tbsp (dry)	0.2	...	34	135	0.4	varies	0.2	480
Low-protein pasta	1 serving	0.2	1	29	125	0.5	varies	...	105
Low-protein rusk	2 slices	0.2	2	20	95	0.3	0.3	0.2	1
Fat	1 tsp	...	5	...	45	...	2	...	1

Carbohydrate supplement	1 serving	...	...	25	100	...	...	1	varies
Beverages	1 cup	...	...	varies	varies	varies	varies	2	240
Salt	1 tsp	...	...	...	...	...	86	...	...

*Values are based on averages for food groups, pages 94-107.
†Figures represent an average of water content and water formed in oxidation of food.
‡Composition values for medium-fat meats are used as an average. Protein content may vary slightly with fat content of the meat.
§Moderately salted during preparation, about 1/4 teaspoon of salt per pound of meat.
**Figures are based on 1/2 cup of half-and-half, which is incorporated into all renal dietary programs containing 30 g or more of protein.
††Moderately salted during preparation of processing, about 1/8 teaspoon of salt per serving.

*SUGGESTED DAILY FOOD EXCHANGES **

Diet	Meat	Milk†	Starches	Vegetables	Fruit	Low-protein Products	Fat	Carbohydrate Supplement	Beverages	Dessert‡	Saltshaker§
0-5 g of protein (30 meq of potassium, 1,200 ml of fluid,** 2,200 calories) Sodium, meq											
40	...	...	...	2††	3	6	6††	8	3	...	
60	...	...	...	2††	3	6	6††	8	3	...	1/4 tsp
90	...	...	...	2††	3	6	6††	8	3	...	5/8 tsp
30 g of protein (45 meq of potassium, 1,500 ml of fluid,** 2,650 calories) Sodium, meq											
40	3 (2††)	1	1††	2	4	6	10††	7	3	...	
60	3 (2††)	1	1††	2††	4	6	10††	7	3	...	
90	3 (2††)	1	1††	2††	4	6	10††	7	3	...	1/4 tsp
40 g of protein (50 meq of potassium, 1,600 ml of fluid,** 2,650 calories) Sodium, meq											
40	4 (3††)	1	2 (1††)	2	4	6	10††	6	3	...	
60	4 (3††)	1	2††	2 (1††)	4	6	10††	6	3	...	
90	4 (3††)	1	2††	2††	4	6	10††	6	3	...	1/8 tsp
50 g of protein# (60 meq of potassium, 1,650 ml of fluid,** 2,350 calories) Sodium, meq											
40	5 (4††)	1	4	2	5	...	10††	7	3	...	
60	5 (4††)	1	4 (1††)	2 (1††)	5	...	10††	7	3	...	
90	5 (4††)	1	4 (3††)	2††	5	...	10††	7	3	...	

100 g of protein (90 meq of potassium, 2,150 ml of fluid,** 2,600 calories)

Sodium, meq

9	4	6	4	5	...	6††	2	3	1
9††	4	6(1††)	4	5	...	6††	2	3	1
9††	4	6(5††)	4	5	...	6††	2	3	1

120 g of protein (95 meq of potassium, 2,200 ml of fluid,** 2,800 calories)

Sodium, meq

11	6	7	3	4	...	6††	1	3	1
11	6	7(3††)	3	4	...	6††	1	3	1
11	6	7††	3	4	...	6††	1	3	1

*See next page for portion sizes. Caloric content of each standard plan may be modified by adding or subtracting foods from the fat, carbohydrate supplement, and low-protein products groups.

†One-half cup of half-and-half is included in all diets (protein, 4 g; fat, 14 g; carbohydrate, 6 g).

‡See "Food Exchange List for Sodium Control," page 77, for listing of desserts.

§In place of the salt allowance, the equivalent in sodium-containing foods may be given.

**Fluid content includes 3 cups (720 ml) of beverage per day.

††Foods salted in preparation or processing.

#In some individual cases, it may be necessary to add low-protein products to the 50-g protein diet. Such addition would increase the caloric content of the diet significantly. The contribution of the protein from the low-protein products should be included. Amount of starches, vegetables, or fruits may be modified according to the patient's preferences.

FOOD EXCHANGE LIST FOR PROTEIN, SODIUM, AND POTASSIUM CONTROL

This food exchange list is intended to be used as a reference tool. For this reason, a more comprehensive list of foods is given than may actually be used for instruction of individuals.

LIST 1:   MEAT EXCHANGES — protein (high biologic value), 7 g*; sodium, 1 meq (unsalted), 3 meq (salted with 1/4 tsp/lb); potassium, 2.5 meq; 73 kcal; fluid, 20 ml

Measure or wt	Gram wt	Lean meat
1 oz	30	Beef: baby beef (very lean), chuck, flank steak, tenderloin, plate ribs, plate skirt steak, round (bottom, top), all rump cuts, spareribs, tripe,† ground (preceding meats trimmed of fat and ground)
1 oz	30	Lamb: leg, rib, sirloin, loin (roast and chops), shank, shoulder
1 oz	30	Pork: leg (whole rump, center shank)
1 oz	30	Veal: leg, loin, rib, shank, shoulder, cutlets
1 oz	30	Poultry (meat without skin): chicken, turkey, cornish hen, guinea hen, pheasant
1 oz	30	Fish, any fresh or frozen
1/4 cup	30	Salmon and tuna: fresh, waterpacked (unsalted)
1 1/2 oz	45	Clams† (8 1/2 g of protein)
1 oz	30	Shrimp,† scallops,† lobster†
2 oz	60	Oysters†
1/4 cup	60	Egg substitutes, fat-free
		Medium-fat meat
1 oz	30	Beef: ground (less than 20% fat), rib eye, round (ground commercial)
1 oz	30	Pork: loin (all tenderloin cuts), shoulder arm (picnic), shoulder blade, Boston butt
1 oz	30	Liver,† heart,† kidney†
1 oz	30	Cheese, low-fat (unsalted)
1	50	Egg‡

LIST 1: MEAT EXCHANGES — protein (high biologic value), 7 g*; sodium, 1 meq (unsalted), 3 meq (salted with 1/4 tsp/lb); potassium, 2.5 meq; 73 kcal; fluid, 20 ml *(Continued)*

Measure or wt	Gram wt	High-fat meat
1 oz	30	Beef: brisket, ground (more than 20% fat), hamburger (commercial), chuck (ground commercial), roasts (rib), steaks (club and rib)
1 oz	30	Lamb, breast
1 oz	30	Pork: spareribs, loin (back ribs), ground
1 oz	30	Veal, breast
1 oz	30	Poultry: capon, duck (domestic),† goose†
1 oz	30	Cheese, unsalted cheddar types
2 tbsp	30	Peanut butter, unsalted
2 tbsp	20	Peanuts, unsalted

Avoid: Salt-cured and kosher meats; salted canned or processed meats, fish, and fowl; bacon; ham; dried beef; corned beef; frankfurters; processed cold cuts; sausages; sardines; salted cheese and cheese foods; salted peanut butter; salted peanuts; commercial casserole mixes; frozen dinners

*The protein content of meat varies with fat content. In calculating diets requiring strict control of protein (≤40 g), the following values may be used: lean meat, 8 g of protein; medium-fat meat, 7 g; high-fat meat, 6 g.

†Limit to 2 servings a week because of higher natural sodium content. Values range from 1 to 5 meq per exchange.

‡Eggs must count as salted meat exchanges.

LIST 2: FAT EXCHANGES — fat, 5 g; protein, trace; potassium, trace; 45 kcal; fluid, 1 ml

Measure	Gram wt	Trace of sodium
		Predominantly polyunsaturated or monounsaturated fats
1 tsp	5	Margarine,* unsalted
1 tsp	5	Mayonnaise, unsalted
2 tsp	10	Mayonnaise-type salad dressing,* unsalted
1 tsp	5	Oil: corn, cottonseed, safflower, soy, sunflower
1 tsp	5	Oil: olive,† peanut†
		Predominantly saturated fats
1 tsp	5	Butter, unsalted
1 tsp	5	Lard
		2 meq of sodium
		Predominantly polyunsaturated or monounsaturated fats
1 tsp	5	Margarine,* salted
1 tsp	5	Mayonnaise,* salted
2 tsp	10	Mayonnaise-type salad dressing,* salted
		Predominantly saturated fats
1 tsp	5	Butter, salted

Note: Nondairy cream substitutes are a source of fat calories. Two tablespoons supply approximately 45 calories; protein content is variable but generally low. A nondairy cream substitute may be consumed freely (up to 1 cup per day), and use should be encouraged because of the calorie contribution.

Avoid: Commercially prepared salad dressing (other than those listed); bacon; salt pork; olives; nuts; commercial gravy and gravy mixes

*Made with corn, cottonseed, safflower, soy, or sunflower oil only.
†Fat content is primarily monounsaturated.

LIST 3: MILK EXCHANGES — protein (high biologic value), 4 g; sodium, 2.5 meq; potassium, 4 meq; calories, variable; fluid, 80 ml

Measure	Gram wt	
1/2 cup	120	Skim milk
1/2 cup	120	2% milk
1/2 cup	120	Whole milk
2 tbsp	15	Nonfat dry milk
2 tbsp	15	Dry whole milk
1/4 cup	60	Evaporated or condensed milk
1/2 cup	120	Chocolate milk
1/2 cup	120	Half-and-half
1/2 cup	120	Sour cream
2/3 cup	160	Whipping cream, light
3/4 cup	180	Whipping cream, heavy
1/3 cup	85	Custard
1/2 cup	130	Pudding
3/4 cup	105	Ice cream, any flavor
2/3 cup	80	Ice milk
1 cup	200	Sherbet
1/2 cup	120	Yogurt, plain or flavored

Avoid: Cultured buttermilk; instant beverage mixes; commercial pudding and custard mixes

LIST 4: STARCH EXCHANGES* – protein, 2 g; potassium, 1.5 meq; 68 kcal; fluid, variable

Measure	Gram wt	Group 1: 1 meq of sodium
		Bread
1 slice	25	Unsalted bread
1	30	Tortilla, 6 in.
		Cereal
2/3 cup	15	Corn flakes, unsalted
1 1/2 cup	20	Puffed wheat or rice, unsalted
1 biscuit	15	Shredded wheat, unsalted
1/2 cup	100	Cooked cereal, no salt
1/2 cup	100	Grits (cooked, no salt)
1/4 cup	50	Rice or barley (cooked, no salt)
1/4 cup	50	Pasta, spaghetti, noodles, macaroni (cooked, no salt)
2 cups	30	Popcorn (popped, no salt, no added fat)
2 tbsp	15	Cornmeal, dry
2 tbsp	15	Flour
		Crackers
4	20	Salt-free soda crackers, 2 1/2 in. sq
		Starchy vegetables
1/3 cup	80	Corn†: fresh, frozen, or canned (low-sodium); cooked
1 small (3 1/2 in.)	100	Corn on the cob†
1/2 cup	100	Parsnips,† cooked
1/4 cup	50	Peas, canned (low-sodium)
1 small	100	Potato,† baked or boiled
1/2 cup	100	Potato,† mashed
8	40	Potatoes,† French fried (no salt)
1/2 cup	100	Winter squash†: acorn, butternut (baked)
1/2 cup	120	Sweet potato,† baked in skin

LIST 4: STARCH EXCHANGES* — protein, 2 g; potassium, 1.5 meq; 68 kcal; fluid, variable
(Continued)

Measure	Gram wt	Group 2: 5 meq of sodium
		Bread
1 slice	25	White, including French and Italian
1 slice	25	Whole wheat
1 slice	25	Rye or pumpernickel
1 slice	25	Raisin
1/2	30	Bagel, small
1/2	30	English muffin, small
1	30	Plain muffin, small
3 tbsp	20	Dried bread crumbs
		Cereal
1 1/2 cup	20	Puffed rice
		Crackers
3	30	Graham, 2 1/2 in. sq
1/2	20	Matzoth, 4 in. by 6 in.
4	20	Melba toast, 3 3/4 in. by 2 in.
3	20	Rye wafers, 2 in. by 3 1/2 in.
		Starchy vegetables
1/3 cup	80	Corn,† regular
1/4 cup	50	Peas, frozen (cooked)
1/2 cup	120	Sweet potato,† canned
		Group 3: 10 meq of sodium
		Bread
1	35	Plain roll
1/2	35	Hamburger bun
1	45	Corn bread, 2 in. by 2 in. by 1 in.

LIST 4: STARCH EXCHANGES* — protein, 2 g; potassium, 1.5 meq; 68 kcal; fluid, variable
(Continued)

Measure	Gram wt	
		Cereal
2/3 cup	20	Wheat, corn, bran, or oat flakes
2/3 cup	20	Puffed oats
1/2 cup	100	Cooked cereal (with 1/8 tsp of salt)
1/2 cup	100	Grits, cooked (with 1/8 tsp of salt)
1/4 cup	50	Rice or barley, cooked (with 1/8 tsp of salt)
1/4 cup	50	Pasta, spaghetti, noodles, macaroni (cooked; with 1/8 tsp of salt)
		Starchy vegetables
1 small or 1/2 cup	100	Potatoes,† cooked (with 1/8 tsp of salt)

Avoid: Salted snack foods; salted crackers; potato chips; corn chips; pretzels; salted popcorn; commercial mixes; commercially frozen convenience foods; canned soups; dried soup mixes; broth; bouillon

*The starch group is subdivided into groups of 1, 5, and 10 meq of sodium. For diets allowing 90 meq of sodium that include foods from both the 5- and the 10-meq groups, basing calculations on an average of 8 meq of sodium per starch exchange may be sufficiently accurate.
†Contains 2 to 10 meq of potassium per serving.

LIST 5: *VEGETABLE EXCHANGES* — protein, 1 g; sodium, 0.5 meq (unsalted*), 12 meq (salted with 1/8 tsp/exchange)

Measure	Gram wt	Group 1: potassium, 3 meq; 15 kcal; fluid, 60 ml
1/4 cup	50	Asparagus: fresh, frozen, or canned
1/4 cup	50	Bean sprouts
1/2 cup	100	Beans, green or wax (canned)
1/4 cup	50	Broccoli, fresh or frozen
1/4 cup	50	Carrots, fresh or canned (cooked)
1/4 cup	50	Cauliflower, fresh or frozen
1/4 cup	50	Collards, frozen
1/4 cup	50	Dandelion greens
20 small leaves	50	Endive
4 large leaves	50	Escarole
1/4 cup	50	Mustard greens, frozen
1/4 cup	50	Okra, fresh or frozen
1/2 cup	100	Onions, cooked
1/2 cup	100	Pepper, green (cooked)
1/4 cup	50	Spinach, canned
1/3 cup	35	Summer squash

LIST 5: *VEGETABLE EXCHANGES* — protein, 1 g; sodium, 0.5 meq (unsalted*), 12 meq
(salted with 1/8 tsp/exchange) *(Continued)*

Measure	Gram wt	Group 2: potassium, 5 meq; 20 kcal; fluid, 80 ml
1/2 cup	100	Beans, green or wax (fresh or frozen)
1/2 cup	100	Beets, fresh or canned
1/2 cup	100	Cabbage, raw or cooked
1/4 cup	50	Carrots, raw
1/4 cup	50	Celery, raw or cooked
1/2 cup	100	Cucumber
1/2 cup	100	Eggplant, raw or cooked
1/4 small head	100	Lettuce
1/4 cup	50	Mushrooms, raw or cooked
1/2 cup	100	Onions, raw
1/3 cup	35	Peppers, green (raw)
1/3 cup	35	Pumpkin, fresh or canned
10 small	100	Radishes
1/2 cup	35	Rutabagas
1/2 cup or 1 small	35	Tomato, fresh or canned
1/2 cup	120	Tomato juice, unsalted
1/3 cup	80	Turnip greens
10 sprigs	50	Watercress

Avoid: Sauerkraut; pickled vegetables; salted tomato juice; seasoned tomato sauces;
commercially frozen vegetable mixes and sauces; dried beans†; any vegetable not
listed

*Unsalted vegetables are those that do not have salt added in preparation or processing, including fresh, frozen (no salt added), and canned (low-sodium) vegetables. Regular canned vegetables and frozen vegetables with salt added in processing are "salted" vegetables; salt should not be added in cooking.
†To be avoided because of higher protein and potassium content.

LIST 6: FRUIT EXCHANGES – protein, 0.5 g; sodium, trace; 70 kcal; fluid, 85 ml

Measure	Gram wt	Group 1: 2.5 meq of potassium
1 small	80	Apple
1/2 cup	120	Apple juice*
1/2 cup	100	Applesauce
1/2 cup	70	Blackberries
1/2 cup	70	Blueberries: fresh, frozen, or canned
1/3 cup	50	Cantaloupe
1/3 cup	80	Cherries: fresh, frozen, or canned
1/2 oz	15	Coconut, fresh
1/2 cup	100	Cranberries, fresh or frozen
2 cups	480	Cranberry juice*
2	15	Dates
1/3 cup or 15	65	Grapes, canned
1/4 cup or 8	50	Grapes, fresh
1 cup	240	Grape juice*
1 cup	240	Grape drink*
1/3 cup	50	Honeydew melon
1/3 cup	80	Loganberries, canned
1/2 cup	120	Orange-apricot drink*
2/3 cup	160	Peach nectar*
1 small	100	Pear, fresh
3/4 cup	150	Pears, canned
3/4 cup	180	Pear nectar*
1 medium	30	Persimmon, native
1/2 cup	100	Pineapple, canned
1/3 cup	80	Pineapple, frozen
2/3 cup	160	Pineapple-grapefruit drink*
2/3 cup	160	Pineapple-orange drink*
2 tbsp	15	Raisins
1/3 cup	40	Raspberries, fresh or frozen
1/2 cup	75	Strawberries, frozen
2 small	80	Tangerines
1/2 cup	85	Watermelon

LIST 6: FRUIT EXCHANGES — protein, 0.5 g; sodium, trace; 70 kcal; fluid, 85 ml
(Continued)

Measure	Gram wt	Group 2: 5 meq of potassium
2 small	80	Apricots, fresh
1/3 cup	80	Apricots, canned
1/2 cup	120	Apricot nectar*
1/8	30	Avocado
1/2 cup	60	Banana
1 large	50	Figs, fresh
1/2 cup	100	Figs, canned
1/2 cup	100	Fruit cocktail, canned
1/2 cup	120	Grape juice,* canned
1/2 medium	100	Grapefruit, fresh
1/2 cup	120	Grapefruit juice*
1/2 cup	100	Grapefruit sections, canned
1/2 cup	120	Lemon juice*
1/2 medium	100	Mango, fresh
1 small	80	Nectarine
1 small	100	Orange
1/2 cup	120	Orange juice*: fresh, frozen, or canned
1/3 cup	80	Papaya, fresh
1 medium	100	Peach, fresh
1/2 cup	100	Peaches, canned or frozen
1/2 cup	100	Pineapple, fresh
1/2 cup	120	Pineapple juice*
2 small	80	Plums, fresh
1/2 cup	100	Plums, canned
1/3 cup	80	Prune juice*
1/3 cup	80	Rhubarb, fresh or frozen
1/2 cup	75	Strawberries, fresh

Avoid: Fruits that have been crystallized, glazed, or dried with a sodium compound; any fruits not listed

*If fluid in the diet is controlled, use must be included in the total fluid allowance.

LIST 7: LOW-PROTEIN PRODUCTS — protein, 0.2 g; sodium, 0.5 meq; potassium, trace; 120 kcal; fluid, variable

Measure	Gram wt	Low-protein...
1 slice (1 1/2 oz)	40	bread
2 slices	20	rusk
1/3 cup, dry; 2/3 cup, cooked	150	ring macaroni
3/4 cup, dry; 1 cup, cooked	130	ribbed macaroni
1 1/2 rolls, dry; 1/2 cup, cooked	120	flat noodles
4 tbsp, dry; 2 cups, cooked	60	hot cereal*
2	30	cookies
1/2 cup	120	gelatin*

*If fluid in the diet is controlled, use must be included in the total fluid allowance.

LIST 8: **CARBOHYDRATE SUPPLEMENTS** — protein, trace; sodium, trace; potassium, 1 meq; 100 kcal; fluid, variable

Measure	Gram wt	Sugar and syrups
2 tbsp	25	Sugar
2 tbsp	40	Honey
2 tbsp	40	Jelly or jam
2 tbsp	40	Syrup (table blends)
		Candy
3	30	Fondant or sugar mints
3 large	30	Gumdrops
6 pieces	30	Hard candy, unfilled
20	30	Jelly beans
1 medium	30	Lollipops, unfilled
		Fruit desserts
2 tbsp	80	Cranberry sauce or relish
2/3 cup	140	Fruit ice*
1 twin bar	130	Popsicle (120 ml of fluid)*
		Flavored beverages*
1 cup (8 oz)	240	Carbonated, fruit-flavored, Kool-Aid, lemonade
		Flour products
1/4 cup	30	Cornstarch or tapioca
		High-calorie beverages*
1/4 cup	60	Cal Power, Hycal liquid, Polycose liquid†
		Other carbohydrate sources
4 tbsp	32	Polycose powder†

Avoid: Chocolate‡ and cream-filled candies; salted-nut candies

*If fluid in the diet is controlled, use must be included in the total fluid allowance.

†Contains 2 meq of sodium per exchange.

‡Chocolate may be included in some diets as considered appropriate; 1 oz of chocolate contains 1 to 2 g of protein, a trace of sodium, and 1 to 4 meq of potassium.

LIST 9: BEVERAGES — nutritive values should be calculated individually

Measure	Gram wt	
1 cup (8 oz)	240	Coffee, decaffeinated coffee, tea — 2 meq of potassium
1 cup (8 oz)	240	Lemonade, limeade — 1 meq of potassium
1 cup (8 oz)	240	Carbonated beverages, Kool-Aid — trace of potassium
1 cup (8 oz)	240	Water*

*Drinking water, either natural or softened, may be a significant source of sodium. Patients on diets of 20 meq of sodium are advised to ask the public health department about the sodium content of the local water supply. If the content exceeds 40 parts per million (2 meq, or 40 mg, of sodium per liter), distilled water should be used. Patients who are limited to 20 meq of sodium in the diet and whose water supply must be softened should have the softener attached only to the hot water line so that cold water used in cooking and for drinking will not contribute to sodium intake.

LIST 10: MISCELLANEOUS

Allow: Spices and herbs; garlic and onion powder; dry mustard; fresh horseradish; flavoring extracts; vinegar

Avoid: Salt (except as allowed); seasoning salts; seasoning mixes; meat tenderizer; monosodium glutamate; catsup; prepared mustard and horseradish; soy sauce; bottled meat and barbecue sauce; olives; pickles; salt substitutes

POTASSIUM CONTROL

GENERAL DESCRIPTION

Potassium is widely distributed in foods but is highest in fruits and vegetables. General guidelines are given for increasing potassium intake.

For restriction of dietary sources of potassium, see "Food Exchange List for Protein, Sodium, and Potassium Control," page 90.

INDICATIONS AND RATIONALE

Hypokalemia is most often associated with use of diuretics but may also be induced by other drugs (such as corticosteroids), gastrointestinal disturbances (such as diarrhea and vomiting), some renal disturbances, and some endocrine disorders. In many instances, use of parenterally or orally administered potassium supplements is warranted.

Treatment of hypokalemia occurring with diuretic therapy for hypertension may consist of (1) restriction of dietary sodium to lessen urinary potassium wastage, (2) substitution of a potassium-sparing diuretic for a potassium-wasting one, (3) use of potassium chloride supplements or potassium chloride salt substitutes, or (4) use of foods high in potassium.

Many potassium chloride supplements are poorly accepted because of their unpleasant taste. Salt substitutes containing potassium chloride may be a reasonable alternative, since they generally cost less and are more palatable than prescription potassium chloride supplements. Although there is some variation among brands of potassium chloride salt substitutes, the usual potassium content is 10 to 13 meq of potassium per gram.* Five grams (1 teaspoon) of these salt substitutes would provide 50 to 65 meq of potassium. A specific daily dose of the potassium chloride salt substitutes should be recommended to the patient. Many dietetic "low-sodium" products use potassium chloride instead of sodium chloride, a substitution that substantially increases the potassium content of these foods.

The usual American diet provides 40 to 100 meq of potassium daily. It is difficult for most patients consistently and reliably to increase dietary intake of potassium beyond this level. A range of 40 to 60 meq of potassium from potassium chloride supplements is a frequently prescribed dose. When a similar increase in potassium is attempted with food, the total intake of calories or sodium (or both) is often also appreciably increased. Attempts to increase dietary potassium may be useful if the patient requires only a very low level of potassium supplementation to prevent hypokalemia, if the patient's usual diet is very low in potassium, or if therapy adjunctive to potassium supplements is required.

---

*Potassium chloride provides 13.4 meq of potassium per gram.

FOOD SOURCES OF POTASSIUM

Low in Calories*	Low in Sodium†	Food	Size, Processing, Preparation	Measure
		5 to 10 meq of potassium per serving		
		Vegetables		
●	●	Asparagus	Fresh or frozen	1/2 cup
	●	Beans, lima	Fresh or frozen, cooked	1/2 cup
●	●	Beets	Fresh, cooked	1/2 cup
●	●	Broccoli	Fresh or frozen, cooked	1/2 cup
●	●	Brussels sprouts	Fresh or frozen	1/2 cup
●	●	Cabbage	Raw	1 cup
●	●	Carrots	Fresh, raw or cooked	1/2 cup
●		Celery	Raw	1 cup
●		Chard, Swiss	Fresh, cooked	1/2 cup
●	●	Cress	Cooked	1/2 cup
●	●	Dandelion greens	Cooked	1/2 cup
●	●	Eggplant	Baked	1/2 cup
●	●	Kale	Fresh, cooked	1/2 cup
●	●	Leeks	Raw	3/4 cup
●	●	Mushrooms	Fresh, cooked	1/2 cup
	●	Parsnips	Cooked	1/2 cup
	●	Peas	Dried, cooked	1/2 cup
●	●	Pumpkin	Fresh	1/2 cup
●	●	Rutabagas	Raw	3/4 cup
●	●	Squash, winter	Frozen, cooked	1/2 cup
●	●	Tomato	Fresh	1 medium
●		Tomato juice	Canned	1/2 cup
●	●	Tomato juice	Low-sodium or fresh, unsalted	1/2 cup
●	●	Turnip	Raw	3/4 cup

FOOD SOURCES OF POTASSIUM (Continued)

Low in Calories*	Low in Sodium†	Food	Size, Processing, Preparation	Measure
		5 to 10 meq of potassium per serving		
		Fruits		
	•	Apple juice	Unsweetened, canned or fresh	1 cup
	•	Apricots	Fresh	2 medium
•	•	Apricots	Canned, unsweetened	1/2 cup
	•	Apricots	Dried	4 halves
	•	Banana		1 small
•	•	Blackberries	Fresh or frozen	1 cup
	•	Grape juice	Unsweetened, canned or fresh	1 cup
	•	Grapefruit juice	Unsweetened, canned or fresh	1 cup
•	•	Orange juice	Unsweetened, fresh or frozen	1/2 cup
	•	Orange, tangerine, mandarin orange	Fresh	1 medium
	•	Pineapple juice	Unsweetened, canned or frozen	1 cup
	•	Prune juice	Unsweetened, canned	1/2 cup
	•	Prunes	Dried	8
•	•	Raspberries	Fresh or frozen	1 cup
•	•	Strawberries	Fresh or frozen	1 cup
		Meats		
		Meat	Cooked	3 oz
		Shrimp	Fresh or cooked	3 1/2 oz
		Tuna	Fresh or canned	3/4 cup
		Milk		
		Skim, 2%, or whole		1 cup

FOOD SOURCES OF POTASSIUM (Continued)

Low in Calories*	Low in Sodium†	Food	Size, Processing, Preparation	Measure
		10 to 15 meq of potassium per serving		
		Vegetables		
●	●	Artichokes	Cooked	1/2 cup
	●	Beans	Dried, cooked	1/2 cup
●	●	Beet greens	Cooked	1/2 cup
●		Chard, Swiss	Chopped	2 cups
●	●	Chard, Swiss	Whole leaves	3 cups
●	●	Cress, garden	Raw	3 cups
●		Dandelion greens	Raw	1 cup
●		Kale	Fresh, whole leaves	3 cups
●		Kale	Chopped	2 cups
●	●	Mushrooms	Fresh	10 small or 4 large
●	●	Mushrooms	Sliced	1/2 cup
	●	Potatoes	Baked or raw	1/2 cup
●		Spinach	Raw, chopped	2 cups
●		Spinach	Raw, whole leaves	3 cups
		Fruits		
●	●	Cantaloupe	6 in. in diameter	1/4
●	●	Honeydew	7 in. in diameter	1/8
		Meats		
		Cod	Cooked	3 1/2 oz
		Flounder	Cooked	3 1/2 oz
		Halibut	Cooked	3 1/2 oz
		Salmon	Fresh or cooked	3 1/2 oz
		Scallops	Cooked	3 1/2 oz
		Miscellaneous		
		Peanuts	Roasted with skins	45
		Walnuts		3/4 cup

*≤50 calories per serving.
†≤2 meq per serving.

SELECTED BIBLIOGRAPHY

Bateson, M.C.: Dietary potassium and diuretic therapy (annotation). Am. Heart J., 88:124-125, 1974.
Sopko, J. A., and Freeman, R. M.: Salt substitutes as a source of potassium. J.A.M.A., 238:608-610, 1977.

DIETARY MANAGEMENT OF THE PATIENT WITH CANCER

INDICATIONS AND RATIONALE

The progressive growth of cancer leads to striking alterations of structure and function in the host organ. All too often, cachexia is the result. This syndrome is characterized by anorexia, weakness, nutritional depletion, and redistribution of host nutrients. Cachexia results from local structural changes due to tumor growth, decreased food intake, maldigestion, malabsorption, and altered metabolism.

Weight loss is one of the common presenting manifestations of cancer and also often occurs later as part of the natural history of cancer. Anorexia is unquestionably one of the common causes of weight loss, although its pathogenesis remains unclear. Interesting findings include alterations of taste perception, increased production of lactate and ketones, and psychologic factors that contribute to the lessening of food consumption. An increased metabolic rate has been reported as a contributing cause of malnutrition in some patients with cancer. A measurement of oxygen consumption* may help decide whether increased calorie expenditure is responsible for weight loss and would aid in setting a goal for calorie intake. Weight loss in cancer patients is associated with loss of body fat and protein. Superimposed on this background of local and systemic effects from cancer in the patient undergoing treatment for the disease may be further alterations in the nutritional state due to surgery, radiation, or chemotherapy.

Oral feeding, enteral nutrition by tube, and parenteral nutrition are all potentially useful in the nutritional management of the cancer patient. Treatment of anorexia and improvement in the patient's nutritional state often lead to an increased sense of well-being, may enhance the likelihood of response to therapy, and diminish the toxicity from therapy.

Oral feedings should be used whenever possible in the nutritional management of the cancer patient. If oral intake is contraindicated or inadequate, tube feedings should be considered as an alternative to supplying nutrients intravenously. The details of tube feeding can be found on page 237.

GENERAL DIETARY RECOMMENDATIONS

Nutritional support of the cancer patient must be individualized. All patients, however, should be helped to understand that nutrition is an integral part of the total management of the disease. The patient must understand that malnutrition is not necessarily an unavoidable consequence of the disease. The dietary modifications depend on the extent to which the patient is experiencing anorexia, taste alterations, easy satiation, nausea, weight loss, and consequences of treatment.

Some general considerations in designing a diet for the cancer patient follow.

1. A detailed diet history should be obtained to determine past food preferences and eating habits, present calorie and protein intake, food likes and dislikes, specific food intolerances, taste abnormalities or altered taste sensations, distribution of feedings throughout the day, number of times the patient eats each day, who does the cooking, and whether the patient eats alone.

2. The diet should be specific in number of calories and amount of protein needed each day. Suggested ranges of protein and calories for nutritional treatment of adult patients with cancer are as follows:

	Calories kcal/kg	Protein g/kg
Maintenance	25 to 35	1 to 1.5
Repletion	40 to 50	1.5 to 2

Information obtained in the diet history should be carefully considered in formulating the diet. For example, if the patient is unable to tolerate red meats, chicken and fish should be suggested.

---

*Milliliters of oxygen consumed per minute multiplied by the factor 7 yields calories expended per 24 hours.

For some patients, nonmeat protein sources, such as milk, cheese, eggs, and peanut butter, should be suggested. In some cases, protein sources described in "Vegetarian Diets," page 16, may be useful.

3. If the patient has been losing weight, the first realistic goal of nutritional intervention may be to prevent further loss of weight. The patient who can maintain present weight with a new diet is more likely to follow later dietary guidelines that will demand even larger amounts of calories and protein to achieve nutritional repletion and weight gain.

4. Recommendations should take into account the patient's strength and ability to prepare food. Ways that the spouse could help to make food available if the patient is alone during part of the day should be suggested.

5. If the patient experiences easy satiation or anorexia, a division of foods into five or six small meals a day is usually well tolerated. Planning larger meals early in the day is often useful, because the patient is less fatigued then and is therefore better able to eat.

6. If the patient is nauseated from the underlying cancer, from radiation, or from chemotherapy, the use of an antiemetic from the phenothiazine class of drugs, such as prochlorperazine (Compazine), can be very helpful. The drug should be given from 30 to 60 minutes before planned meals. Likewise, if pain hinders eating, systematic administration of analgesics will enhance the patient's willingness and desire to eat.

7. The necessity of changing lifetime meal and snack patterns should be frankly explained to the patient. For example, the patient who was conditioned to omitting snacks or desserts to avoid gaining weight before the diagnosis of cancer should be told that this routine is no longer appropriate.

8. The patient should be given dietary guidelines in writing and be encouraged to eat the suggested foods in the suggested amounts.

9. Food should fill the diet prescription whenever possible. Sometimes, supplementation with high-calorie, high-protein liquid feedings is necessary (see page 242). Chemically defined diets should be used only if specifically indicated.

10. A therapeutic multiple vitamin and mineral supplement should be given to patients who are not able to ingest a well-balanced diet or who have specific deficiencies.

11. The patient's progress should be evaluated at regular intervals to determine whether the nutritional state is improving. Follow-up also offers a means of support and reinforcement, so that the diet prescription can be advanced or modified in response to treatment.

Methods to treat cancer may induce other nutrition-related problems. If surgery is performed on the digestive tract, symptoms interfering with ingestion, digestion, or absorption of foods may occur. They should be treated as they would for any patient undergoing a similar procedure, except that the other problems the cancer patient is experiencing must be recognized.

Radiation and chemotherapy may result in a temporary loss of taste sensations, in dry mouth, or in sore mouth, which may discourage eating. Artificial saliva (glycerin and lemon juice) may be useful. Sauces, gravy, melted butter, salad oil, and syrup may make foods easier to swallow. Eating hard candies or gumdrops may alleviate dry mouth between meals, but this practice should not be encouraged if it interferes with intake of other nutrients. Texture and appearance of the food must be considered to encourage eating.

Obesity is common in patients with breast cancer. Skeletal metastasis may cause more problems, such as pathologic fractures, in the overweight person. Evidence suggests that the cancer recurrence rate is adversely affected by the patient being overweight. Therefore, obesity should be treated by gradual weight reduction through moderate calorie control.

Nutritional support to the cancer patient is most effective if dietary guidelines are designed in the light of that patient's problems. The patient should be seen at regular intervals so that emotional support can be given and changes necessitated by therapy can be made in the diet prescription.

SELECTED BIBLIOGRAPHY

Bozzetti, F., Pagnoni, A. M., and Del Vecchio, M.: Excessive caloric expenditure as a cause of malnutrition in patients with cancer. Surg. Gynecol. Obstet., 150:229-234, 1980.

Conference on Nutrition and Cancer Therapy. Cancer Res., 37:2321-2471, 1977.

Donegan, W. L., Hartz, A. J., and Rimm, A. A.: The association of body weight with recurrent cancer of the breast. Cancer, 41:1590-1594, 1978.

DIETARY MANAGEMENT OF ANOREXIA NERVOSA

INDICATIONS AND RATIONALE

Anorexia nervosa occurs chiefly in adolescent girls shortly after the onset of puberty. It may begin just before puberty or later in adolescence, less commonly after the age of 20. It occurs 10 times more frequently in girls than in boys. The disorder is characterized by self-imposed dieting, refusal to eat, hyperactivity, and extreme loss of weight. Psychologic characteristics include misperception of the body image, with the patient seeing herself as being fatter than she is, the fear of becoming fat, and denial of fatigue. Physiologic accompaniments consist of the somatic changes associated with starvation, notably lowered basal metabolic rate, and reduced gonadotropin production resulting in the cessation of menses in girls.

A primary form of anorexia nervosa in which relentless pursuit of thinness is the driving motivation has been differentiated from atypical forms in which the patients are concerned about the weight loss but may use it as a means of controlling others.

Treatment involves medical care by a pediatrician, internist, or psychiatrist or collaborative treatment by a psychiatrist and a general physician. Requirements for medical treatment vary greatly, depending on the age of the patient, duration and severity of starvation, and degree of dehydration or other complications. The diet history, whether bulimia and vomiting are present, and abuse of medications (including laxatives and diuretics) influence the approach to treatment. Restoring normal physiologic function by correction of starvation and associated changes is the initial aim of treatment. Too rapid reversal of the hypometabolic state by rapid refeeding may cause excessive peripheral edema, but some edema is to be expected during refeeding and should not be cause for alarm. Nearly all patients should be able to resume oral intake of small amounts of regular food. This approach is much preferable to liquid food substitutes given orally or to tube feeding, because the aim is for the patient to resume normal eating habits. Usually only small quantities of food can be tolerated in the beginning because of postprandial discomfort. Fear of becoming fat is often a major obstacle to eating. A frank explanation of the physiologic changes associated with starvation and careful explanation of the treatment are essential before treatment is begun. The long-term aim, beyond restoring normal eating patterns, is for the patient to become an effective, independently functioning individual.

Treatment of patients with anorexia nervosa, particularly the primary form, can be exceedingly difficult and time-consuming. Hospitalization is often necessary, with long-term, intensive psychotherapy the focus of treatment. Some patients require only brief hospitalization, and others can be managed entirely as outpatients.

In any case, effective treatment requires a planned program and a well-coordinated treatment team experienced in dealing with anorectic patients. Treatment goals must be set with the patient, yet there should be flexibility in implementing the program. A goal weight based on standard growth charts and the patient's history may be determined. At first, dependence on the therapist and the program is fostered; in time, there is gradual movement toward greater responsibility and autonomy for the patient.

Clinical judgment dictates whether dietary instruction should be avoided entirely. Some patients do best when external pressure is removed from eating and the normal drive to eat is allowed to reassert itself. In other instances, rational diet instruction can be helpful at first in structuring the process and in resolving decisions about eating. Care must be taken not to reinforce the compulsive rituals and preoccupation with food existing in many patients. Principles rather than rigid plans should be conveyed.

DIETARY RECOMMENDATIONS

Whether hospitalization or outpatient treatment is utilized, those planning treatment for patients with anorexia nervosa must plan a cohesive program to assure a consistent approach. No specific protocol is suitable for every patient or for all treatment centers. Thus, each center must develop its own program. One approach is referred to in the bibliography (Lucas et al., 1976).

The dietary management of the patient with anorexia nervosa should include a detailed diet history of the patient's current and past food intake, an estimation of the calorie content of the present diet, the selection of calorie levels for both the initial treatment diet and the maintenance diet when goal weight has been reached, a discussion with the patient of the concept of a balanced diet, an initial diet prescription that accounts for the patient's preferences, a realistic plan for increasing calorie content of the diet during treatment, a discussion of weight gain, and, finally, the establishment of guidelines for a weight maintenance diet.

Diet History. The initial diet history should determine current calorie and protein intake, foods or categories of foods omitted, food preferences, frequency and types of snacks, and family eating patterns. It investigates, as accurately as possible, the patient's eating pattern before she began to reduce her food intake. In the diet history, the dietitian tries to differentiate between true dislike of a food and avoidance of a food as a part of the patient's dietary manipulations.

Determination of Calorie Level. The basal calorie requirement for the patient's present weight calculated by means of the nomogram is compared with current calorie intake obtained from the diet history. Usually, the former is greater than the latter. If the basal calorie requirement is 300 to 400 calories greater than current intake, the dietitian may select the basal calories as the level for the initial diet, since this amount is as much as the patient is likely to tolerate. If the figures are nearly equal, the patient may be able to tolerate an initial diet that exceeds basal calories by 300 to 400 calories. If the initial calorie level is set too high, the patient may feel overwhelmed rather than challenged. It is appropriate to increase calories slowly.

Early in the dietary program, it is useful to determine and discuss with the patient the calorie level needed for weight maintenance at the goal weight. The patient must also understand that this calorie level may have to be exceeded during the treatment program to reach goal weight.

It is essential that the patient understand the relationship between food (energy intake) and activity (energy expenditure) for weight control. It is useful to illustrate this concept by comparing the patient's present calorie needs with her intake and to show her how the calorie progression of the diet allows for weight gain and how the weight maintenance calorie level will allow for maintenance of goal weight. If the patient is still in the growth phase, she should understand that weight gain will occur until growth ceases.

Frequently, the patient fears that if she begins eating and gaining weight, she will lose control and become overweight. It is important that the patient understand the relationship between energy intake and expenditure and that she be constantly reassured that the diet will be carefully monitored first for appropriate weight gain and then for weight maintenance.

Concept of Balanced Diet. The dietitian should thoroughly explain the body's need for nutrients for growth and development and tissue maintenance and how these needs can be met both quantitatively and qualitatively by food.

The initial treatment diet is designed to include foods from each of the basic food groups; portions are increased as calorie increases are made in the diet. Although the calorie content of the initial stages of the diet in anorexia nervosa is equivalent to that of the weight reduction diet, these diets are not equivalent. The low-calorie weight reduction diet emphasizes foods of lower caloric density to help satisfy the overweight patient's desire to eat by increasing bulk in the diet. The low-calorie diet for the anorexia nervosa patient includes foods from all food groups, with emphasis on the calorically concentrated foods. This patient usually is able to tolerate only small feedings and therefore should not be given bulky foods, especially in the first stages of dietary progression.

If, during the first dietary history, the patient reveals a desire to increase calories by eating more sweet desserts or snack foods or wishes to continue to omit a particular group of foods, the need for a varied diet to obtain all the required nutrients should be reemphasized.

Designing the Diet. The diet plan should be formulated to reflect the patient's food preferences within the structure of a well-balanced diet. It generally includes three conventional meals, but often the same amount of food can be tolerated more comfortably if divided into three smaller meals and between-meal and bedtime snacks. The patient must understand that she will feel uncomfortable at first after eating the prescribed amount of food but that her capacity for food will increase as she consistently eats the prescribed diet.

Keeping diet records helps most patients adhere to the plan. Diet records aid the dietitian in judging how well the patient is fulfilling the dietary recommendations and where the greatest difficulties are occurring and in determining when the next dietary progression can be made. The record keeping should be discontinued when eating becomes more comfortable and spontaneous.

The patient is encouraged to measure the foods in the diet at first to ensure that she is taking adequate portions, hence adequate calories. If foods are not measured and the patient determines portions in relation to her present appetite and desire for food, adequate intake will not be achieved.

The patient should understand that the diet is designed as a minimum guideline; she may eat more of anything on the diet but should not omit any of the recommended food items. Nonetheless, many patients continue to consider it as a maximum guideline, or the amount they may "safely" eat.

Dietary Progression. The progression of the calorie content of the diet is individual for each patient. The increase in calories should be realistic yet challenging for the patient. In general, an increase of 250 calories per week in the early stages of treatment and greater increments later are reasonable. When calorie increases are made, the diet records are reviewed and progress in food consumption is discussed with the patient. Such discussion enables the patient to see the next step as less difficult and more attainable.

Weight Gain Expectations. The patient should be told what she might expect in terms of weight gain at the outset and as the treatment program progresses. During the first 1 to 2 weeks of refeeding, rapid weight gain may occur because of retention of water through expansion of extracellular water, retention of electrolytes, and repletion of liver and muscle glycogen stores. This stage may be followed by several weeks of stable weight during which accumulation of fat and repair of depleted protein structures, such as muscle, are being balanced by loss of water. This period is followed by slower, more consistent weight gain of body fat and protein. It is especially important that the patient understand that the initial rapid weight increase shown by the scales is a consequence of rehydration; otherwise, she may think the weight gain represents fat or that she will continue to gain weight indefinitely at this rate. If the patient does not understand this concept and have it reinforced several times during the first days of treatment, she may stop eating, fearing that her weight gain will continue at this rate. The patient may require repeated reassurance that the postprandial discomfort, "bloating," and water retention during the early stage of weight gain will ultimately resolve.

One should not expect a particular number of pounds to be gained each week. In general, as long as progress continues to be made, first by the stopping of weight loss and then by consistent increases in weight, dietary treatment can be considered adequate. For some patients, the physician may choose to state weekly weight gain goals.

Constipation is a frequent complaint during the early stages of treatment, when caloric intake is minimal. The patient is advised that it will be relieved as food intake becomes more normal.

Maintenance Diet. The patient needs frequent reassurance that when she achieves her goal weight, dietary guidelines will be given to allow her to maintain this weight without causing further weight gain. This phase of treatment is much easier for the patient and the dietitian if a high-quality diet has been followed throughout the treatment program.

If the patient again keeps diet records during the early stages of weight maintenance, the dietitian can more accurately assess the patient's food choices and offer appropriate suggestions.

PHYSICIANS: HOW TO ORDER DIETS

The diet order should indicate **low-calorie diet for anorexia nervosa**. The dietitian will determine content and calorie level according to the principles outlined above.

SELECTED BIBLIOGRAPHY

Berkman, J. M.: Anorexia nervosa: The diagnosis and treatment of inanition resulting from functional disorders. Ann. Intern. Med., 22:679-691, 1945.

Bruch, H.: Eating Disorders: Obesity and Anorexia Nervosa. New York, Basic Books, Publishers, 1973.

Keys, A. B., Brozek, J., Henschel, A., et al.: The Biology of Human Starvation. Vol. 1 and 2. Minneapolis, University of Minnesota Press, 1950.

Lucas, A. R.: On the meaning of laboratory values in anorexia nervosa (editorial). Mayo Clin. Proc., 52:748-750, 1977.

Lucas, A. R., Duncan, J. W., and Piens, V.: The treatment of anorexia nervosa. Am. J. Psychiatry, 133:1034-1038, 1976.

DIETARY MANAGEMENT OF UROLITHIASIS

GENERAL DESCRIPTION

Adequate fluid intake is recommended in the management of all types of stone disease. Other diet modifications are based on the type of stone disease and are generally directed at reduction of excessive intake of a particular dietary constituent.

INDICATIONS AND RATIONALE

The major components of urinary stones are calcium, oxalate, phosphate, uric acid, and cystine. Chemical analysis of the stones can determine the predominant components. Recommendations for or contraindications to dietary modification are discussed for each of these constituents and for other nutritional factors affecting urolithiasis.

Fluid. Dilution of urine is of primary importance. Fluid intake should be sufficient to maintain a urine volume of at least 2,500 ml/24 hours. The amount of fluid that must be consumed is greater in warm climates. In moderate climates, the patient should be advised to drink 250 to 300 ml (8 to 10 oz) of fluid per hour while awake and on each occasion during the night that the patient arises to void. At least half the fluid ingested should be water.

Calcium. In normal persons, urinary calcium excretion has little correlation with calcium consumption, since intestinal absorption of calcium decreases when dietary intake is excessive. In idiopathic calcium lithiasis, 40 to 60% of the patients with normal calcium intake have hypercalciuria (excretion of more than 300 mg of calcium in 24 hours). In most of them, increased excretion is the consequence of increased intestinal absorption of calcium. Although the mechanism is unknown, it has been suggested that the increased absorption of calcium is the result of increased production of 1,25-dihydroxyvitamin D_3. Hypercalciuria can be reduced in these patients (especially if intake of calcium is high) by reduction of dietary calcium to about 600 mg (see page 119). Restriction of calcium to less than 600 mg yields no additional clinical benefit and is not usually recommended, since a calcium intake below this level may cause a negative calcium balance.

Oxalate. Oxalic acid or oxalate is the end product of both glyoxylic acid and ascorbic acid metabolism. Normal urinary excretion of oxalate is less than 40 mg/24 hours, of which less than 10% comes from oxalate in the diet. Dietary calcium intake and intestinal oxalate absorption are inversely related. Calcium normally combines with oxalate in the intestinal lumen and makes it less available for absorption. Therefore, a diet very low in calcium may increase urinary oxalate excretion.

Urine is commonly supersaturated with calcium oxalate, since this compound is poorly soluble. Small increases in urinary oxalate concentration have a great effect on crystal formation. Control of dietary oxalate (see page 121) may be of benefit to some patients, since there may be increased urinary excretion of oxalate after ingestion of high-oxalate foods. Urinary oxalate levels in normal persons taking perhaps 4 g or more of ascorbic acid may be high enough to put them at risk for stone formation.

Patients with ileal disease, ileal resection, or jejunoileal bypass may have increased urinary oxalate excretion due to enhanced absorption of dietary oxalate. Oxalate is normally sequestered by calcium in the intestinal lumen and is poorly absorbed. In ileal disease and resection, malabsorbed fatty acids bind with calcium, so that oxalate is more available for absorption. The malabsorbed fatty acids and bile salts may also increase colonic permeability to oxalate. Foods high in oxalate (see page 121) should be avoided. These patients should also avoid taking greater than physiologic amounts of vitamin C. A low-fat diet (see page 145) may be warranted if steatorrhea is significant. Calcium restriction is contraindicated because of the mechanisms of increased oxalate absorption. In fact, calcium supplements may be recommended.

Phosphate. Attempts to control the formation of phosphate-containing stones through use of a low-phosphate diet and phosphate-binding agents have been largely unsuccessful.

Cystine. Cystinuria is an inherited disorder involving gastrointestinal and renal transport of the amino acids cystine, lysine, arginine, and ornithine. The only major complication in this disorder is the tendency to form cystine stones because of the low urinary solubility of cystine. Cystine is the end product of methionine metabolism. Urinary excretion of cystine can be lowered by reducing dietary intake of methionine, and this can be accomplished by decreasing the total protein content of the diet. Stringent restriction of protein is rarely recommended, since the patients do not see immediate benefit from the diet and therefore are less likely to adhere to it.

Uric Acid. Uric acid stones may develop as a result of hyperuricuria, dehydration, or excessive acidity of the urine. Uric acid is the end product of purine metabolism. Foods high in purines generally have a high acid ash content and tend to acidify the urine in addition to increasing urinary excretion of uric acid. Exclusion of foods very high in purines may be helpful.

Acid Ash and Alkaline Ash Diets. Dietary manipulations that alter the pH of the urine may be useful in the management of urinary stones. Foods that render the urine acid are spoken of as "acid ash" foods, since the ash remaining after their combustion is acid in reaction. Foods that leave an alkaline ash after combustion under laboratory conditions cause the urine to become alkaline. Both the acid ash and the alkaline ash diets tend to become monotonous, so that compliance by the patient is often poor. Since these diets are generally considered to be supplemental to acidifying or alkalinizing medications, advising the patient simply to avoid excessive use of particular foods may be sufficient.

CALCIUM CONTROL

GENERAL DESCRIPTION

Calcium intake can be controlled by avoiding or limiting milk and foods containing large amounts of milk. The calcium content of a diet that includes a variety of foods but no milk products can be estimated as 500 to 600 mg/day.* Specified amounts of milk or milk products can be added to achieve the desired level of calcium.

INDICATIONS AND RATIONALE

Restriction of calcium intake may be advisable if hypercalciuria is present or is thought to be a contributory cause of calcium-containing stones. The diet should not contain more than about 600 mg of calcium per day.

As a precaution against hypercalciuria and urolithiasis in patients immobilized by spinal cord injury, current practice is to advise limitation of calcium intake to about 800 mg per day during the first 3 to 6 months after injury or until there is weight-bearing activity. Need for continuation of diet controls should be assessed on an individual basis. Maintaining urinary volume by generous intake of fluid is thought to be the primary defense against stone formation and should be emphasized in addition to restriction of dietary calcium.

A high intake of protein has been said to favor hypercalciuria and a negative calcium balance, but there is probably no advantage to restricting protein intake to less than conventional levels.

---

*Based on the calcium content of sample diets of 1,500 to 2,500 calories.

PHYSICIANS: HOW TO ORDER DIETS

The diet order should indicate the level of calcium (either **600 mg** or **800 mg of calcium**) *or* indicate **low calcium**. If "low calcium" is indicated, the dietitian will determine the appropriate level of calcium from the guidelines given.

DIET CONTAINING 600 mg OF CALCIUM

Avoid milk and milk beverages, yogurt, cottage cheese, other cheese, ice cream, sherbet, custard, and pudding.

DIET CONTAINING 800 mg OF CALCIUM

Allow the following foods in limited amounts.*

300 mg of calcium

Whole milk	1 cup
Chocolate milk	1 cup
Evaporated milk	1/2 cup
Nonfat dry milk	1/3 cup
Skim milk	1 cup
Buttermilk	1 cup
Yogurt	1 cup

200 mg of calcium

Cheese	1 oz
Cheese spreads	1 oz
Cheese foods	1 oz

100 mg of calcium

Cottage cheese	1/2 cup
Ice cream	1/2 cup
Pudding	1/2 cup
Custard	1/3 cup
Cream pie	1/6 of 9-in. pie
Half-and-half or cream	1/3 cup

---

*Some other foods—sardines, fish canned with bones, quick-cooking cereals, quick breads, sweet potato, beet greens, Swiss chard, collards, dandelion greens, kale, mustard greens, okra, spinach, turnip greens, endive, escarole, rhubarb, and dried fruits—may contribute a substantial amount of calcium to the diet if used frequently and in large amounts. It is not necessary to restrict these foods unless a diet history reveals a high frequency of use and the situation warrants their exclusion.

OXALATE CONTROL

GENERAL DESCRIPTION

Oxalic acid occurs primarily in foods of plant origin. The diet excludes foods that are very high in oxalates and is intended to provide less than 50 mg of oxalate per day.

PHYSICIANS: HOW TO ORDER DIETS

The diet order should indicate **low-oxalate diet**. Any other diet modifications needed, such as a low-fat diet, should be included in the diet order.

FOODS TO ALLOW AND FOODS TO AVOID *

Food Groups	Allow	Avoid
Beverage	Coffee (limit to 3 cups a day); noncola carbonated beverages; artificially flavored fruit drinks (not fortified with vitamin C)	Tea; cola beverages; chocolate flavored beverages; Ovaltine
Meat	All except peanut butter and peanuts	Peanut butter; peanuts
Fat	All except nuts	Nuts
Milk	Milk and milk beverages (limit to 2 to 3 cups/day)	None
Starch	All except those in "Avoid" column	Sweet potato; pumpkin; parsnips; wheat germ
Vegetable	Onions (use only as a seasoning; limit to 1 to 2 tbsp/day); all others except those in "Avoid" column	Beets; carrots; celery; chives; green beans; greens: beet, collards, dandelion, kale, mustard, spinach, Swiss chard, turnip; okra; parsley; tomatoes; tomato juice, sauce, and paste
Fruit	All except those in "Avoid" column (limit juice of allowed fruits to 1/2 cup/day)	Currants; figs; gooseberries; grapefruit; oranges; plums; prunes; raspberries; rhubarb; tangerines; cranberry juice†; grape juice†; grapefruit juice; orange juice; orange and lemon peel

FOODS TO ALLOW AND FOODS TO AVOID* (Continued)

Food Groups	Allow	Avoid
Soup	Any containing allowed foods	All others
Dessert	Any containing allowed foods	Any with nuts, chocolate, or disallowed fruits
Sweets	All except those in "Avoid" column	Marmalade; any with nuts, chocolate, or disallowed fruits
Miscellaneous	Tomato-based condiments, such as catsup and chili sauce (use only as a seasoning; limit to 1 to 2 tbsp/day); all other foods except those in "Avoid" column	Chocolate; cocoa; beer

Medications: Pharmacologic levels of ascorbic acid supplementation may increase urinary oxalate excretion. Therefore, the patient should be advised to avoid ascorbic acid supplements unless approved by the physician.

*Data available on the average oxalate content of foods vary greatly, in part because of differences among and inaccuracies in analytic methods. The oxalate content of a particular food is also variable and seems to be related to variety of plant, season, age of plant, variation from one part of the plant to another, climate, and soil conditions. The exact oxalate content of specific foods or the total diet is difficult to verify. For practical purposes, the diet is designed to prohibit or limit foods that tend to be high in oxalate.

†Although grapes and cranberries are not extremely high in oxalate, juices from them are excluded because they are concentrated and may therefore be a substantial source of oxalate.

PURINE CONTROL

GENERAL DESCRIPTION

Foods high in purines are specific kinds of meats and meat extracts.

INDICATIONS AND RATIONALE

Persons with disorders affecting purine metabolism, such as gout and urinary uric acid lithiasis (see page 119), may be advised to avoid excessive intake of any kind of meat, fish, or poultry, since all contain moderate amounts of purine, and to avoid specific foods that are very high in purines. Weight control is particularly important for persons with gout.

FOODS HIGH IN PURINES

Organ meats, such as liver, heart, tongue, kidneys, sweetbreads, brains
Anchovies, sardines
Meat extracts, gravy, broth, bouillon

PHYSICIANS: HOW TO ORDER DIETS

The diet order should indicate **purine control**. If indicated, a weight reduction diet should be ordered.

ACID-ASH AND ALKALINE-ASH DIETS

INDICATIONS AND RATIONALE

Description of foods as either "acid-ash" or "alkaline-ash" is based on the reaction of the ash remaining after combustion of foods under laboratory conditions. Acid-ash foods tend to promote a more acidic urine. Conversely, alkaline-ash foods tend to promote a more alkaline urine.

A strict dietary regimen is rarely necessary. Since diet is generally considered an auxiliary measure to acidifying or alkalinizing medications, simply avoiding excessive use of particular foods may be sufficient. For example, if medical treatment is directed at acidifying the urine, the diet should not contain large amounts of alkaline-ash foods; complete avoidance of all alkaline-ash foods, however, would probably not yield any further benefit and is unwarranted.

ACID-BASE REACTION OF FOODS

Potentially Acid or Acid-Ash Foods

Meat	Meat; fish; fowl; shellfish; eggs; all types of cheese; peanut butter; peanuts
Fat	Bacon; nuts (Brazil nuts, filberts, walnuts)
Starch	All types of bread (especially whole wheat), cereals, and crackers; macaroni; spaghetti; noodles; rice
Vegetable	Corn; lentils
Fruit	Cranberries; plums; prunes
Dessert	Plain cakes; cookies

Potentially Basic or Alkaline-Ash Foods

Milk	Milk and milk products; cream; buttermilk
Fat	Nuts (almonds, chestnuts, coconut)
Vegetable	All types (except corn, lentils), especially beets, beet greens, Swiss chard, dandelion greens, kale, mustard greens, spinach, turnip greens
Fruit	All types (except cranberries, prunes, plums)
Sweets	Molasses

Neutral Foods

Fats	Butter; margarine; cooking fats; oils
Sweets	Plain candies; sugar; syrup; honey
Starch	Arrowroot; corn; tapioca
Beverages	Coffee; tea

PHYSICIANS: HOW TO ORDER DIETS

The diet order should indicate **acid-ash** or **alkaline-ash diet.**

SELECTED BIBLIOGRAPHY

(for dietary management of urolithiasis; calcium, oxalate,
and purine control; and acid-ash and alkaline-ash diets)

Earnest, D. L., Johnson, G., Wiliams, H. E., et al.: Hyperoxaluria in patients with ileal resection: An abnormality in dietary oxalate absorption. Gastroenterology, 66:1114-1122, 1974.

Kahn, H. D., Panariello, V. A., Saeli, J., et al.: Effect of cranberry juice on urine. J. Am. Diet. Assoc., 51:251-254, 1967.

Maynard, F. M., and Imai, K.: Immobilization hypercalcemia in spinal cord injury. Arch. Phys. Med. Rehabil., 58:16-24, 1977.

Nordin, B. E. C.: Metabolic Bone and Stone Disease. Baltimore, Williams & Wilkins Company, 1973, pp. 206-243.

Ozog, L. S., and Tomskey, G. C.: Diagnosis and treatment of cystinuria. Urology, 3:197-199, 1974.

Smith, L. H., Van Den Berg, C. J., and Wilson, D. M.: Nutrition and urolithiasis. N. Engl. J. Med., 298:87-89, 1978.

Stauffer, J. Q.: Hyperoxaluria and calcium oxalate nephrolithiasis after jejunoileal bypass. Am. J. Clin. Nutr., 30:64-71, 1977.

Thomas, W. C., Jr.: Renal Calculi: A Guide to Management. Springfield, Illinois, Charles C Thomas, Publisher, 1976, pp. 20-30.

Urinary calcium and dietary protein. Nutr. Rev., 38:9-10, 1980.

Zarembski, P.M., and Hodgkinson, A.: The oxalic acid content of English diets. Br. J. Nutr., 16:627-634, 1962.

COPPER CONTROL

GENERAL DESCRIPTION

The diet is designed to achieve either of two levels of copper control—strict (not more than 1 mg of copper per day) and low (less than 2 mg of copper per day). Copper is widely distributed in foods and does not occur exclusively in a particular category of foods.

NUTRITIONAL ADEQUACY

Neither level of low-copper diet is so restrictive that there is danger of nutritional inadequacy. However, if use of a vitamin supplement is warranted, it should be free of copper.

INDICATIONS AND RATIONALE

A low-copper diet may be indicated in the treatment of Wilson's disease and primary biliary cirrhosis, both of which are associated with excessive accumulation of copper in various tissues.

Wilson's disease (hepatolenticular degeneration) is an inherited disorder of copper metabolism characterized by abnormal transport and storage of copper. Copper accumulates primarily in the liver, brain, kidney, and cornea and has a toxic effect on these tissues. The primary metabolic defect is in the liver, where copper accumulates in lysosomes as the disease progresses; a block of lysosomal copper excretion may explain the decrease in biliary copper excretion. Also, incorporation of copper into ceruloplasmin, the main copper transport, decreases. Initial symptoms include hepatic, neurologic, and psychiatric dysfunction. If untreated, Wilson's disease causes progressive deterioration.

Long-term therapy consists primarily of use of a copper chelating agent, such as D-penicillamine, in association with a diet very low in copper (not more than 1 mg/day). The purpose of treatment is to reduce copper stores by keeping the patient in negative copper balance. This means of treatment usually improves neurologic and hepatic function. Furthermore, treatment of asymptomatic patients with Wilson's disease usually prevents occurrence of signs and symptoms.

Primary biliary cirrhosis, or cholangiolitic hepatitis, is also associated with excessive storage of copper. Excessive concentrations of copper are found in the liver, spleen, and kidney but not, as in Wilson's disease, in the brain. Primary biliary cirrhosis is a chronic disease of unknown cause characterized by progressive destruction of the interhepatic bile ducts, which leads eventually to cirrhosis. The initial clinical findings are usually pruritus and jaundice. Previously, treatment was directed primarily at alleviation of symptoms.

Attempts to deplete liver stores of copper in patients with primary biliary cirrhosis are fairly recent. The rationale for this line of treatment is that specific treatment for primary biliary cirrhosis is lacking, D-penicillamine and the low-copper diet are effective in Wilson's disease, and the two diseases have similar degrees of hepatic copper elevation. Furthermore, D-penicillamine probably reduces levels of circulating immune complexes; a disturbance of immune mechanisms may be a contributing cause of primary biliary cirrhosis. The copper-mobilizing therapy includes use of a chelating agent, such as D-penicillamine, and a low-copper diet (less than 2 mg of copper per day). Although in primary biliary cirrhosis the copper-mobilizing therapy reduces liver stores of copper and maintains cupresis, the long-term effects are unknown.

DIET VERY LOW IN COPPER (≤1 mg/day)

Allow only foods of low copper content. Avoid all foods listed as having moderate or high copper content.

DIET LOW IN COPPER (<2 mg/day)

Allow foods of low copper content. Foods of moderate copper content may be used in limited amounts. Allow only 1 serving from each food group per week. Avoid foods of high copper content.

COPPER CONTENT OF FOODS*

Food Groups	High	Moderate	Low
Beverage	Tea; cocoa; Ovaltine		Coffee; decaffeinated coffee; lemonade; carbonated beverages (allow only one 12-oz can/day)
Meat	All organ meats, including liver, brain, heart, and kidney; all shellfish, including oysters, scallops, shrimp, clams, and crab; goose; duck; meat gelatin	All other fish, including tuna and salmon; peanut butter	All other meats; cheese; cottage cheese; eggs; cold cuts and frankfurters (check label; should not contain any organ meats)
Fat	All nuts; avocado	Olives	All others
Milk	Chocolate milk		All others
Starch	Wheat germ; bran products; dried beans	Commercially prepared English muffins, sugar wafers, French fries, and potato chips; corn; parsnips; peas	Other breads, cereals, crackers, and potatoes; pasta; rice

COPPER CONTENT OF FOODS* (Continued)

Food Groups	High	Moderate	Low
Vegetable	Lentils; mushrooms	Asparagus; beets; spinach; squash; tomatoes, tomato juice, and all tomato products	All others
Fruit	Dried fruit; avocado; coconut	Applesauce; bananas; all berries; cherries; mango; pear	All others
Soup	Broth; bouillon; dehydrated soup mixes	Commercial canned soups	Cream-based soups
Dessert	Any containing chocolate, coconut, or nuts		All others
Sweets	Chocolate; licorice; molasses; syrups		Sugar; honey; jam; jelly; other candy
Miscellaneous	Curry powder; water† with high copper content; all alcoholic beverages‡	Pepper (limit to ≤1/2 tsp/day); catsup (limit to ≤1 tbsp/ day); pickles (limit to 1 serving/week)	Salt; other spices; other herbs; flavoring extract; mustard; horse-radish; vinegar

*Data available on the average copper content of foods vary greatly. There is disagreement on the copper content of the usual American diet, with estimates ranging from 1 mg of copper a day to 2 to 5 mg a day. The concentration of copper in foods is affected by many factors, including soil conditions, geographic location, species, diet, processing method, and contamination in processing. The exact copper content of the foods listed or the diets given here is difficult to verify. For practical purposes, the diets are designed to prohibit or limit foods that tend to have a higher copper content than other foods, and the total copper content of the diet is given only as a rough estimate.

†A water sample from the patient's home water supply should be analyzed for copper content. Demineralized water should be used if the water contains more than 100 μg per liter.

‡Although not necessarily high in copper, alcoholic beverages are not allowed because of their action as a hepatotoxin.

PHYSICIANS: HOW TO ORDER DIETS

The diet order may specify the diet modification, such as **strict** ($\leq$1 mg of copper/day) or **low** (<2 mg of copper/day) **copper control**, *or* indicate the disorder, such as **Wilson's disease** or **primary biliary cirrhosis**. If the disorder is indicated, the dietitian will determine the appropriate level of copper according to the guidelines given.

SELECTED BIBLIOGRAPHY

Berry, W. R., Aronson, A. E., Darley, F. L., et al.: Effects of penicillamine therapy and low-copper diet on dysarthria in Wilson's disease (hepatolenticular degeneration). Mayo Clin. Proc., 49:405-408, 1974.

Deering, T. B., Dickson, E. R., Fleming, C. R., et al.: Effect of D-penicillamine on copper retention in patients with primary biliary cirrhosis. Gastroenterology, 72:1208-1212, 1977.

Fleming, C. R., Dickson, E. R., Baggenstoss, A. H., et al.: Copper and primary biliary cirrhosis. Gastroenterology, 67:1182-1187, 1974.

Fleming, C. R., Dickson, E. R., Wahner, H. W., et al.: Pigmented corneal rings in non-Wilsonian liver disease. Ann. Intern. Med., 86:285-288, 1977.

Goldstein, N. P., and Owen, C. A., Jr.: Introduction: Symposium on copper metabolism and Wilson's disease. Mayo Clin. Proc., 49:363-367, 1974.

Hook, L., and Brandt, I. K.: Copper content of some low-copper foods. J. Am. Diet. Assoc., 49:202-203, 1966.

Pennington, J. T., and Calloway, D. H.: Copper content of foods. J. Am. Diet. Assoc., 63:143-153, 1973.

Schaffner, F.: Primary biliary cirrhosis. Clin. Gastroenterol., 4:351-366, 1975.

Sternlieb, I., and Feldmann, G.: Effects of anticopper therapy on hepatocellular mitochondria in patients with Wilson's disease: An ultrastructural and stereological study. Gastroenterology, 71:457-461, 1976.

Zook, E. G., and Lehmann, J.: Mineral composition of fruits. II. Nitrogen, calcium, magnesium, phosphorus, potassium, aluminum, boron, copper, iron, manganese, and sodium. J. Am. Diet. Assoc., 52:225-231, 1968.

CARBOHYDRATE CONTROL

LACTOSE CONTROL

GENERAL DESCRIPTION

The diet limits the disaccharide lactose contained in milk and milk products to the amount tolerated by the individual.

NUTRITIONAL ADEQUACY

The diet may be low in calcium, riboflavin, and vitamin D, depending on the degree of lactose restriction and the age of the person receiving the diet.

INDICATIONS AND RATIONALE

A lactose-controlled diet may be of benefit to persons deficient in the intestinal enzyme lactase. Lactase deficiency occurs as a primary disorder or as a complication of disorders affecting the absorptive surface of the gastrointestinal tract. Primary lactase deficiency is seen less often in Caucasian than in non-Caucasian persons. In children, transient lactase deficiency occurs most commonly after viral gastroenteritis.

In the lactase-deficient individual, much of dietary lactose is not hydrolyzed in the small bowel. Lactose that passes into the large bowel is broken down by bacterial action into substances of lower molecular weight. These substances, by irritating the colonic mucosa, cause increased motility and, by raising the osmolality of intestinal contents, interfere with reabsorption of fluid. Symptoms may include abdominal pain, flatulence, and diarrhea after ingestion of lactose, but some lactase-deficient persons can tolerate moderate amounts of milk without difficulty. Fermentation of lactose by bacteria in the colon tends to produce hydrogen, which is absorbed into the blood and exhaled in the breath, and acidic stool.

The following methods are used to detect lactose intolerance (positive findings are in parentheses): small bowel biopsy (decreased lactase activity in mucosa), measurement of capillary plasma glucose after oral ingestion of 50 g of lactose (increase of less than 20 mg/dl), analysis of the breath after ingestion of lactose (detection of hydrogen), trial of a lactose-restricted diet (relief of symptoms), and obtaining a diet history (symptoms occurring consistently after ingestion of lactose-containing foods).

GENERAL DIETARY RECOMMENDATIONS

Most persons with lactase deficiency can tolerate the amount of lactose in 1/2 cup of milk (6 g of lactose) each day, and many can tolerate more.* Low-lactose milk and soy milk may be tolerated in larger quantities. Fermented milk products (for example, yogurt, aged cheese, and cottage cheese) may be tolerated better than nonfermented milk products (Gallagher et al., 1974).

---

*A person with lactase deficiency is not likely to have complete intolerance to lactose. However, if it is necessary to eliminate even trace amounts of lactose from the diet, the galactose-controlled diet (see page 132) can be used.

LACTOSE CONTENT OF MILK AND SELECTED MILK PRODUCTS

The following foods in the measures given contain an amount of lactose equivalent to 1/2 cup of milk.

1/2 cup	Milk: whole, low-fat, skim, buttermilk
2 tbsp	Condensed milk
1/4 cup	Evaporated milk
3 oz	Processed cheese food or cheese spread
1/2 cup	Cream: half-and-half, whipped, sour
1/2 cup	Yogurt
1/2 cup	Ice cream
1/2 cup	Ice milk

The following foods contain small amounts of lactose and are generally well tolerated.

Butter

Cottage cheese

Soft cheeses (cream cheese, Neufchâtel)

Aged cheese (Swiss, American, and others)

Commercial foods processed with small amounts
of milk, milk products, milk solids, or lactose

LACTOSE CONTENT PER SERVING IN COMMON PORTIONS*

11 to 15 g	5 to 6 g	1 to 3 g	0.5 to 1 g	<0.5 g
Milk, 1 cup	Ice cream, 1/2 cup	Pudding, 1/2 cup	Processed American cheese, 1 oz	Butter, 1 tsp
Yogurt, 1 cup	Ice milk, 1/2 cup	Sherbet, 1/2 cup	Cottage cheese, 1/4 cup	Cream cheese, 1 tbsp
		Processed cheese spread,† 1 oz	Sour cream, 2 tbsp	Aged cheese, 1 oz
		Half-and-half, 2 tbsp		

*Content may vary with brand names.
†Processed cheese spreads and cheese foods may have added nonfat dry milk solids, which increase the lactose content.

PHYSICIANS: HOW TO ORDER DIETS

The diet order should indicate lactose intolerance. The dietitian will determine modifications according to the guidelines given and tolerances of the patient.

SELECTED BIBLIOGRAPHY

Bayless, T. M.: Disaccharidase deficiency. J. Am. Diet. Assoc., 60:478-482, 1972.
Feeley, R. M., Criner, P. E., and Slover, H. T.: Major fatty acids and proximate composition of dairy products. J. Am. Diet. Assoc., 66:140-146, 1975.
Gallagher, C. R., Molleson, A. L., and Caldwell, J. H.: Lactose intolerance and fermented dairy products. J. Am. Diet. Assoc., 65:418-419, 1974.
Greenberger, N. J., and Winship, D. H.: Gastrointestinal Disorders: A Pathophysiologic Approach. Chicago, Year Book Medical Publishers, 1976, pp. 151-152.
Newcomer, A. D., McGill, D. B., Thomas, P. J., et al.: Prospective comparison of indirect methods for detecting lactase deficiency. N. Engl. J. Med., 293:1232-1236, 1975.
Turner, S. J., Daly, T., Hourigan, J. A., et al.: Utilization of a low-lactose milk. Am. J. Clin. Nutri., 29:739-744, 1976.

GALACTOSE CONTROL

GENERAL DESCRIPTION

Galactose is a monosaccharide derived primarily through hydrolysis of lactose in milk. The diet essentially eliminates milk in all forms. All foods to which milk products or lactose are added in processing must be identified and eliminated.

NUTRITIONAL ADEQUACY

Adequacy of the diet depends primarily on the use of lactose-free milk substitutes appropriate to age. Supplemental calcium, riboflavin, and vitamin D may need to be prescribed for adults not using milk substitutes or for children using less than the equivalent of 3 cups of milk a day.

INDICATIONS AND RATIONALE

A galactose-restricted diet is the mainstay of the management of galactosemia. The diet may also be used in severe lactase deficiency, since it is based on the elimination of lactose.

Galactosemia is a hereditary disease, transmitted by an autosomal recessive gene, in which the ability to metabolize galactose normally is adversely affected. Accumulation of galactose metabolites (primarily galactose-1-phosphate) in body tissues is considered to be the cause of damage to the developing brain, liver, lens of the eye, and other organs.

The limits of tolerance to galactose are difficult to define precisely, since they may vary among persons and with age. Poor adherence to diet and late initiation of dietary management are associated with a greater incidence and severity of mental handicaps. Dietary control can be monitored by checking the level of accumulation of galactose-1-phosphate in the erythrocytes every 2 or 3 months.

PHYSICIANS: HOW TO ORDER DIETS

The diet order should indicate **galactose control.**

FOODS TO ALLOW AND FOODS TO AVOID

Food Groups	Allow	Avoid
Beverage	Coffee; tea; carbonated beverages	Milk; hot cocoa; Ovaltine; malt; malted milk; any containing milk products or lactose, such as instant coffee and powdered soft drink mixes
Meat	Pure meat, fish, fowl, and eggs; peanut butter; legumes* and lentils*	Organ meats†; cheese; cottage cheese; creamed meats; any containing milk products or lactose, such as commercially breaded meats and meat dishes, sausage, cold cuts, and frankfurters
Fat	Milk-free margarine; oil; shortening; bacon; water-based gravies; olives; nuts	Butter; cream; cream cheese; milk-based gravies; any containing milk products or lactose, such as margarine, salad dressings, and nondairy cream substitutes
Milk	Soybean milk‡; lactose-free formulas	All milk and milk products; whole, low-fat, skim, chocolate, dry powdered, evaporated, and sweetened condensed milk; buttermilk; yogurt
Starch	French bread; Italian bread; any bread products and cereals prepared without milk; lentils*; potato; rice; popcorn	Any item containing milk products or lactose, such as commercially prepared baked goods and mixes, dry cereals, instant cooked cereals, crackers, snack foods, zwieback, French fried potatoes, instant potatoes, and pastas
Vegetable	All except those with butter, cream, or cheese sauce	Any with butter, cream, or cheese sauce
Fruit	All except those processed with lactose	Any processed with lactose, such as frozen or canned fruits
Soup	Broth; bouillon; broth-based soups	Cream soups; any containing milk products or lactose, such as commercial canned soup and packaged dehydrated soup
Dessert	Gelatin; fruit ice; puddings made with fruit juice; any other prepared without milk	Ice cream; sherbet; pudding; custard; any containing milk products or lactose, such as commercially prepared cakes, cookies, and mixes

FOODS TO ALLOW AND FOODS TO AVOID (Continued)

Food Groups	Allow	Avoid
Sweets	Sugar; honey; jelly; corn syrup; pure sugar candy; marshmallows; bittersweet, semisweet, and unsweetened chocolate; carob	Cream candy; milk chocolate; peppermints; butterscotch candy; caramels; toffee; any containing milk products or lactose, such as chocolate syrup, artificial sweeteners, and flavored syrups
Miscellaneous	Salt; pepper; pure spices	Any containing milk products or lactose, such as mixed spices, monosodium glutamate, soy sauce, chewing gum, dried coconut, and food colorings
	Alcoholic beverages except cordials and liqueurs; beer; wine	Cordials; liqueurs
Medications:	Some drugs and vitamin preparations contain lactose.	
Food labeling:	The patient should be advised to read product labels carefully and to avoid milk and milk products, milk solids, filled milk, cheese and cheese products, cream and cream products, curds, whey and whey solids, casein, and lactose. Lactate, lactic acid, lactalbumin, and calcium compounds do not contain lactose and are permissible.	

*Legumes and lentils contain galactose in the form of oligosaccharides (raffinose and stachyose), which are not completely utilized. These items are acceptable if monitoring is done every 2 to 3 months. Legumes and lentils do not need to be avoided by those following the diet because of lactose intolerance.

†Organ meats do not need to be avoided by those following the diet because of lactose intolerance.

‡Soy protein is lower in methionine than is milk. Careful growth records should be kept on infants.

SELECTED BIBLIOGRAPHY

Department of Nutrition, University of California, Davis, California, and Maternal and Child Health Branch, California Department of Health: Parents' guide to the galactose restricted diet, Oct. 1976.

Hsia, D. Y.: Galactosemia. Springfield, Illinois, Charles C Thomas, Publisher, 1969.

Isselbacher, K. J.: Clinical and biochemical observations in galactosemia. Am. J. Clin. Nutr., 5:527-532, 1957.

Koch, R., Acosta, P., Ragsdale, N., et al.: Nutrition in the treatment of galactosemia. J. Am. Diet. Assoc., 43:216-222, 1963.

Mayer, J.: Galactosemia and nutrition. Postgrad. Med., 35:647-651, 1964.

DISACCHARIDE CONTROL

In general, the diet is a graduated one for patients who cannot utilize the disaccharides lactose, sucrose, isomaltose, and maltose. Intolerance to ingestion of the disaccharides may be congenital or the result of acute or protracted trauma to the gastrointestinal tract. In congenital saccharidase deficiencies, it is often sufficient to restrict only the one offending saccharide. The most common secondary saccharidase deficiency is diarrhea due to a bacterial or viral infection. In the severe stages, only glucose and fructose are tolerated. As the patient's condition improves, the diet may become more liberal; starches, sucrose-containing foods, and, finally, lactose-containing foods are added gradually. A carbohydrate-free formula prepared with the addition of a tolerated form of carbohydrate should be used during the progression (see pages 228 and 242).

PHYSICIANS: HOW TO ORDER DIETS

The diet order should indicate **low-disaccharide diet**. If only a specific disaccharide is not tolerated, this fact should be indicated in the diet order.

FOODS TO ALLOW*

Food Group	Low-disaccharide	Starches Tolerated	Sucrose Tolerated	Milk Solids Tolerated
Beverages	Kool-Aid or tea sweetened with dextrose; special formula containing monosaccharides (Pregestimil, Cho-Free with dextrose)	Soft drinks containing corn syrup solids (e.g., 7-Up)	Beverages containing sucrose if it has been found to be tolerated	Milk
Breads	None	Breads made with dextrose but without sugar or milk; crackers that do not contain added sugar or milk	Breads and crackers that do not contain milk	Any
Cereals	None	Farina; infant oat and rice cereals; oatmeal; puffed rice; shredded wheat	Any that do not contain milk solids	Any
Desserts	Gelatin flavored with Kool-Aid and dextrose	Dextrose-sweetened lemon pudding	Any that do not contain milk or milk products	Any
Eggs	Any preparation to which milk is not added			
Fats	Butter; vegetable oils; margarine without milk solids	Butter; vegetable oils; margarine without milk solids	Butter; vegetable oils; margarine without milk solids	Any
Fruits, fruit juices	Juice of allowed fruits; unsweetened fresh, frozen, or canned fruits; fruits sweetened with dextrose: apples, boysenberries, cranberries, currants, cherries, figs, Concord grapes, Malaga grapes, lemons, loganberries, loquats, papayas, pears, damson plums, pomegranates, raspberries, strawberries		Other fruits as tolerated	Any
Meat, fish, poultry, cheese	Fresh beef; chicken; lamb; liver; pork; turkey; fish and seafood that do not contain fillers, breading, lactose, or sucrose	Any that do not contain sucrose or milk solids	Any that do not contain milk solids	Any
Potatoes or substitutes	None	Boiled or baked white potatoes; hominy; macaroni; noodles; spaghetti; rice	Sweet potato	Others

FOODS TO ALLOW* (Continued)

Food Group	Low-disaccharide	Starches Tolerated	Sucrose Tolerated	Milk Solids Tolerated
Soups	Any made from allowed vegetables	Any made from allowed foods		Any
Sugar, sweets	Dextrose; fructose		Sucrose	
Vegetables, vegetable juices	Asparagus; green and wax beans; cabbage family; carrots; celery; cucumber; pumpkin; lettuce; rutabaga; squash; tomato; juices from allowed vegetables	Corn; lima beans	Others	Any
Miscellaneous	Herbs (read labels for other foods not listed above)			

*Modified from Dietary Department, University of Iowa Hospitals and Clinics: Recent Advances in Therapeutic Diets. Third edition. Ames, Iowa, Iowa State University Press, 1979.

SELECTED BIBLIOGRAPHY

Cornblath, M., and Schwartz, R.: Disorders of carbohydrate metabolism in infancy. Major Probl. Clin. Pediatr., 3:1-501, 1976.

Dietary Department, University of Iowa Hospitals and Clinics: Recent Advances in Therapeutic Diets. Third edition. Ames, Iowa, Iowa State University Press, 1979.

Hardinge, M. G., Swarner, J. B., and Crooks, H.: Carbohydrates in foods. J. Am. Diet. Assoc., 46:197-204, 1965.

Lee, C. Y., Shallenberger, R. S., and Vittum, M. T.: Free sugars in fruits and vegetables. N.Y. Food Life Sci. Bull., 1:1-12, Aug. 1970.

FIBER AND RESIDUE CONTROL
HIGH-FIBER DIET

GENERAL DESCRIPTION

The diet essentially emphasizes use of whole grain bread and cereal products, fruits, and vegetables.

INDICATIONS AND RATIONALE

Discussion of fiber is associated with a number of problems. Difficulties arise in defining fiber, quantitating fiber in foods, and determining the physiologic functions of fiber.

Fiber has been commonly referred to as roughage, bulk, nonnutritive residue, and unavailable carbohydrate. Dietary fiber is defined in physiologic terms as all food residue that is resistant to hydrolysis by digestive enzymes. However, most food composition tables report crude fiber rather than dietary fiber. Crude fiber is defined as the residue of plant materials left after sequential extraction with solvents of dilute acid and dilute alkali. Crude fiber is composed primarily of cellulose and some hemicellulose and lignin, whereas dietary fiber includes cellulose, hemicellulose, lignin, pectins, gums, and nondegradable animal tissues, such as mucopolysaccharides and the exoskeleton of crustaceans. The amount of dietary fiber in a diet can be roughly estimated to be five times (range, 2 to 10) that of the crude fiber content.

The crude fiber content of the present American diet is estimated to be 2 to 5 g/day, whereas a range of 18 to 35 g/day is reported to exist in some other cultures (Raymond et al., 1977).

Fiber has the physical properties of water binding, cation exchange, and gel formation. There may be differences in the degree to which the various components of dietary fiber exhibit these properties.

Epidemiologic evidence has implicated low consumption of dietary fiber in the causation of a number of diseases, for example, coronary heart disease, diabetes mellitus, cancer of the colon, appendicitis, and dental caries. The contribution of high-fiber diets to the prophylaxis or therapy of many of these disorders is speculative. Evidence now exists that a high-fiber diet does not alter intestinal absorption of cholesterol or have a significant effect on lipid metabolism in man (Raymond et al., 1977).

High-fiber diets are useful in the treatment of chronic constipation. Although the evidence is not conclusive, increased intake of fiber also appears to benefit some persons with diverticular disease and irritable bowel syndrome. Fiber affects function by bringing about increased stool volume, decreased intracolonic pressure, and altered transit time. Increased intake of fiber tends to normalize transit time (that is, transit time becomes slower in persons with initially rapid transit time and more rapid in those with initially slow transit time). For most persons with chronic constipation and for some with diverticulosis or irritable bowel syndrome, increased intake of fiber may lead to more regular bowel habits and partial relief of symptoms. Increased intake of high-fiber foods also is encouraged in the rehabilitation unit, especially in bowel training for paraplegics.

For some individuals, a high-fiber diet initially may produce some unpleasant effects, such as increased flatulence and borborygmi. Flatulence and borborygmi are likely to be less intense with gradual increase in intake of high-fiber foods and after the person has become accustomed to the diet. A high-fiber diet may have some detrimental effect, however, because of the potential of fiber to bind to, and thus impair absorption of, calcium, iron, zinc, and possibly other trace minerals.

GENERAL DIETARY RECOMMENDATIONS

A high-fiber diet is generally considered to consist of at least 5 to 6 g of crude fiber (about 30 g of dietary fiber) per day. The goal of the diet is to increase the intake of fiber rather than to attain a precise level of intake. An optimal level of fiber in the diet has not been established. Most persons, except those following weight reduction diets, can attain a level of 5 to 6 g of crude fiber. This level of intake can be accomplished by use of:

1. More vegetables and fruits (preferably fresh, dried, or slightly cooked).
2. Whole grain breads, cereals, and flours.
3. One-fourth to 1/2 cup (1/2 to 1 oz) of bran daily.

Patients should be advised to increase their intake of high-fiber foods gradually.

PHYSICIANS: HOW TO ORDER DIETS

The diet order should indicate **high-fiber diet**.

CRUDE FIBER CONTENT OF SELECTED FOODS*

	Grams Per Serving			
	<0.2	0.2 to 1 (avg, 0.6)	1 to 2 (avg, 1.5)	>2
Fruit (1/2 cup or 1 medium)	Juice	Applesauce Apricots Banana Cantaloupe Cherries Fruit cocktail Grapefruit Grapes Honeydew melon Nectarine Orange Peaches Pears without skin Pineapple Plums Raisins Strawberries Watermelon	Apples with skin Avocado Blueberries Dates Figs Pears with skin Prunes Raspberries	Blackberries
Vegetables (1/2 cup)	Juice	Asparagus Bean sprouts Beets Cabbage Carrots Cauliflower Celery Collards Corn Cucumber Dandelion greens Eggplant Green pepper Kale Kohlrabi Lettuce Mushrooms Mustard greens Okra Onions Potatoes Radishes Sauerkraut Spinach Split peas String beans: green, yellow Summer squash Sweet potatoes Tomatoes Turnip greens Turnips	Baked beans Beet greens Black beans Broccoli Brussels sprouts Chick-peas Kidney beans Lentils Lima beans Parsnips Peas Pinto beans Pumpkin Rutabaga Winter squash	Artichoke
Bread† (1 slice)	Cracked wheat French Rye White	Pumpernickel Raisin Whole wheat		

CRUDE FIBER CONTENT OF SELECTED FOODS* (Continued)

	Grams Per Serving			
	<0.2	0.2 to 1 (avg, 0.6)	1 to 2 (avg, 1.5)	>2
Cereals, cooked (1/2 cup)	Cream of Rice Cream of Wheat Farina Maltex	Oatmeal Wheatena		
Cereals, ready-to-eat (1 oz = 1/4 to 1 1/4 cup)	Puffed corn Puffed rice	Cornflakes Granola Raisin bran Shredded wheat Wheat flakes Wheat germ	Bran flakes	100% bran cereals
Crackers (20 g = 2 to 4 crackers)	Saltines Soda crackers	Graham crackers Rye wafers Whole wheat crackers		
Snack foods	Popcorn (1 cup) Pretzels (10 medium)	Corn chips (10 medium) Potato chips (10 medium)		
Other starches (1/2 cup)	Grits Macaroni Noodles Spaghetti White rice	Barley Brown rice		
Flours (1 cup)	Wheat, cake or pastry	Cornmeal, degermed Rye, light Wheat, all purpose	Cornmeal, whole, ground	Whole rye Whole wheat
Nuts and seeds (1/4 cup)		Almonds Cashews Peanuts Pecans Pumpkin seeds Walnuts	Brazil nuts Coconut Roasted soybeans Sunflower seeds	

*Based on data from Watt, B. K., and Merrill, A. L.: Composition of Foods: Raw, Processed, Prepared (Agriculture Handbook No. 8). Washington, D.C., United States Department of Agriculture, United States Agricultural Research Service, 1963. These are the most recent and nearly complete data available.

†Several so-called high-fiber breads are on the market. Generally, they contain added cellulose and have a crude fiber content of 1.5 to 2 g, whereas whole wheat bread contains approximately 0.4 g of crude fiber per slice.

SELECTED BIBLIOGRAPHY

Connell, A. M.: Natural fiber and bowel dysfunction. Am. J. Clin. Nutr., 29:1427-1431, 1976.
Connell, A. M.: Wheat bran as an etiologic factor in certain diseases. J. Am. Diet. Assoc., 71:235-239, 1977.
Cummings, J. H.: Progress report: Dietary fibre. Gut, 14:69-81, 1973.
Fifth Annual Marabou Symposium: "Food and Fibre." Nutr. Rev., 35 No. 3:1-72, 1977.
Ismail-Beigi, F., Faraji, B., and Reinhold, J. G.: Binding of zinc and iron to wheat bread, wheat bran, and their components. Am. J. Clin. Nutr., 30:1721-1725, 1977.
Kelsay, J. L.: A review of research on effects of fiber intake on man. Am. J. Clin. Nutr., 31:142-159, 1978.
Mendeloff, A. I.: Dietary fiber and human health. N. Engl. J. Med., 297:811-814, 1977.
Raymond, T. L., Connor, W. E., Lin, D. S., et al.: The interaction of dietary fibers and cholesterol upon the plasma lipids and lipoproteins, sterol balance, and bowel function in human subjects. J. Clin. Invest., 60:1429-1437, 1977.
Symposium on Role of Dietary Fiber in Health. Am. J. Clin. Nutr., 31 Suppl.:1-291, 1978.

LOW-FIBER DIET

GENERAL DESCRIPTION

The diet recommends use of refined bread and cereal products, cooked fruits and vegetables, and juices.

INDICATIONS AND RATIONALE

The diet may be indicated during exacerbations of chronic ulcerative colitis, ileitis, or other inflammatory bowel disease. Rationale for use of the diet is to attempt to avoid a large fecal volume that might distend the bowel and further aggravate inflamed tissue.

The crude fiber content of the present American diet is estimated to be 2 to 5 g of crude fiber per day.

GENERAL DIETARY RECOMMENDATIONS

A low-fiber diet contains approximately 2 g* of crude fiber per day. (See page 140 for the fiber content of foods.) This level of intake can be accomplished by:

1. Avoiding fresh or dried fruits and vegetables and using juices and cooked fruits and vegetables.

2. Avoiding whole grain bread and cereal products and using refined wheat or light rye breads.

3. Avoiding nuts, seeds, and legumes.

PHYSICIANS: HOW TO ORDER DIETS

The diet order should indicate **low-fiber diet**.

---

*A diet containing less than 2 g of crude fiber a day and allowing a variety of foods is difficult to plan.

MINIMUM-RESIDUE DIET

GENERAL DESCRIPTION

The diet consists of foods that are low in crude fiber. Foods omitted include those of moderate and high content of fiber and foods that are believed to increase fecal residue despite low content of fiber.

NUTRITIONAL ADEQUACY

The diet may be low in a number of nutrients. It is intended to be used for a short period only. If long-term use of a low-residue diet is indicated, a chemically defined low-residue formula or parenteral nutrition should be considered (see page 237).

INDICATIONS AND RATIONALE

The diet may be used before surgery or temporarily in disorders, such as partial obstruction, affecting the lower portion of the small bowel or the large bowel.

The term "residue" refers to unabsorbed dietary constituents (such as fiber), sloughed cells from the gastrointestinal tract, intestinal bacteria, and some of the metabolic products of bacteria. The purpose of the diet is to minimize fecal volume. The effect of fiber on stool volume is well established. Some foods, such as milk and the connective tissue of meats, that are low in crude fiber may also affect stool volume. However, restriction of these so-called residue-producing foods is based more on tradition than on substantiated scientific evidence.

GENERAL DIETARY RECOMMENDATIONS

1. Avoid whole fruits and vegetables. Use fruit and vegetable juices (except prune juice).
2. Avoid whole grain bread and cereal products. Use refined wheat or light rye breads.
3. Avoid potatoes, legumes, seeds, and nuts. Use pasta made from refined flours and white rice.
4. Avoid meat and shellfish with tough connective tissue.
5. Limit use of milk to 1 cup or less per day.
6. Limit use of foods containing milk, such as ice cream, pudding, cottage cheese, and other cheese, to 2 servings or less per day.

PHYSICIANS: HOW TO ORDER DIETS

The diet order should indicate **minimum-residue diet**.

SELECTED BIBLIOGRAPHY
(Low-fiber and Minimum-residue Diets)

Beyer, P. L., and Flynn, M. A.: Effects of high- and low-fiber diets on human feces. J. Am. Diet. Assoc., 72:271-277, 1978.

Fischer, J. E., and Sutton, T. S.: Effects of lactose on gastro-intestinal motility: A review. J. Dairy Sci., 32:139-162, 1949.

Goldstein, F.: Diet and colonic disease. J. Am. Diet. Assoc., 60: 499-503, 1972.

Kramer, P.: The meaning of high and low residue diets (editorial). Gastroenterology, 47:649-652, 1964.

Watts, J. H., Graham, D. C. W., Jones, F., Jr., et al.: Fecal solids excreted by young men following the ingestion of dairy foods. Am. J. Dig. Dis., n.s. 8:364-375, 1963.

Weinstein, L., Olson, R. E., Van Itallie, T. B., et al.: Diet as related to gastrointestinal function. J.A.M.A., 176:935-941, 1961.

FAT CONTROL

GENERAL DESCRIPTION

Guidelines are given for three levels of low-fat diets (30, 50, and 70 g of fat). Fat restriction implies that both visible fats and fats incorporated into foods are limited.

Dietary supplements of medium-chain triglycerides may be indicated in some situations. Rationale for use of medium-chain triglycerides and guidelines for incorporating them into the diet are given on page 147.

INDICATIONS AND RATIONALE

Several disorders can interfere with the normal processes for utilizing dietary fat.* A low-fat diet is likely to be indicated in the treatment of (1) malabsorption due to inadequate intraluminal digestion or absorption of fat, (2) disorders involving a defect in the lymphatic transport of fat, and (3) type I hyperlipoproteinemia, which is caused by abnormal metabolism of fat.

Malabsorption. Fat malabsorption or steatorrhea is defined as a stool fat content of more than 7 g per 24 hours after ingestion of a diet containing 100 g of fat.† Expressed another way, the efficiency of fat absorption should be equal to or greater than 93%. Causes of malabsorption include disorders of the stomach (rapid emptying and excessive production of acid, as in gastric resection and the Zollinger-Ellison syndrome, respectively), liver (impaired production or secretion of bile acid), pancreas (inadequate lipase), small bowel (sprue, for example), and lymphatics (delayed transport caused by obstruction or lymphoma).

---

*Dietary fats are composed primarily of long-chain triglycerides, which have a carbon chain length greater than 14 carbon atoms.

†See page 258 for a test diet for steatorrhea.

Hepatobiliary disease may result in insufficient production of bile or obstruction to bile flow. Bile salts are necessary for normal micelle formation, an important step in the absorption of fatty acids. Diminished bile flow, therefore, lessens emulsification of fatty acids in the intestinal contents.

Ileal resection or disease decreases the area available for active absorption of bile acid and diminishes the bile salt pool. When bacterial overgrowth occurs in the small intestine (as in an afferent loop after gastric resection), bile salts are deconjugated and are no longer effective in causing dispersion of fatty acids.

Pancreatic lipase is the enzyme responsible for hydrolysis of most dietary fat. Lipase insufficiency occurs in pancreatitis, cystic fibrosis, and pancreatic carcinoma and after radical pancreatectomy. Lipase concentration has been reduced 90% (in response to stimulation by cholecystokinin and pancreozymin) before steatorrhea of pancreatic origin appears.

Primary disease of the small bowel, such as celiac sprue or Whipple's disease, reduces the absorptive surface and leads to fat malabsorption. In such cases, other therapy (for example, gluten restriction in sprue and antibiotics in Whipple's disease) is usually sufficient to correct the malabsorption. Patients with short bowel syndrome have malabsorption related to decreased mucosal surface and decreased transit time. Recommendations for nutritional therapy depend on the location and degree of resection and the condition of the remaining bowel. The dietitian and physician should be aware of the possibility of disaccharidase deficiency and fecal loss of protein, vitamins, minerals, and electrolytes. Analysis of stools for nitrogen, fat, sodium, and potassium aids in setting goals for intake of calories, fat, protein, and electrolytes.

This discussion of potential causes of fat malabsorption is not intended to be all-inclusive. Diagnosis of one of these disorders does not always necessitate a fat-controlled diet. By lessening diarrhea, restriction of fat reduces symptoms and lengthens transit time; increased time favors absorption of other nutrients. The level of fat prescribed generally is based on the symptomatic response. Mild diarrhea may be satisfactorily controlled by a diet of 70 g of fat, whereas a diet of 50 g of fat may only partly relieve symptoms in severe malabsorption.

Defects in Lymphatic Transport of Fat. Several uncommon disorders are associated with abnormal drainage of lymph into the urinary tract, pleural or peritoneal spaces, or the intestinal lumen. There is loss of chylous lymph, which contains chylomicrons derived from dietary fat. A low-fat diet aids in management of these disorders by decreasing chylomicron formation and lymph flow.

Type I Hyperlipoproteinemia. A diet very low in fat ($\leqslant$30 g for adults and $\leqslant$15 g for children under 12 years) is recommended in the management of type I hyperlipoproteinemia, or hyperchylomicronemia (see pages 52 and 54). Hyperchylomicronemia is the result of a defect in the catabolism of chylomicrons by lipoprotein lipase. The clinical features include eruptive xanthomas, hepatosplenomegaly, and pancreatitis. Dietary treatment is directed at alleviating symptoms by minimizing chylomicron formation.

Medium-Chain Triglycerides (MCT). Medium-chain triglycerides oil (MCT oil) is derived from coconut oil through a process of fractionation and reesterification of the medium-chain fatty acids with glycerol. MCT oil contains fatty acids primarily of 8 to 10 carbon atoms, whereas the usual dietary fats contain fatty acids of 16 to 18 carbon atoms. At room temperature, MCT oil is a thin, clear, light yellow, odorless liquid with a bland taste.

MCT are available in two principal forms, MCT oil and formulas containing MCT oil (see page 228). MCT oil provides 8.3 kcal/g. One tablespoon weighs 14 g and provides 116 calories.

MCT oil is a special-purpose food for use as supportive nutritional therapy. It may be used in addition to a low-fat diet or for almost total replacement of fat in infant formulas. The primary purposes of MCT oil are to increase the caloric value and improve the palatability of a low-fat diet.

Rationale for the use of MCT is based on differences in digestion, absorption, transport, and catabolism between MCT and long-chain triglycerides (LCT). Although MCT are rapidly hydrolyzed by pancreatic lipase, absorption can occur before hydrolysis. Bile salts and micelle formation are not required for dispersion or absorption of MCT. MCT are transported across the mucosal cell more rapidly than LCT. MCT do not enter the lymph system but are transported through the portal venous system as albumin-bound free fatty acids. They are not incorporated into chylomicrons and therefore do not require lipoprotein lipase for oxidation. MCT may be used as a dietary supplement in most disorders in which a low-fat diet is indicated.

The amount of MCT oil used should be small at first and then be gradually increased to the desired level. Usually, 20 to 60 g is well tolerated. Unpleasant side effects, such as nausea, vomiting, abdominal pain, abdominal distention, and diarrhea, may occur with rapid introduction of MCT into the diet or excessively high levels of intake. Some of the side effects may be related to the hyperosmolar solution that is produced by rapid hydrolysis of MCT. Although the mechanisms are not clearly understood, it may be that interaction or competition between LCT and MCT causes increased malabsorption and diarrhea when MCT are added to a diet already high in LCT or when excessively large amounts of MCT are incorporated into the diet.

MCT oil can be taken as a medication or incorporated into foods, whichever the patient prefers. The following suggestions may be helpful to the patient.

1. Combine MCT oil and skim milk. Add 1 to 2 teaspoons of MCT oil to 1/2 cup of milk and serve with cereal. Combine 1/3 cup of nonfat dry milk powder, 2/3 cup of water, and 2 to 4 teaspoons of MCT oil. Mix with an electric mixer or blender. Add sugar and flavoring, such as vanilla, lemon, maple, chocolate, coffee, or strawberry, if desired.

2. Combine 1 to 2 teaspoons of MCT oil with fruit juice or a carbonated beverage.

3. Substitute MCT oil for vegetable oils in recipes for salad dressings, mayonnaise, and sauces.

4. Use MCT oil for frying or grilling meats. Moderately low heat should be used, since MCT oil has a low smoking point.

5. Use MCT oil in preparing vegetables. Combine vegetables, a small amount of water, 1 to 2 teaspoons of MCT oil, and seasonings in a tightly covered skillet. Cook over very low heat, stirring occasionally until vegetables are tender (5 to 15 minutes). MCT oil may also be used to sauté vegetables for casserole dishes.

6. Use MCT oil in baking. MCT oil may be substituted for vegetable oil in some baked goods, such as muffins, pancakes, and waffles. Egg whites should be substituted for whole eggs, when possible, and skim milk should be substituted for whole milk. Since the baking characteristics of MCT oil and the method of incorporation into some foods differ from those of other fats, special recipes may be helpful for baked goods, such as cakes, cookies, piecrust, and biscuits, and for frozen desserts, such as ice cream.

7. Special recipes may be obtained from the manufacturer. Write for "Recipes Using MCT Oil and Portagen," Mead Johnson & Company, Evansville, IN 47721.

PHYSICIANS: HOW TO ORDER DIETS

The diet order should either (1) indicate **low-fat diet** or **low-fat diet with MCT** (the dietitian will determine the appropriate amounts) *or* (2) specify the **level of fat** (for example, 70g of fat) or the **level of fat and MCT** (for example, 50 g of fat, 30 g of MCT).

SAMPLE DAILY FOOD EXCHANGES*

Food Groups†	30 g of Fat		30 g of Fat with MCT		50 g of Fat		50 g of Fat with MCT		70 g of Fat	
	Unrestricted Calorie Intake	2,000 kcal	Unrestricted Calorie Intake	2,000 kcal	Unrestricted Calorie Intake	2,000 kcal	Unrestricted Calorie Intake	2,000 kcal	Unrestricted Calorie Intake	2,000 kcal
Meat‡	6	6	6	6	7	7	7	7	6–8	8
Fat, LCT	None	None	None	None	3	3	3	3	5–7	5
Fat, MCT	. . .	. . .	20–60	40	. . .	. . .	20–60	30	. . .	. . .
Milk, nonfat	Ad lib	2	Ad lib	2	Ad lib	2	Ad lib	2	Ad lib	2
Vegetable	Ad lib	2	Ad lib	2	Ad lib	2	Ad lib	2	Ad lib	2
Fruit, sweetened	Ad lib	4	Ad lib	4	Ad lib	3	Ad lib	3	Ad lib	3
Starch	Ad lib	9	Ad lib	7	Ad lib	9	Ad lib	7	Ad lib	8
Dessert, low-fat	Ad lib	2	Ad lib	1	Ad lib	2	Ad lib	1	Ad lib	1
Sweets	Ad lib	4	Ad lib	3	Ad lib	3	Ad lib	3	Ad lib	2

*Planning a palatable diet low in fat may be difficult if the patient needs more than 2,000 calories. In this case, attempting to keep the percentage of calories from fat similar to that in the 2,000-calorie diet may be more practical than attempting to maintain a precise level of fat. The percentages of calories from fat for the diets of 30, 50, and 70 g of fat are 12, 22, and 32, respectively.

†See the exchange list on page 36 to determine the serving portion.

‡Calculations are based on values for medium-fat meats. Lean meats should be used as much as possible, especially in the diets limited to 30 and 50 g of fat.

FOODS TO ALLOW AND FOODS TO AVOID

Food Groups	Allow	Avoid
Beverage	Coffee; tea; decaffeinated coffee; cereal beverage; carbonated beverage	Hot chocolate mixes
Meat	Lean and medium-fat meats (trimmed of visible fat); fish; shellfish; fowl (without skin); eggs; cheese made with low-fat or skim milk (sapsago; dry, 1%, and 2% cottage cheese); medium-fat cheese (creamed cottage cheese, mozzarella, ricotta, Neufchâtel, Parmesan, farmer, pot, hoop, and baker's cheeses)	High-fat meats, including cold cuts, frankfurters, sausage, canned meats, corned beef, spareribs, ground beef with more than 20% fat, commercially prepared hamburgers, capon, duck, goose; skin of fowl; any fried meat; any containing sauces, gravies, added fat, or oil; cheddar types of cheese; peanut butter
Fat	Any included in fat allowance	Any, including avocado, nuts, coconut, and olives, *unless* included in fat allowance
Milk	Milk and milk products containing no more than 1%, or 1 g/serving, of butterfat: skim milk, nonfat dry milk, buttermilk made from skim milk, yogurt made from skim milk	Milk and milk products containing 1% or more butterfat: whole milk, 2% milk, 1% milk, evaporated milk, sweetened condensed milk, buttermilk made from whole or low-fat milk, yogurt made from whole or low-fat milk, chocolate milk
Starch	Any product containing less than 1 g of fat per serving: white or whole grain breads, rolls, and cereals; plain crackers; starchy vegetables; popcorn; pasta	Any product containing 1 g or more of fat per serving: pancakes, waffles, biscuits, muffins, other quick breads, doughnuts, variety or butter types of snack crackers, French fries, potato and corn chips, wheat germ
Vegetable	Any prepared without fat	None
Fruit	Any	None
Soup	Any fat-free soup or any containing less than 1 g of fat per serving: bouillon, fat-free broth, soups with base of skim milk, packaged dehydrated soups	Any with added fat or containing 1 g or more of fat per serving: commercial canned soups, cream soups, soups containing whole milk products

FOODS TO ALLOW AND FOODS TO AVOID (Continued)

Food Groups	Allow	Avoid
Dessert	Angel food cake; gelatin; fruit ice; meringues; sherbet, ice milk, and puddings made with skim milk; low-fat cookies (gingersnaps, vanilla wafers, commercial fig bars)	Any other homemade or commercially prepared desserts or mixes containing added fat, whole milk, cream, chocolate, coconut, or nuts
Sweets	Sugar; honey; jam; jelly; syrup; plain sugar candies (hard candy, gumdrops, jelly beans, marshmallows)	Any containing added fat, whole milk, cream, chocolate, coconut, or nuts
Miscellaneous	Salt; pepper; herbs; spices; pickles; relishes; catsup; mustard; meat sauces and extracts; vinegar; cocoa powder; carob powder; flavoring extracts; fat-free butter flavoring; nonstick vegetable pan sprays	Any product containing ingredients that must be avoided

SELECTED BIBLIOGRAPHY

Alfin-Slater, R. B., and Aftergood, L.: Fats and other lipids. *In* Goodhart, R. S., and Shils, M. E., eds.: Modern Nutrition in Health and Disease: Dietotherapy. Fifth edition. Philadelphia, Lea & Febiger, 1973, pp. 117-141.

Greenberger, N. J., and Skillman, T. G.: Medium-chain triglycerides: Physiologic considerations and clinical implications. N. Engl. J. Med., 280:1045-1058, 1969.

Hines, C., Jr.: Vitamins: Absorption and malabsorption. Arch. Intern. Med., 138:619-621, 1978.

Holt, P. R.: Medium chain triglycerides. D. M., June 1971, pp. 1-30.

Schizas, A. A., Cremen, J. A., Larson, E., et al.: Medium-chain triglycerides–use in food preparation. J. Am. Diet. Assoc., 51:228-232, 1967.

Senior, J. R.: Medium Chain Triglycerides. Philadelphia, University of Pennsylvania Press, 1968.

DIETARY MANAGEMENT OF OTHER GASTROINTESTINAL DISORDERS

Some of the diets for gastrointestinal disorders have been extensively revised since the previous edition of this manual. The diets included in this section are less precise and are based more on individual tolerances than they were in the past. In some cases, such as the bland ulcer diet, guidelines are given rather than a definite regimen. Diets for gastrointestinal disorders that require control of specific food constituents are listed elsewhere in the manual.

Dietary regimens for inflammatory bowel disease and chronic liver disease are not included. The diets in these conditions should be determined by the stage of the disease and the nutritional state of the patient. Although an important consideration, dietary management should be based on control of nutrients (for example, protein, fat, and calorie levels) and other dietary constituents (for example, lactose and residue) according to individual assessment.

GLUTEN CONTROL

GENERAL DESCRIPTION

The diet restricts the vegetable protein gluten, a constituent of cereal grains such as wheat, oats, rye, and barley. The diet is intended to minimize intake of gluten.

NUTRITIONAL ADEQUACY

Because many persons with sprue have severe demineralization of their bones and may not tolerate milk well, calcium supplementation may be necessary to replete the calcium deficit.

INDICATIONS AND RATIONALE

A gluten-controlled diet is the primary means of treatment for nontropical sprue, also termed "celiac disease," gluten-sensitive enteropathy, and idiopathic steatorrhea. Nontropical sprue is a disease in which the mucosa of the small intestine is sensitive to toxic effects of gliadin, the alcohol-soluble fraction of gluten. Although the details of this effect are not clear, the cause appears to be an immunologic defect.

Nontropical sprue may be associated with generalized malabsorption. Symptoms and other findings may include diarrhea, steatorrhea, weight loss, anemia, edema, tetany, bone pain, hypocalcemia, and hypophosphatemia. Radiologic studies of the skeleton may show osteomalacia. There is a characteristic lesion of the small intestine, which is seen as flattening of the mucosal villi.

A definitive diagnosis requires relief of symptoms and improvement in abnormalities of intestinal structure after exclusion of gluten from the diet. Although nontropical sprue is associated with exacerbations and remissions, the disease is not transient and requires lifelong diet therapy.

The patient should be cautioned against resuming use of gluten-containing products when symptoms subside. Periodic review of the diet and update on special products are important for compliance. A diet history may help the physician determine whether dietary indiscretions or a coexisting disorder is responsible for symptoms.

Two rare forms of nontropical sprue, termed "collagenous sprue" and "ulcerative ileojejunitis," respond inconsistently and often poorly to dietary restriction of gluten.

Dermatitis herpetiformis is a chronic inflammatory disease of the skin. In about 70% of persons, it is accompanied by lesions of the mucosa of the small intestine that appear to be identical to those of nontropical sprue. The degree of mucosal involvement and steatorrhea is much more variable and tends to be less severe in dermatitis herpetiformis than in nontropical sprue. In most cases, the malabsorption associated with dermatitis herpetiformis can be controlled with a gluten-restricted diet. The histologic appearance of the jejunum returns toward normal, and the skin lesions may improve somewhat.

PHYSICIANS: HOW TO ORDER DIETS

This diet may be ordered as **gluten control**.

FOODS TO ALLOW AND FOODS TO AVOID

Food Groups	Allow	Avoid
Beverage	Coffee; tea; decaffeinated coffee; pure instant coffee*; carbonated beverages; artificially flavored fruit drinks	Cereal beverage; coffee beverages containing cereal grains; root beer†
Meat	Pure meat, fish, fowl, and eggs; guaranteed pure meat cold cuts,* frankfurters,* and sausage*; aged cheese; cottage cheese; cream cheese; peanut butter; soybeans; peanuts	Commercially prepared meat and egg products,† breaded meats, meat loaf, and meat patties; processed cheese†; cheese foods† and dips†; texturized or hydrolyzed vegetable protein products†
Fat	Butter; margarine; cream; vegetable oil; shortening; nuts; olives; mayonnaise; gravies and sauces made with allowed thickening agents	Nondairy cream substitutes†; commercial salad dressing†; commercially prepared gravies and sauces
Milk	Milk; yogurt	Commercial chocolate milk; malted milk; instant milk drinks†; hot cocoa mixes†
Starch	Specially prepared bread and other baked products made with the following flours: corn, rice, potato, soybean, wheat starch	Any homemade or commercially prepared baked goods or mixes containing wheat (except wheat starch), oats, rye, graham, barley, buckwheat pancakes†, bran, or wheat germ; commercially prepared and corn muffins†; gluten bread
	Corn and rice cereals‡	Cereals containing wheat, oats, rye, barley, bran, wheat germ, graham, bulgur, or millet
	Potatoes; rice; hominy grits; low-protein wheat starch pastas	Commercial rice mixes; pasta, noodle, spaghetti, and macaroni products
	Snack foods, chips, and wafers made only of rice, corn, or potato; corn tortillas; popcorn	Crackers, chips,† and other snack foods†
	Thickening agents: corn flour, cornstarch, cornmeal, potato flour, potato starch, wheat starch, soybean starch, arrowroot starch, tapioca, gelatin	All others

FOODS TO ALLOW AND FOODS TO AVOID (Continued)

Food Groups	Allow	Avoid
Vegetable	All except those in "Avoid" column	Any commercially prepared with cheese sauce† or cream sauce; canned baked beans
Fruit	All except those in "Avoid" column	Commercially prepared pie fillings†; thickened fruit†
Soup	Homemade broth, vegetable, or cream soups thickened with allowed flours or starches	Commercially prepared soup,† soup mixes,† bouillon,† and broth†; any containing barley, pasta, or noodles
Dessert	Gelatin; meringues; custard; corn-starch, rice, and tapioca puddings; specially prepared desserts made of allowed flours and cereal-free baking powder; junket	Commercially prepared desserts and mixes: cookies, cakes, pie, piecrust, pastries, pudding; ice cream†; sherbet†; ice cream cones
Sweets	Sugar; honey; jelly; jam; molasses; corn syrup; pure maple syrup; pure baking chocolate; pure cocoa; coconut	Flavored syrups†; chocolate and other commercial candies†
Miscellaneous	Salt; pepper; other spices and herbs; dry yeast; food coloring and extracts	Prepared catsup,† mustard,† and horseradish†; bottled meat sauces†; soy sauce†; pickles†; seasoning mixes†; cake yeast†; chewing gum†; baking powder†
	Wine; rum; brandy; vermouth; cognac	Beer; ale; alcoholic beverages distilled from cereal grains
Food labeling:	The patient should be advised to read product labels carefully and avoid sources of gluten: wheat, oats, rye, barley, bran, wheat germ, bulgur, millet, graham, durham, and malt. Possible sources of gluten in processed foods include stabilizers, emulsifiers, cereal additives, and vegetable protein. If there is any doubt, the product should be avoided until absence of gluten is verified by the manufacturer or by a brand name list prepared by the research unit of a hospital or university.	

*Check label carefully to be sure gluten is not an ingredient.

†Avoid unless absence of gluten is verified by the manufacturer or by special brand name product lists.

‡Ready-to-eat corn and rice cereals may contain a small amount of malt as flavoring, but the amount usually is well tolerated.

SELECTED BIBLIOGRAPHY

Alexander, J. O.: Dermatitis herpetiformis. Major Probl. Dermatol., 4:1-338, 1975.
Collagenous sprue. Br. Med. J., 2:65-66, 1971.
Harrington, C. I., and Read, N. W.: Dermatitis herpetiformis: Effect of gluten-free diet on skin IgA and jejunal structure and function. Br. Med. J., 1:872-875, 1977.
Heading, R. C., Paterson, W. D., McClelland, D. B. L., et al.: Clinical response of dermatitis herpetiformis skin lesions to a gluten-free diet. Br. J. Dermatol., 94:509-514, 1976.
Katz, A. J., and Falchuk, Z. M.: Current concepts in gluten sensitive enteropathy (celiac sprue). Pediatr. Clin. North. Am., 22 No. 4:767-785, 1975.
Strober, W. (Moderator): The pathogenesis of gluten-sensitive enteropathy (NIH Conference). Ann. Intern. Med., 83:242-256, 1975.
Strober, W.: Gluten-sensitive enteropathy. Clin. Gastroenterol., 5 No. 2:429-452, 1976.
Weiser, M. M., and Douglas, A. P.: An alternative mechanism for gluten toxicity in coeliac disease. Lancet, 1:567-569, 1976.

DIETARY MANAGEMENT OF PEPTIC ULCER DISEASE

GENERAL DESCRIPTION

Guidelines are given to avoid extreme elevations of gastric acid secretion. A regular diet with only slight modification is recommended in most cases.

INDICATIONS AND RATIONALE

Various bland and ulcer diets with progressive levels of intake have been used in the treatment of peptic ulcer disease. In some instances, the rationale for these diets has been physiologically inappropriate and the food restrictions have been unwarranted. There is evidence that bland and ulcer diets are no more effective than a more general diet in speeding the rate of ulcer healing and reducing gastric acid secretion. Bland and ulcer diets probably are not detrimental to most persons if used for a short time and may be of psychologic benefit to some. However, prolonged adherence to these regimens is not necessary and is not recommended.

Milk has been an important part of ulcer diets because it was believed to neutralize gastric contents. This belief has been found to be only partly true. Any type of food in the stomach first causes a decrease in gastric acidity and then stimulates secretion of hydrochloric acid and pepsin. Protein has a greater potential than either carbohydrates or fats to buffer gastric contents but also produces a greater rebound stimulation. Neutralization by milk is a transient effect that is followed by hypersecretion of gastric acid. Frequent milk feedings are not encouraged.

Rough or coarse food has previously been excluded from bland diets on the presumption that it irritates the gastric mucosa. This effect has not been found to be true.

Various spices and seasonings are thought to irritate the gastric mucosa, but their effect appears to vary greatly among individuals. The spices most often implicated are black pepper, chili powder, cloves, nutmeg, garlic, other spices, pickles, meat extracts, gravies, and chocolate. Restriction of spices and other foods should be determined by individual tolerances.

Potent stimulators of hydrochloric acid secretion should be avoided. Coffee, tea, decaffeinated coffee, caffeine, alcohol, and calcium-containing antacids stimulate gastric secretion. Alcohol and some medications (for example, aspirin and corticosteroids) decrease mucosal barriers to back-diffusion of gastric acid secretion. The adverse effect of these substances is much less when they are consumed with food. Cigarette smoking decreases secretion of pancreatic bicarbonate, the normal buffer of gastric acid in the duodenum. A very large meal may be an additional stimulus to gastric acid secretion. Small-volume, frequent feedings have not been found to be more effective than three meals a day in long-term treatment of peptic ulcer disease. However, some patients claim relief of symptoms with frequent feedings, especially during acute stages.

The guidelines given here are based on physiologic responses of the gastrointestinal tract. Other dietary modifications should be determined by assessment of individual tolerances. For some patients, such as the hospitalized patient with acute peptic ulcer disease, temporarily following a definite dietary regimen may be of symptomatic benefit. The soft diet (see page 12) provides some modification in texture, types of food, and seasonings. Requests for small, frequent feedings or milk feedings may be specified in the diet order.

GENERAL DIETARY RECOMMENDATIONS

Avoid:

1. Coffee, tea, decaffeinated coffee, and colas and other carbonated beverages containing caffeine.
2. Alcoholic beverages.
3. Other foods according to individual tolerances.
4. Very large meals. Small-volume, frequent feedings may benefit some patients.

PHYSICIANS: HOW TO ORDER DIETS

This diet order should either indicate the disorder — **peptic ulcer** — *or* specify diet modification — **soft** (or **general**) **diet, no gastric stimulants.**

SELECTED BIBLIOGRAPHY

American Dietetic Association: Position paper on bland diet in the treatment of chronic duodenal ulcer disease. J. Am. Diet. Assoc., 59:244-245, 1971.
Cohen, S., and Booth, G. H., Jr.: Gastric acid secretion and lower-esophageal-sphincter pressure in response to coffee and caffeine. N. Engl. J. Med., 293:897-899, 1975.
Ippoliti, A. F., Maxwell, V., and Isenberg, J. I.: The effect of various forms of milk on gastric-acid secretion: Studies in patients with duodenal ulcer and normal subjects. Ann. Intern. Med., 84:286-289, 1976.
Welsh, J. D.: Diet therapy of peptic ulcer disease. Gastroenterology, 72:740-745, 1977.

DIETARY MANAGEMENT OF ESOPHAGEAL REFLUX

GENERAL DESCRIPTION

Guidelines are given to prevent esophageal reflux and to reduce symptoms. A specific dietary regimen is rarely necessary unless reflux is associated with other disorders.

INDICATIONS AND RATIONALE

Esophageal reflux refers to regurgitation of gastric contents into the esophagus. The most common symptom is heartburn (substernal pain or discomfort). Esophageal reflux usually is a mild condition that can be managed medically. However, chronic reflux may lead to esophagitis and subsequently to ulceration, hemorrhage, and stricture, which may even necessitate surgical treatment.

The esophagus ordinarily is protected from reflux of gastric contents by contraction of the lower esophageal sphincter. It is generally held that the lower esophageal sphincter is incompetent in persons with chronic esophageal reflux. The mean sphincter pressure tends to be lower in these persons, so that the likelihood of reflux is increased.

Factors predisposing to reflux are recumbent body position, obesity, and increased intra-abdominal pressure. Nocturnal reflux may be reduced by elevating the head of the bed and avoiding late evening snacks. Obesity and constricting garments may increase intra-abdominal pressure. Regression of symptoms is likely to accompany weight loss (see page 50 for weight reduction diet). Large meals should be avoided, since they may increase gastric pressure on the lower esophageal sphincter.

Changes in lower esophageal sphincter pressure normally occur in response to hormonal, mechanical, drug, and dietary factors. Some of the factors that reduce this pressure and therefore increase chances of reflux are cigarette smoking and ingestion of coffee, decaffeinated coffee, alcohol, a high-fat meal, chocolate, peppermint oil, and spearmint oil. Caffeine has a minimal effect on sphincter pressure but increases gastric secretion. Persons with esophageal reflux tend to experience discomfort with ingestion of citrus and tomato juices. These foods have not been found to consistently decrease lower esophageal sphincter pressure, but it is speculated that their mild acidity may irritate the esophageal mucosa, produce esophageal spasm, and delay clearing of refluxed gastric contents. Some persons associate reflux symptoms with spicy foods. Spices are not believed to affect esophageal mucosa or lower esophageal sphincter pressure but are often eaten with high-fat or tomato-base foods.

Antacids will likely reduce reflux symptoms. Antacids increase lower esophageal sphincter pressure and neutralize gastric contents, so that any reflux is less likely to damage esophageal mucosa.

GENERAL DIETARY RECOMMENDATIONS

1. Achieve and maintain ideal weight.
2. Avoid very large meals. Eat three normal (or slightly smaller than normal) meals and midmorning and midafternoon snacks (if at ideal weight). Avoid snacks before bedtime.
3. Avoid:
   - High-fat foods: fried foods, cream sauces, high-fat meats, pastries (limit use of butter, margarine, cream, oil, and salad dressings)
   - Coffee, tea, decaffeinated coffee, colas and other carbonated beverages containing caffeine
   - Chocolate: cocoa, hot chocolate, desserts or candies made with chocolate
   - Alcoholic beverages
   - Peppermint oil and spearmint oil
   - Other foods according to individual tolerance

PHYSICIANS: HOW TO ORDER DIETS

This diet order should indicate the disorder — **esophageal reflux**.

SELECTED BIBLIOGRAPHY

Castell, D. O.: Diet and the lower esophageal sphincter. Am. J. Clin. Nutr., 28:1296-1298, 1975.
Cohen, S., and Booth, G. H., Jr.: Gastric acid secretion and lower-esophageal-sphincter pressure in response to coffee and caffeine. N. Engl. J. Med., 293:897-899, 1975.
Hutcheon, D. F., and Hendrix, T. R.: Esophageal reflux: Diagnosis and therapy. Postgrad. Med., 61:131-137, Feb. 1977.

DIETARY MANAGEMENT OF POSTGASTRECTOMY DUMPING SYNDROME

GENERAL DESCRIPTION

Dietary management of postgastrectomy dumping syndrome is aimed at alleviating symptoms. Individual tolerances vary greatly, and most patients quickly learn which modifications best suit their needs. Guidelines for initial use are given. In general, the diet restricts simple sugars, recommends small and frequent meals, and limits fluid intake between meals.

INDICATIONS AND RATIONALE

Dumping syndrome, or postgastrectomy syndrome, is a possible complication of partial or total gastric resection. Symptoms and signs — weakness, pallor, abdominal distress, tachycardia, sweating, and in some instances, syncope — usually occur from 10 to 15 minutes after meals. Weight loss is common.

Because of gastric resection, the capacity of the stomach has been reduced, so that food enters the intestine in larger quantities and more rapidly. It is believed that when a hyperosmolar mixture is rapidly introduced into the small intestine, plasma water shifts into the intestine to equalize intraluminal osmotic pressure and that of body water. Withdrawal of fluid from the blood reduces blood volume and pressure, and reduction may produce signs of hypovolemia and dumping syndrome.

Research suggests that serotonin and bradykinin also may contribute to early postprandial dumping syndrome. A hyperosmolar solution and increased intraluminal pressure due to distention of the small intestine cause excessive output, from the small intestine mucosa, of serotonin and bradykinin, which enter the circulation and may produce the characteristic symptoms. Fluids taken with the meal may contribute to symptoms, perhaps by distending the upper portion of the small intestine.

Patients experiencing dumping symptoms generally lose weight because of a reluctance to eat rather than malabsorption. In some cases, milk and milk products must be omitted because of lactose intolerance. The caloric level should be determined by the need for weight gain or maintenance.

In some postgastrectomy patients, symptoms begin 2 to 4 hours after a meal. This disorder has been referred to as "late postprandial dumping syndrome." For a discussion of dietary management, see page 170.

GENERAL DIETARY RECOMMENDATIONS

1. Simple carbohydrates, such as sugar, honey, and foods with added sugar, are kept to a minimum to prevent the formation of a hyperosmolar solution. The total amount of carbohydrate in the diet varies with the calorie level.

2. Protein and fat are increased to provide sufficient calories. A relatively high fat content also retards gastric emptying.

3. Fluids should not be taken with meals but may be taken 30 to 60 minutes before or after meals.

4. Small, frequent meals (five or six) are recommended to prevent distention.

5. Very hot and cold foods may be restricted according to individual tolerance. Extremes in temperature produce symptoms in some persons.

PHYSICIANS: HOW TO ORDER DIETS

This diet order should either indicate the disorder — **dumping syndrome** (the dietitian will modify the diet according to the guidelines given and to the tolerances of the patient) — *or* specify the diet modifications needed, such as **small, frequent feedings; no free sugars; no fluids with meals.**

SELECTED BIBLIOGRAPHY

Buchwald, H.: The dumping syndrome and its treatment: A review and presentation of cases. Am. J. Surg., 116:81-88, 1968.

Fein, H. D.: Nutrition in diseases of the gastrointestinal tract. Section A. Nutrition in diseases of the stomach. *In* Goodhart, R. S., and Shils, M. E., eds.: Modern Nutrition in Health and Disease: Dietotherapy. Fifth edition. Philadelphia, Lea & Febiger, 1973, pp. 780-782.

Lieber, H.: The jejunal hyperosmolic syndrome (dumping) and its prophylaxis. J.A.M.A., 176:208-211, 1961.

Woodward, E. R.: The early postprandial dumping syndrome: Clinical manifestations and pathogenesis. Major Probl. Clin. Surg., 20:1-12, 1976.

DIETARY MANAGEMENT OF GASTRIC RETENTION

GENERAL DESCRIPTION

The diet includes liquids and solid foods that become liquid at room temperature. Small meals are served every 2 hours from 8 a.m. to 8 p.m. The diet is identical to the full liquid diet (see page 10), but greater emphasis is placed on smaller and more frequent feedings.

INDICATIONS AND RATIONALE

The diet may be indicated in cases of gastric retention caused by partial obstruction at the outlet of the stomach or of the small bowel. The purpose of the diet is to provide foods that can pass by a partial obstruction before or during absorption. Small feedings are given to prevent excessive distention of the stomach. A mechanial soft diet (see page 14) may be tolerated in instances of lesser obstruction. A diet low in residue (see pages 143 and 242) may be necessary if the obstruction is located lower in the gastrointestinal tract.

PHYSICIANS: HOW TO ORDER DIETS

This diet may be ordered as **full liquid diet with frequent feedings.**

DIETARY MANAGEMENT OF ALLERGY

Diets used in the management of allergies have been developed largely through experience. In some instances, there is biochemical evidence of specific allergies (such as serum antibodies to food proteins). More often, there is no precise biochemical or symptomatic means of identifying the allergen. The diets are often used first in identification of the allergen and second in treatment.

By analyzing a diet history recall or a record of daily food intake, the dietitian may help determine which foods cause allergic responses. The trial and evaluation method of dietary restriction sometimes is necessary because of imperfections in other diagnostic methods.

An unflavored elemental diet (see page 242) may be useful in diagnosis of multiple food allergies. The elemental diet has the advantage of being a hypoallergenic base to which suspected foods can be added as challenge tests.*

FOOD SENSITIVITY ELIMINATION DIET

GENERAL DESCRIPTION

The diet consists of elimination of specific foods from the person's usual diet. It was formerly called "diet with common irritants omitted" (CIO).

NUTRITIONAL ADEQUACY

Although the diet is similar to the general hospital diet, it should not be used for an extended period without medical supervision. The physician will tell the patient when to include foods eliminated.

INDICATIONS AND RATIONALE

The diet may be useful in the treatment of chronic urticaria and in some cases of atopic reactivity. The purpose of the diet is to eliminate foods that are most often found to cause urticaria. In many instances, sensitivity to foods is not accurately identified by testing the skin. It is often more practical to try an elimination diet.

PHYSICIANS: HOW TO ORDER DIETS

The diet order should indicate **food sensitivity elimination diet.**

---

*Galant, S. P., Franz, M. L., Walker, P., et al.: A potential diagnostic method for food allergy: Clinical application and immunogenicity evaluation of an elemental diet. Am. J. Clin. Nutr., 30:512-516, 1977.

FOODS TO AVOID

(Any foods not listed are allowed.)

Beverage	Coffee; cola beverages; chocolate-flavored beverages
Meat	Fish; shellfish; fresh pork; corned beef; highly seasoned meats (such as cold cuts); peanut butter; fermented cheese and cheese spreads; eggs*
Fat	All nuts
Milk	Chocolate milk; hot cocoa; eggnog
Vegetable	Tomato; tomato products
Fruit	Fresh or frozen: apples, cherries, berries†; fresh, frozen, dried, or cooked: bananas, grapes, mangoes, papayas, pineapple, rhubarb, raisins

---

*Egg in all forms and amounts should be avoided when the diet is ordered for children. Adults, however, may have small amounts of cooked egg, such as those in most desserts. The allergenic protein in eggs is denatured by cooking.

†Cooking denatures some allergens; therefore, cooked apples, cherries, and berries may be used. Other fruits to be eliminated may be extremely allergenic in some patients, and cooking does not denature the allergens.

SELECTED BIBLIOGRAPHY

Winkelmann, R. K.: Chronic urticaria. Proc. Staff Meet. Mayo Clin., 32:329-334, 1957.

PENICILLIN-FREE AND MOLD-FREE DIET

GENERAL DESCRIPTION

The diet is intended to eliminate penicillin and molds. Milk and all dairy products are to be avoided, since they may contain penicillin as a contaminant. Food sources of molds may be categorized as (1) mold foods (such as mushrooms), (2) mold-containing foods, including foods to which molds are added to develop a particular flavor (such as cheese, sour cream, buttermilk, bacon, sausage, ham), and (3) mold-acquiring foods, including foods likely to act as a substrate for mold growth (such as jams, jellies, tea, spices).

NUTRITIONAL ADEQUACY

The diet is low in calcium and riboflavin. If the diet is to be followed for an extended period, a supplement should be prescribed.

INDICATIONS AND RATIONALE

The diet may be useful in the treatment of some types of chronic urticaria or other forms of allergic response due to penicillin hypersensitivity. The mechanism of action is thought to be the contribution of the metabolic products of penicillin to the formation of antibodies. Penicillin may also contribute nonspecifically to the exacerbation of chronic atopic urticaria.

Contamination of milk occurs when animals with bovine mastitis are treated with penicillin. Although the sale of milk from these animals is legally prohibited for a certain period, small amounts of penicillin may nevertheless be present. Processing of milk is not likely to destroy all penicillin, and it is possible that the degradation products are as sensitizing as penicillin itself, if not more so. Therefore, no dairy products may be used in any form.

Food sources of molds are restricted on the basis that *Penicillium* is one of the most commonly occurring molds. Other molds may produce a reaction similar to that of penicillin.

An acceptable level of penicillin in the diet has not been determined. The diet is intended to be as free of penicillin and molds as possible.

The diet is likely to be used in the treatment of chronic urticaria if there is a history of hypersensitivity to injection or oral administration of penicillin. The diet should not be followed for a prolonged period without adequate medical supervision and evaluation of symptomatic response.

PHYSICIANS: HOW TO ORDER DIETS

The diet order should indicate **penicillin-free and mold-free diet**.

FOODS TO ALLOW AND FOODS TO AVOID

Food Groups	Allow	Avoid
Beverage	Coffee; decaffeinated coffee; cereal beverage; carbonated beverage; soft drink mixes	Tea; cocoa; hot chocolate; beverage mixes containing milk products
Meat	All except those in "Avoid" column	Ham; sausage; cottage cheese; cheese; cheese spreads; processed cheese; cold cuts; frankfurters
Fat	Nondairy cream substitutes; all others except those in "Avoid" column	Bacon or bacon drippings; butter; cream cheese; half-and-half; cream; sour cream; whipping cream; margarines containing milk products; salad dressings containing milk products, cheese, or vinegar; gravy containing milk
Milk	Soybean milk	All milk and milk products: whole milk, low-fat milks, skim milk, buttermilk, evaporated milk, condensed milk, dry powdered milk, yogurt
Starch	Any not containing milk products; potatoes; rice; noodles; spaghetti	Any breads, cereals, crackers, or prepared foods containing milk products
Vegetable	All except those in "Avoid" column	Any prepared with milk products; mushrooms; truffles; morels
Fruit	All except dried fruit	Dried fruit
Soup	All except those in "Avoid" column	Cream soups; any made with milk products
Dessert	Fruit ices; gelatin; others made with allowed foods	Ice cream; ice milk; sherbet; any containing milk, including commercial mixes, bakery products, and homemade foods
Sweets	Sugar; pure sugar candy	Jams; jellies; honey; syrup; molasses; any containing milk products
Miscellaneous	Salt	Pepper; herbs; spices; seasonings and flavorings containing milk products; chocolate; cocoa; beer; wine; distilled alcoholic beverages
Food labeling:	The patient should be advised to read product labels carefully and to avoid dairy products (that is, milk and milk products, cheese and cheese products, cream and cream products, milk solids, casein and lactalbumin, and curds and whey).	
Medications:	Antibiotics related to penicillin may have the same effect as penicillin itself. Caution should be exercised in the prescription and administration of medications.	

SELECTED BIBLIOGRAPHY

Rosanove, R.: Contamination of milk with penicillin. Minn. Med., 43:306-309, 1960.
Warin, R.P., and Champion, R. H.: Major Probl. Urticaria. Dermatol., 1:34-39, 1974.

YEAST-FREE DIET

GENERAL DESCRIPTION

The diet attempts to eliminate food sources of yeast and some yeastlike molds. These sources include bread products leavened with yeast, enriched flours and fortified cereals containing vitamins derived from yeast, yeast-forming foods (such as fermented beverages, vinegar, malt), mold foods (such as mushrooms), and mold-containing foods (such as cheese).

NUTRITIONAL ADEQUACY

Although the diet is similar to the general hospital diet, it should not be used for an extended period without medical supervision. If a vitamin supplement is needed, it should not contain vitamins derived from yeast. This information is available from the manufacturer.

INDICATIONS AND RATIONALE

The diet may be useful in the treatment of some types of chronic urticaria.

The role of yeasts in urticaria is not clearly established. Sensitivity to yeasts is more common among persons who are hypersensitive to *Candida albicans,* an organism that is often present in the gastrointestinal tract. There may be a cross-reaction between the *Candida* organism and food yeasts. Another hypothesis is that yeasts cause release of tyramine or similar amines, which may have a nonspecific effect in the exacerbation of chronic urticaria.

An acceptable level of yeast in the diet has not been established. The diet is designed to be as free of yeasts as possible. Since the tolerance level may vary among individuals, the initial diet should be yeast-free. Modification allowing trace amounts of yeast derivatives may be made later, depending on individual tolerance.

The diet is likely to be used if there is a positive response to prick tests or challenge tests with *Candida* or food yeasts. The diet should not be followed for a prolonged period without medical supervision and evaluation of symptomatic response.

PHYSICIANS: HOW TO ORDER DIETS

The diet order should indicate **yeast-free diet.**

FOODS TO ALLOW AND FOODS TO AVOID

Food Groups	Allow	Avoid
Beverage	Coffee; decaffeinated coffee; cereal beverages; other carbonated beverages; artificially flavored fruit drink.	Black tea; root beer; ginger ale
Meat	Pure meat, fish, fowl, and eggs; peanut butter	Cold cuts; frankfurters; aged and processed cheese; cottage cheese; hamburger (unless pure meat); commercially prepared meat products; meat loaf; breaded meats; meat patties; croquettes; omelets
Fat	Butter; margarine; cream; bacon; vegetable oil; shortening; nuts; gravies and sauces made with allowed thickening agent	Nondairy cream substitutes*; cream cheese; sour cream; commercially prepared gravies and cream sauces; olives; commercially prepared salad dressings
Milk	All except those in "Avoid" column	Buttermilk; yogurt; malted milk
Starch	Baked products leavened with baking powder or baking soda: biscuits, muffins, quick breads, pancakes, waffles, corn bread	Baked products leavened with yeast: bread, rolls, buns; commercially prepared baked goods,* mixes,* muffins,* biscuits,* pancakes,* and waffles*; cereals containing malt; vitamin-fortified cereals*
	Flours not vitamin enriched: rice flour, cornmeal and corn flour, potato flour, soy flour, low-protein wheat-starch flour; unenriched wheat, graham, and rye flours	Flours enriched with vitamins derived from yeast: wheat,* graham,* rye*
	Potatoes; rice; hominy grits; starchy vegetables; low-protein wheat-starch pasta; popcorn	Commercial rice mixes; pasta*; noodles* and macaroni* products; crackers*; pretzels*; snack foods* and chips*
Vegetable	All except those in "Avoid" column	Mushrooms; truffles; morels; sauerkraut; pickled vegetables
Fruit	Freshly prepared fruit juices; all fruits and fruit products except those in "Avoid" column	Dried fruit; frozen and canned fruit juices; commercially prepared pie filling*
Soup	Homemade broth, vegetable soup, and cream soups thickened with allowed flours	Commercially prepared soup,* soup mixes,* and bouillon*
Dessert	Meringues; plain gelatin; custard; cornstarch, rice, or tapioca pudding; specially prepared desserts made with allowed flours and leavening agents	Commercially prepared desserts and mixes; cookies*; cakes*; piecrust*; pastries*; ice cream cones*; gelatin with added vitamins; puddings*; ice cream*; sherbet*

FOODS TO ALLOW AND FOODS TO AVOID (Continued)

Food Groups	Allow	Avoid
Sweets	Sugar; honey; jelly; jam; molasses; corn syrup; pure maple syrup; pure baking chocolate; pure cocoa; coconut	Flavored syrups*; chocolate and cream candies*
Miscellaneous	Salt; all spices and herbs except those in "Avoid" column	Pepper; curry powder*; vinegar; catsup; mustard; bottled meat sauces; soy sauce; horseradish; pickles; seasoning mixes*; yeast tablets; beer; wine; distilled alcoholic beverages

*Check label carefully. Avoid if ingredients include substances that may contain yeast or yeast derivatives.

FOOD LABELING

The patient should be advised to read product labels carefully.

If the list of ingredients includes	the product should be avoided unless the manufacturer verifies that
"enriched" or "fortified" flour or cereal grains	yeast is not the source of added vitamins
"leavening"	yeast is not the leavening agent
"stabilizers," "emulsifiers," or "thickening agents"	it does not contain vitamin-enriched flour

SELECTED BIBLIOGRAPHY

Brown, D. W., Jr.: Mold allergy affecting the ears, nose, and throat. Otolaryngol. Clin. North Am., 4:491-505, 1971.

James, J., and Warin, R. P.: An assessment of the role of *Candida albicans* and food yeasts in chronic urticaria. Br. J. Dermatol., 84:227-237, 1971.

Karvonen, J., and Hannuksela, M.: Urticaria from alcoholic beverages. Acta Allergol. (Kbh.), 31:167-170, 1976.

Warin, R. P., and Champion, R. H.: Urticaria. Major Probl. Dermatol., 1:50-60, 1974.

SALICYLATE-FREE AND TARTRAZINE-FREE DIET

GENERAL DESCRIPTION

The diet is designed to minimize* intake of tartrazine or both salicylates and tartrazine. Salicylates occur naturally in some foods, predominantly in the fruit group. Other sources of salicylates are acetylsalicylic acid (in aspirin and aspirin-containing medications) and methyl salicylate or salicin (wintergreen or mint flavoring added to foods, drugs, and cosmetics). It is the intention of this diet to exclude all forms of the salicylate radical.

Tartrazine (FD&C Yellow No. 5) is a certified coloring dye used in foods, drugs, and cosmetics. Manufacturers are not currently required to identify tartrazine on food product labels. Regulations have been proposed that would mandate the listing of tartrazine on all food products containing this color dye. At the time of writing of this manual, however, the issue is unresolved and food labeling of tartrazine is generally not practiced. Foods listed under the "may contain tartrazine" category on pages 167 and 168 are the foods most likely to contain tartrazine. A product is acceptable only if it has been established that it does not contain tartrazine. This information is usually available, on request, from the manufacturer and in the future may be listed on product labels.

NUTRITIONAL ADEQUACY

Although the diet is similar to the general hospital diet, it should not be used for an extended period without medical supervision.

INDICATIONS AND RATIONALE

In this institution, a diet that restricts both salicylates and tartrazine is currently used in the treatment of specific types of chronic urticaria. The mechanism by which salicylates and tartrazine induce or aggravate urticaria has not been clearly established. It has been hypothesized that the salicylate radical, by acting as an antigen in the development of the allergic reaction or by enhancing the effect of histamine on the skin, produces urticaria. Some persons with salicylate hypersensitivity may also have a hypersensitivity to the azobenzene dye tartrazine. The similarity between the symptoms produced by tartrazine and salicylate hypersensitivities suggests that a similar biochemical abnormality is present or that there is partial cross-reactivity between the two substances. The salicylate-free and tartrazine-free diet is likely to be used to treat chronic urticaria if there is a history of aspirin hypersensitivity and analysis of plasma indicates that salicylate is present.

In some patients with asthma, particularly those with nasal polyps, the ingestion of aspirin may cause severe asthmatic reactions. In a small percentage of these patients, asthmatic attacks may also follow ingestion of tartrazine. Patients sensitive to aspirin or tartrazine, however, often can ingest salicylates other than aspirin without difficulty. Food sources of salicylates and tartrazine are listed separately so that the diet can be adjusted to meet the particular need of the patient.

PHYSICIANS: HOW TO ORDER DIETS

The diet order should indicate either **salicylate-free and tartrazine-free diet** *or* **tartrazine-free diet.**

---

*Available data do not quantify the salicylate or tartrazine content of foods. The diet is intended to be as free of salicylates or tartrazine (or both) as possible.

FOOD SOURCES OF TARTRAZINE AND SALICYLATES

Food Groups	May Contain Tartrazine*	Contain Salicylates	Allowed
Beverage	Carbonated beverages; soft drinks and soft drink mixes	Tea; root beer; birch beer	Coffee; decaffeinated coffee; cereal beverage
Meat	Sausage; frankfurters; cheese-flavored foods	Corned beef; meat processed with vinegar	All other meats, fish, and fowl; eggs; peanut butter; other cheese
Fat	Nondairy cream	Salad dressing; mayonnaise; avocado; olives	Butter; margarine; vegetable oil; cream and cream products; nuts; other fats
Milk	Yogurt; hot chocolate and cocoa mixes		All others
Starch	Ready-to-eat cereals; variety crackers; noodles; commercial mixes	White potato	Bread; spaghetti; macaroni; rice; most commercially prepared breads and rolls
Vegetable		Cucumbers; green bell and other peppers; tomatoes	All others
Fruit		Apples; apple cider; apricots; blackberries; boysenberries; cherries; currants; dewberries; gooseberries; huckleberries; maraschino cherries; grapes; melon; nectarines; peaches; raisins; raspberries; prunes; plums	Banana; blueberries; cranberries; dates; figs; grapefruit; lemon; lime; loganberries; oranges; mango; papaya; pear; pineapple; rhubarb; strawberries; tangerines
Soup	Commercial soups and soup mixes		All others made from allowed foods
Dessert	Gelatin; sherbet; ice cream; ice milk; fruit ice; commercially prepared desserts and mixes, including cakes, frostings, puddings, and gingerbread		All others made from allowed foods

FOOD SOURCES OF TARTRAZINE AND SALICYLATES (Continued)

Food Groups	May Contain Tartrazine*	Contain Salicylates	Allowed
Sweets	Commercially prepared jams, jelly, and candy; any colored yellow, orange, pink, green, or brown; chewing gum	Any mint- or wintergreen-flavored	Sugar; honey; syrup; all others
Miscellaneous	Cocoa and hot chocolate mixes; flavoring extracts	Cloves; pickles; catsup; tartar sauce; Tabasco sauce; cider vinegar; wine vinegar; beer; wine; distilled alcoholic beverages (except vodka)	Salt; pepper; other spices; herbs; distilled white vinegar; cocoa powder; pure chocolate

*These foods are likely to contain tartrazine. If the manufacturer states that a specific brand does not contain tartrazine or FD&C Yellow No. 5, it may be used. This information is usually available from the company's consumer service department.

SELECTED BIBLIOGRAPHY

Ashoor, S., and Chu, F. S.: Analysis of salicylic acid and methyl salicylate in fruits and almonds (unpublished data). University of Wisconsin, 1978.

Juhlin, L., Michaëlsson, G., and Zetterström, O.: Urticaria and asthma induced by food-and-drug additives in patients with aspirin hypersensitivity. J. Allergy Clin. Immunol., 50:92-98, 1972.

Moore-Robinson, M., and Warin, R. P.: Effect of salicylates in urticaria. Br. Med. J., 4:262-264, 1967.

Noid, H. E., Schulze, T. W., and Winkelmann, R. K.: Diet plan for patients with salicylate-induced urticaria. Arch. Dermatol., 109:866-869, 1974.

Settipane, G. A., Chafee, F. H., Postman, I. M., et al.: Significance of tartrazine sensitivity in chronic urticaria of unknown etiology. J. Allergy Clin. Immunol., 57:541-546, 1976.

Smith, L. J., and Slavin, R. G.: Drugs containing tartrazine dye. J. Allergy Clin. Immunol., 58:456-470, 1976.

Zlotlow, M. J., and Settipane, G. A.: Allergic potential of food additives: A report of a case of tartrazine sensitivity without aspirin intolerance. Am. J. Clin. Nutr., 30:1023-1025, 1977.

DIETARY MANAGEMENT OF HYPOGLYCEMIA

GENERAL DESCRIPTION

For hypoglycemia resulting from islet cell tumors and other neoplasms, idiopathic hypoglycemia of childhood, and ketotic hypoglycemia, food is given at frequent intervals in amounts necessary to prevent symptoms. Sugars need not be specifically avoided and are particularly useful for rapid correction of symptoms.

For reactive hypoglycemia, free sugars should be avoided. The meal plan can be that for diabetes. If three regular meals are not well tolerated, smaller feedings at intervals of 2 to 3 hours may, by trial, be tolerated better.

INDICATIONS AND RATIONALE

Hypoglycemia may result from many causes; classifications have been published (Service, 1976). Only those categories involving dietary factors are discussed here.

Hypoglycemia occurring with islet cell tumors and with some extrapancreatic tumors is elicited by deprivation of food and tends to become progressively more severe with increasing duration of fasting. *Treatment is surgical. Trials of diet as definitive therapy are inappropriate.* While the patient awaits arrangements for surgery or if surgery has not succeeded in removing the tumor, feedings should be given often enough to prevent symptoms. Although gain in weight is not characteristic of such patients, obesity could become a problem if frequent, large feedings are continued for a substantial period. The carbohydrate and protein content of the diet should be emphasized, since fat is largely ineffective in correcting hypoglycemia and would contribute additional calories. Sugars rapidly correct symptoms and need not be avoided. Carbohydrates that are more slowly absorbed than sugar may be preferable for preventing symptoms, since they may extend the intervals between feedings.

Idiopathic hypoglycemia of infancy and ketotic hypoglycemia occur in infants and in children up to about 5 years of age. Food appropriate for the child's age should be given frequently. Again, sugars need not be specifically avoided. Ketotic hypoglycemia tends to resolve spontaneously, but idiopathic hypoglycemia of infancy may require subtotal pancreatectomy or drugs, such as diazoxide.

Hypoglycemia occurring 1 to 3 hours after a meal and resolving spontaneously can be termed "reactive hypoglycemia." "Reactive hypoglycemia" is a diagnosis often mistakenly made in persons with anxiety to explain different symptoms occurring throughout the day but having some relation to meals. Commonly, the patient feels somewhat better on a high-protein diet designated to be for hypoglycemia. The patient considers partial relief of symptoms to confirm the diagnosis of "hypoglycemia," whereas the real cause of the symptoms is anxiety, and the apparent response to the diet may be the result of suggestion. Symptoms of anxiety and of hypoglycemia are qualitatively similar, since both are mediated by release of epinephrine.

The diagnosis of reactive hypoglycemia severe enough to cause significant symptoms can be established if plasma glucose levels of less than 40 mg/dl after ordinary meals are associated with symptoms of epinephrine release, such as tachycardia and feelings of apprehension and anxiety. Symptoms should either spontaneously abate in an hour or less or be relieved promptly, consistently, and completely by the ingestion of carbohydrate. A rapid decrease in glucose concentration itself does not provoke epinephrine release and cannot be invoked as a cause for symptoms if the glucose level is well above 40 mg/dl at the time of symptoms. Plasma glucose levels of less than 40 mg/dl may occur in normal, asymptomatic persons during the course of the oral glucose tolerance test. Epinephrine-release symptoms coinciding with the nadir of plasma glucose concentration in the glucose tolerance test is only circumstantial evidence that symptoms occurring after ordinary meals are hypoglycemic in origin, since the glucose tolerance test is a challenge to glucose homeostasis in excess of that posed by ordinary meals.

Documented reactive hypoglycemia with significant symptoms is rare. The disorder sometimes occurs in persons who have had gastric surgery, but the symptoms of "dumping" (see page 157) should be clearly distinguished from those of hypoglycemia. Hypoglycemia occurring at the fourth hour or later in the glucose tolerance test is sometimes said to predict the later occurrence of diabetes.

Dietary management of reactive hypoglycemia consists of avoiding free sugars. If several larger feedings of protein, fat, and slowly absorbed carbohydrate tend to cause distress, small feedings will be appropriate. The frequency of feedings may need to be increased to provide the necessary calorie intake. Restriction of slowly absorbed carbohydrate generally does not relieve symptoms. The meal plans for diabetes offer a reasonable general guide to diet planning in reactive hypoglycemia.

PHYSICIANS: HOW TO ORDER DIETS

The diet order may specify the diet modification, such as **no free sugar,** *or* indicate the disorder, such as **reactive hypoglycemia.** If the disorder is indicated, the dietitian will determine the appropriate modifications according to the guidelines given and tolerances of the patient.

SELECTED BIBLIOGRAPHY

Fajans, S. S., and Floyd, J. C., Jr.: Fasting hypoglycemia in adults. N. Engl. J. Med., 294:766-772, 1976.
Johnson, D. D., Dorr, K. E., Swenson, W. M., and Service, J.: Reactive hypoglycemia. J.A.M.A., 243:1151-1155, 1980.
Service, F. J.: Hypoglycemias. Compr. Ther., 2:27–31, 1976.
Special report: Statement on hypoglycemia. Diabetes, 22:137, 1973.

SECTION 4

DIET DURING PREGNANCY AND LACTATION

DIET DURING PREGNANCY AND LACTATION

GENERAL DESCRIPTION

Dietary intake of all nutrients should be increased for optimal pregnancy outcome. Caloric intake should be increased by an average of 300 kcal/day to achieve an appropriate gain in weight. A level of 30 g/day of protein in excess of Recommended Dietary Allowances for the nonpregnant state is advised to provide the amino acids needed for fetal and placental growth, for expansion of blood volume, and for increase in size of breasts and uterus. The Food and Nutrition Board of the National Research Council has recommended 5 additional milligrams of zinc during pregnancy, which the increase in protein helps to provide. From the beginning of pregnancy, the diet should also provide an increase of 400 mg (for a total of 1,200 mg) of calcium above that amount required for the nonpregnant woman. The Recommended Dietary Allowance for iron for women of childbearing age is 18 mg/day; during pregnancy, a supplement of 30 to 60 mg of iron (equal to 150 to 300 mg of USP ferrous sulfate*) is advised. Dietary sources of folic acid are inadequate to achieve the amount required for pregnancy, and a daily supplement of 400 to 800 μg should be provided.

Some day-to-day variation in nutrient intake is likely, depending on the food items selected. This is of little concern if the *average* intake of essential nutrients is adequate.

RATIONALE

The diet during pregnancy is intended to provide the nutrients and energy needed for growth of the fetus and placenta and for increases in maternal tissues such as the uterus, breasts, blood, and fat.

NORMAL PREGNANCY

An average weight gain of about 11 kg is commensurate with a better-than-average course and outcome of pregnancy; the gain should be 0.75 kg to 1.4 kg during the first trimester and 0.4 kg per week during the rest of the pregnancy (Committee on Maternal Nutrition, National Research Council, 1970; Hytten and Leitch, 1971). The Food and Nutrition Board has recommended that caloric intake be 300 kcal/day more than that required to maintain ideal weight† in the nonpregnant state. A maternal gain in weight of much less than 11 kg tends to be associated with low birth weight of the fetus and increased perinatal mortality. If a woman enters pregnancy 10% or more underweight, she should gain at a greater than average rate. Those entering pregnancy overweight should gain weight at the usual recommended rate.

Because of uncertainties about protein needs during pregnancy, an additional 30 g of protein of high biologic value is desirable (Food and Nutrition Board, National Research Council, 1980). Since protein-rich foods are good sources of several nutrients and since the Recommended Dietary Allowances for some of the trace elements are difficult to meet, it seems prudent to plan pregnancy diets around a level of protein content for which abundant and reliable data are available (Calloway, 1974).

---

*Ferrous sulfate is the form of iron most commonly used for correction of iron deficiencies. The USP form contains 7 mol of water of crystallization. A 325-mg (5-grain) tablet contains 65 mg of elemental iron. Administration with a dietary source of ascorbic acid facilitates absorption.

†Individual caloric needs may be determined by use of the food nomogram (see page 282) and the patient's ideal weight, with increments of 20 to 30% for activity and of 300 calories per day for the caloric cost of pregnancy.

The gestational iron requirement is about 750 mg (Pitkin, 1977b) and is needed for expansion of maternal blood volume and for synthesis of fetal and placental tissues. This requirement cannot be met by the habitual diet, and it is recommended that the physician prescribe 30 to 60 mg of iron per day as a simple ferrous salt (150 to 300 mg of USP ferrous sulfate).

The requirements for folic acid during pregnancy are greatly increased. Although megaloblastic anemia due to folate deficiency is infrequent, routine supplementation with folic acid appears to be desirable, particularly in patients who have had previous pregnancies or who have recently taken oral contraceptive agents (Hillman and Goodhart, 1973). The National Research Council recommends an additional 400 μg of folic acid per day to protect the fetus and to maintain maternal stores.

Sodium is retained in pregnancy as a normal physiologic adjustment (4 meq per day in early pregnancy and 8 meq per day near full term) (Pike and Gursky, 1970). The common practice of routinely restricting salt is perhaps intended to prevent toxemia of pregnancy; however, the causes and mechanisms of toxemia are controversial, and routine restriction of dietary sodium in healthy pregnant women is not justified. Any sodium limitations should be determined on an individual basis.

ADOLESCENT PREGNANCY

The number of pregnant adolescent girls, specifically those younger than 17 or less than 5 years past menarche, continues to increase. The decrease in menarcheal age in the United States has been from 4 to 6 months per decade, but this age currently is remaining steady at 12 years. During adolescence, the nutritional stresses of pregnancy are superimposed on the nutritional needs of growth and maturation.

Teenage girls tend to have poor eating habits, so that the nutritional state at the onset of pregnancy may be inadequate. Dietary preferences are often unusual, and intakes of iron, calcium, vitamin A, and ascorbic acid tend to be particularly low. The average birth weight of infants born to girls 17 years of age or younger is substantially lower than that of infants born to older mothers, and infant mortality is higher.

In the ever-present environment of fashionable slimness, many teenagers consume too few calories, and if they become pregnant, they may persist in consuming too few calories. However, adequate energy intake is critical for support and growth during adolescence. Because energy expenditure is variable, the best assurance of adequate calorie intake is a desirable gain in weight. This should be accomplished by individual dietary counseling on the basis of estimates of activity. Allowances must meet not only pregnancy requirements but also individual needs of patients at different stages of growth.

The most conclusive recent study indicates that pregnant teenagers need at least 1.25 g of protein per kilogram of body weight to meet the usual needs of pregnancy and to allow some growth of lean body mass (King et al., 1973; Calloway, 1974).

DIABETES AND PREGNANCY

Nutritional requirements for the diabetic pregnant woman are not different from those for the nondiabetic (Younger, 1975). See page 28 for general guidelines for planning a diet for diabetes. Control of the rate of weight gain should be emphasized, the goal for total weight gain being the same as that in the nondiabetic patient. In nondiabetic pregnancy, the endocrine changes are reflected by a state of relative insulin resistance. In a pregnant diabetic woman, these changes are manifested by a progressive increase in the insulin requirement as the pregnancy advances.

It is important to distribute meals and between-meal feedings in a fairly even pattern throughout each day in an attempt to match the action of injected insulin; some shifting of food from one time of day to another may serve to minimize hyperglycemia or hypoglycemia tending to occur at a particular hour. A bedtime feeding should be given routinely; between-meal feedings may be helpful.   An even distribution of food intake serves to minimize ketogenesis and to lessen the chance of uncomfortable and potentially hazardous hypoglycemic episodes. A pregnant woman with unstable diabetes may have significant loss of calories as glucose in the urine.

Good control of diabetes during pregnancy favors a good outcome. Poor control with much glycosuria and ketonuria is associated with miscarriage and increased perinatal mortality. The occurrence of frank ketoacidosis increases the risk of fetal death.

It is necessary to distinguish between *starvation* ketosis and *diabetic* ketoacidosis. Fetal glucose uptake accelerates the normal ketogenic response to starvation, as shown by blood ketone levels two to three times those in the nonpregnant state after an overnight fast (Coniff and Maeder, 1976). The distinction between starvation ketosis and diabetic ketosis can usually be made by measurement of plasma glucose.   A low or normal glucose value indicates that ketonuria is primarily the consequence of lack of carbohydrate, whereas an elevated level indicates that ketonuria is mainly the result of a need for insulin. If ketosis from lack of insulin is severe enough, the condition is designated "diabetic ketoacidosis." The finding of starvation ketosis suggests that the diet is not supplying enough carbohydrate or that feedings are spaced at too long an interval.

There appears to be a significant reduction in intelligence quotient in offspring of nondiabetic mothers with starvation ketosis in pregnancy. The importance of recognizing and preventing ketosis should not be minimized (Churchill and Berendes, 1969).

OBESITY AND PREGNANCY

It is recommended that weight gain for the overweight pregnant woman be kept near the average (9 to 11 kg) and follow a normal curve (Simpson et al., 1975; Pitkin, 1977a and 1977b). Attempts to correct obesity during pregnancy by undue restriction of calories may have an adverse effect on fetal survival, perhaps through induction of ketosis or protein catabolism.

It has been recommended that the diet in pregnancy should supply no less than 1,600 calories (Stein and Susser, 1975), 150 g of carbohydrate (Felig, 1977), and 80 g of protein. Because of the accelerated tendency for ketosis during pregnancy, fasting periods should be avoided by means of an even distribution of food throughout the day.

Pregnancy is an excellent time to reinforce the principles of good nutrition. Energy intake above normal pregnancy needs results in deposition of excessive fat and can contribute to the development of long-term obesity. Efforts to limit excessive weight may be warranted to prevent initiation of lifelong obesity in the mother, but these efforts should be directed toward bringing the rate of gain close to normal. It is safer to approach weight reduction after delivery.

LACTATION

During pregnancy, the estimated average increase in body fat of about 4 kg represents an energy store of some 35,000 kcal, or enough to subsidize lactation for 4 months at the rate of 300 kcal daily. The Recommended Dietary Allowances specify a 500-calorie increase per day in the diet to normalize body composition progressively and to provide for adequate lactation (Committee on Nutrition of the American College of Obstetricians and Gynecologists, 1974; Food and Nutrition Board, National Research Council, 1980). For the reference woman, this would be a daily intake of 2,200 kcal. In the weight reduction diet for the obese lactating woman, 500 kcal should be allowed for lactation.

This diet, in addition, should continue to supply an increase of 20 g of protein of high biologic value above the usual Recommended Dietary Allowance of 44 to 46 g. Vitamin and mineral needs ordinarily will be supplied from these additional foods.

For milk formation, the lactating mother should be counseled to drink generous amounts of water and other fluids. Human milk contains about 1.2% protein; an average daily secretion of 850 ml contains about 10 g of protein. Secretion of as much as 1,200 ml per day is not unusual. Dietary protein is converted to milk protein with about 70% efficiency; therefore, an additional 20 g of protein per day is sufficient for the upper range of milk production (Shank, 1970; Thomson et al., 1970; Calloway, 1974). The calcium intake of 1,200 mg per day advised for pregnancy should be continued through lactation.

SMOKING AND ALCOHOL

Both smoking and drinking alcoholic beverages can adversely affect a woman's nutritional state (Committee on Maternal Nutrition, National Research Council, 1970; Corruccini and Cruskie, 1975). Women who smoke are known to have infants of lower birth weight than those of nonsmokers. Alcoholic beverages can become a problem when they replace necessary amounts of food in the diet, and numerous nutritional deficiencies can result. Thiamine deficiency may occur because of impaired intestinal absorption of this vitamin. Infants with fetal alcohol syndrome, characterized by malformations and mental retardation, have been born to alcoholic mothers (Ouellette and Rosett, 1977).

SELECTED BIBLIOGRAPHY

Calloway, D. H.: Recommended dietary allowances for protein and energy, 1973. J. Am. Diet. Assoc., 64:157-162, 1974.

Churchill, J. A., and Berendes, H. W.: Intelligence of children whose mothers had acetonuria during pregnancy. Sci. Publ. Pan Am. Health Organ., No. 185, 1969, pp. 30-35.

Committee on Maternal Nutrition, National Research Council: Maternal Nutrition and the Course of Pregnancy. Washington, D.C., National Academy of Sciences, 1970.

Committee on Nutrition of the American College of Obstetricians and Gynecologists: Nutrition in Maternal Health Care. Chicago, 1974.

Committee on Nutrition of the Mother and Preschool Child, Food and Nutrition Board, National Research Council: Laboratory Indices of Nutritional Status in Pregnancy. Washington, D.C., National Academy of Sciences, 1978.

Coniff, R. F., and Maeder, E. C., Jr.: Management of the pregnant diabetic. Minn. Med., 59:772-778, 1976.

Corruccini, C. G., and Cruskie, P. E.: Nutrition during pregnancy and lactation. Sacramento, Maternal and Child Health Unit, California Department of Health, 1975, pp. 12-13.

Emerson, K., Jr., Saxena, B. N., and Poindexter, E. L.: Caloric cost of normal pregnancy. Obstet. Gynecol., 40:786-794, 1972.

Felig, P.: Maternal and fetal fuel homeostasis in human pregnancy. Am. J. Clin. Nutr., 26:998-1005, 1973.

Felig, P.: Body fuel metabolism and diabetes mellitus in pregnancy. Med. Clin. North Am., 61:43-66, 1977.

Food and Nutrition Board, National Research Council: Recommended Dietary Allowances. Ninth revised edtion. Washington, D.C., National Academy of Sciences, 1980.

Hillman, R. W., and Goodhart, R. S.: Nutrition in pregnancy. In Goodhart, R. S., and Shils, M. E., eds.: Modern Nutrition in Health and Disease: Dietotherapy. Fifth edition. Philadelphia, Lea & Febiger, 1973, pp. 647-658.

Hytten, F. E., and Leitch, I.: The Physiology of Human Pregnancy. Second edition. Oxford, Blackwell Scientific Publications, 1971.

King, J. C., Calloway, D. H., and Margen, S.: Nitrogen retention, total body ^{40}K and weight gain in teenage pregnant girls. J. Nutr., 103:772-785, 1973.

Moghissi, K. S., and Evans, T. N., eds.: Nutritional Impacts on Women: Throughout Life With Emphasis on Reproduction. Hagerstown, Maryland, Harper & Row, Publishers, 1977, pp. 86-106.

Ouellette, E. M., and Rosett, H. L.: The effect of maternal alcohol ingestion during pregnancy on offspring. *In* Moghissi, K. S., and Evans, T. N., eds.: Nutritional Impacts on Women: Throughout Life With Emphasis on Reproduction. Hagerstown, Maryland, Harper & Row, Publishers, 1977, pp. 107-120.

on Reproduction, Hagerstown, Maryland, Harper & Row, Publishers, 1977, pp. 107-120.

Pike, R. L., and Gursky, D. S.: Further evidence of deleterious effects produced by sodium restriction during pregnancy. Am. J. Clin. Nutr., 23:883-889, 1970.

Pitkin, R. M.: Nutrition during pregnancy: The clinical approach. *In* Winick, M., ed.: Current Concepts in Nutrition. Vol. 5. Nutritional Disorders of American Women. New York, John Wiley & Sons, 1977a, pp. 27-36.

Pitkin, R. M.: Nutritional influences during pregnancy. Med. Clin. North Am., 61:3-15, 1977b.

Position Statement on Nutrition and Pregnancy, The American College of Obstetricians and Gynecologists, December 1972.

Rosso, P.: Maternal nutrition, nutrient exchange, and fetal growth. *In* Winick, M., ed.: Current Concepts in Nutrition. Vol. 5. Nutritional Disorders of American Women. New York, John Wiley & Sons, 1977, pp. 3-25.

Shank, R. E.: A chink in our armor. Nutr. Today, 5:2-11, 1970.

Simpson, J. W., Lawless, R. W., and Mitchell, A. C.: Responsibility of the obstetrician to the fetus. II. Influence of prepregnancy weight and pregnancy weight gain on birthweight. Obstet. Gynecol., 45:481-487, 1975.

Stein, Z., and Susser, M.: The Dutch famine, 1944-1945, and the reproductive process. II. Interrelations of caloric rations and six indices at birth. Pediatr. Res., 9:76-83, 1975.

Thomson, A. M., Hytten, F. E., and Billewicz, W. Z.: The energy cost of human lactation. Br. J. Nutr., 24:565-572, 1970.

Weiss, W., and Jackson, E. C.: Maternal factors affecting birth weight. Sci. Publ. Pan Am. Health Organ., No. 185, 1969, pp. 54-59.

Younger, D.: Management of diabetes and pregnancy. *In* Sussman, K. E., and Metz, R. J. S., eds.: Diabetes Mellitus. Fourth edition. New York, American Diabetes Association, 1975, p. 138.

SECTION 5

NORMAL NUTRITION AND THERAPEUTIC DIETS FOR INFANTS AND CHILDREN

MEETING NUTRITIONAL NEEDS IN THE FIRST YEAR

As an infant grows, both energy and protein needs decrease in proportion to body weight. During the first 6 months of life, an infant needs 100 to 120 kcal/kg of body weight per day. By the end of the second 6 months, daily needs have decreased to 90 to 100 kcal/kg. In the course of these two time spans, daily protein needs decrease from 2.2 to 2 g/kg. There is a recognized need for iron, which must be supplied no later than the age of 4 months, at levels approximating 1 mg/kg per day.

Human milk* is ideally suited for the human infant. The immune factors in human milk are especially protective to the baby. The fat of human milk is better absorbed than is the butterfat of cow's milk; human milk contains more polyunsaturated fatty acids than does whole cow's milk. The sodium content of human milk is low, and the amount of protein is appropriate for the infant. Allergic reactions to human milk are few or nonexistent.

Cow's milk,† on the other hand, has a high protein and mineral content that increases the risk of dehydration and hypernatremia whenever diarrhea or other conditions increase the demand for water. It can also cause allergic reactions in susceptible infants and, on the basis of curd formation, is difficult to digest.

Infant formulas‡ are made to simulate human milk and are different from cow's milk in important ways. The protein in formulas has been partially denatured to make it more digestible than that in whole cow's milk. Formulas also have levels of calcium, phosphorus, and other minerals more in keeping with infants' needs and physiologic capabilities. Infant formulas are essentially cholesterol-free, whereas cow's milk contains about 20 mg/dl and human milk, 30 mg/dl. However, commercial formulas do not have the immune properties of human milk.

The recommended fluoride supplementation for breast-fed infants is 0.25 mg/day. Supplementation for formula-fed infants is based on the fluoride content of the drinking water: 0.25 mg per day if the fluoride concentration of the water supply is less than 0.3 ppm and no supplement if the fluoride concentration of the water supply is more than 0.3 ppm (Fomon et al., 1979).

Although weaning to whole milk may occur by 9 months, delay until 1 year is preferable. In the older infant being fed whole milk, intake should be limited to 1 to 1½ pints a day to help control intake of calories and minimize the risk of nutritional iron deficiency.

DISTRIBUTION OF CALORIES

The caloric distribution for protein, fat, and carbohydrate for full-term infants should be patterned after the distribution found in human milk. Commercial formulas as now constituted meet this criterion. This caloric distribution is compatible with the physiologic needs of the full-term infant and neither imposes an excess protein load nor provides a ketogenic diet.

---

*Vitamin D and iron supplementation desirable.
†Vitamin C and iron supplementation desirable.
‡Should be selected from those fortified with iron so that supplementation is not needed.

The caloric distributions* provided by a typical commercial formula and three kinds of milk are as follows:

	% of Total Energy		
	Protein	*Fat*	*Carbohydrate*
Human milk	8	55	37
Commercial formula (milk-based)	9	49	42
Whole cow's milk	21	45	34
Skim milk	40	3	57

*Adapted from: A continuing dialogue on infant nutrition. *In* Filer, L. J., ed.: Dialogues in Infant Nutrition: A Foundation for Lasting Health? Bloomfield, New Jersey, Health Learning Systems, Vol. 1, No. 1, April 1977. By permission.

Cow's milk provides a higher intake of protein (20% of total energy) than necessary, an amount that can be considered excessive. Skim milk provides a highly excessive intake of energy as protein and falls far short of providing sufficient energy in the form of fat.

The primary problem with the use of skim milk during the first year of life is its low caloric density. Skim milk provides about 35 kcal/dl. In contrast, human milk and commercial formulas provide 67 kcal/dl. Skim milk also is inappropriate because of its inadequate content of iron, ascorbic acid, and essential fatty acids. Without question, the prolonged feeding of skim milk may result in anemia and essential fatty acid deficiency.

If 2% milk is fed, the percentage of calories from protein is likely to be substantially above the desirable range and the percentage of calories from fat, below the desirable range. Also, the intake of essential fatty acids is probably less than advisable.

No wide clinical experience is available to indicate the safety of distributions of calories differing greatly from the recommendation of 7 to 16% of calories from protein, 35 to 55% from fat, and the rest from carbohydrate.

INTRODUCTION OF SOLID FOODS

Although solid foods should be introduced when the infant approaches 6 months of age, a more realistic time may be between 4 and 6 months. It is reasonable to delay the introduction of solid foods because of the cost and the potential for overfeeding.

If solid foods are introduced early, the infant may be fed a diet that varies strikingly from the recommended caloric distribution—even though the recommendation is fairly wide. As foods other than human milk or formula are introduced, composition of the total diet must be considered. For example, if certain strained foods (fruit juices, plain or creamed vegetables, soups, or dinners) are substituted for human milk or formula, the infant may receive fewer calories than if human milk or formula were fed. On the other hand, the early introduction of solids without a concomitant decrease in formula can result in an overweight infant.

A reasonable schedule* for the introduction of solid foods is as follows:

	Human Milk (or Commercial Formula) Plus					
	No Solid Food	Cereal	Fruit	Vegetables	Meat	Finger Foods
Age (months)	Birth to 6	6 to 7	7 to 8	8 to 9	9 to 10	10 to 12
Interval (months)	6	1	1	1	1	2

*Adapted from: The feeding transitions in the first year. *In* Barness, L. A., ed.: Dialogues in Infant Nutrition: A Foundation for Lasting Health? Bloomfield, New Jersey, Health Learning Systems, Vol. 1, No. 2, July 1977.

Simple foods are introduced singly, so that if the infant reacts adversely, the offending food can be readily spotted. By about 1 year of age, the infant can begin whole milk and table foods.

SELECTED BIBLIOGRAPHY

A continuing dialogue on infant nutrition. *In* Filer, L. J., Jr., ed.: Dialogues in Infant Nutrition: A Foundation for Lasting Health? Bloomfield, New Jersey, Health Learning Systems, Vol. 1, No. 1, April 1977.
Committee on Nutrition: Fluoride supplementation: Revised dosage schedule. Pediatrics, 63:150-152, 1979.
Fomon, S. J.: Skim Milk in Infant Feeding (DHEW Publication No. [HSM] 73-5608). United States Department of Health, Education, and Welfare, January 1973.
Fomon, S. J.: Infant Nutrition. Second edition. Philadelphia, W. B. Saunders Company, 1974.
Fomon, S. J., Filer, L. J., Jr., Anderson, T. A., et al.: Recommendations for feeding normal infants. Pediatrics, 63:52-59, 1979.
The feeding transitions in the first year. *In* Barness, L. A., ed.: Dialogues in Infant Nutrition: A Foundation for Lasting Health? Bloomfield, New Jersey, Health Learning Systems, Vol. 1, No. 2, July 1977.

NUTRITIONAL REQUIREMENTS OF EARLY CHILDHOOD

The 1-year-old begins to show a decided change in appetite and in interest in food. This change should not be interpreted as a "poor" appetite but rather as the normal appetite for that age. The cause in large measure is a decrease in growth rate and, therefore, in the amount of food needed.

Protein needs for growth of muscles and other tissue are high during this period, whereas caloric needs from 1 to 3 years are low. To ensure that the diet is adequate in other nutrients, one must select the toddler's food carefully. A varied menu (see the guidelines below) provides an adequate intake of vitamins and minerals, with the possible exception of iron, if the toddler's appetite permits the food to be consumed.

See the Appendix for the Recommended Dietary Allowances for 1- to 3-year-olds.

SERVING GUIDELINES

How much is a child-sized serving? Guidelines* for children between the ages of 1 and 6 are as follows:

Basic Four Food Groups	Size of One Serving	Number of Servings per Day
Meat		
Including meat; fish; poultry; eggs; dried beans, peas, and lentils; and peanut butter	1 oz of lean meat, fish, or poultry	2 or more plus 1 egg
Fruits and vegetables		
Every day: include a citrus fruit or other good source of vitamin C	1/4 cup of juice, 1/2 fruit, or 1/4 cup of cooked vegetable	4 or more
Every other day: include a dark green or deep yellow vegetable for vitamin A		
Cereals and breads		
Including whole-grain enriched or fortified foods, such as cereal, bread, cornmeal, macaroni, noodles, rice, and spaghetti	1/2 slice of bread, 1/4 cup of cooked cereal, or about 1/2 cup of ready-to-eat cereal	4 or more
Milk		
Including cheese, yogurt, milk beverages, and milk desserts	1 cup (8 oz)	2 or more

*Adapted from Mitchell, H. S., Rynbergen, H. J., Anderson, L., et al.: Nutrition in Health and Disease. Sixteenth edition. Philadelphia, J. B. Lippincott Company, 1976, p. 266.

Foods in the basic groups above need to be supplemented by different amounts of butter or margarine, salad dressings, jams, jellies, desserts, and, occasionally, other sweets to meet the energy needs of different age groups. The foods in the guidelines for children aged 1 through 6 are also essential, but in increased quantities, for children older than 6 and for adolescents.

NUTRITIONAL REQUIREMENTS OF CHILDREN

The Recommended Dietary Allowances (see Appendix, page 266) for children from age 4 through age 10 are the same for boys and girls. There is a gradual increase in growth, and, therefore, in the recommended amounts for most nutrients throughout childhood. If the guidelines for children on page 184 are followed and servings are matched to age group, the Recommended Dietary Allowances for children will be met.

NUTRITIONAL NEEDS OF ADOLESCENTS

Although nutritional needs during adolescence vary individually and according to sex, they closely parallel velocity of growth in all persons. That is, the period of greatest nutritional need coincides with the peak rate of growth during the adolescent growth spurt.

One can therefore roughly define the periods of greatest nutritional need in adolescence as those between 10 1/4 and 13 1/2 years for girls and 11 3/4 and 14 1/2 years for boys (PHS publications, 1973). Others emphasize the limitations of determining an individual's nutritional needs by chronologic age alone, because the onset of puberty varies so widely. Since the growth spurt and the sequence of sexual development are related, it is useful to consider an adolescent's state of maturation to assess nutritional needs accurately.

Because few studies have been done on adolescent nutritional requirements, the Recommended Dietary Allowances (see the Appendix, page 266) for this group have been extrapolated from findings on the needs of children and adults. Thus, their accuracy is open to question.

A varied diet (see the guidelines, page 184) provides an adequate intake of vitamins and minerals, with the possible exception of iron. Whether or not a given adolescent's nutritional needs are being met is probably best determined by assessing the adequacy of that person's growth rate.

SELECTED BIBLIOGRAPHY

Betty Crocker's How to Feed Your Family to Keep Them Fit & Happy. . .No Matter What. Minneapolis, General Mills, 1972.

Daniel, W., Jr., et al.: Nutrition in Adolescence: Final Report (Research Grant #MC-R-010209-02-0). United States Department of Health, Education and Welfare, 1974.

Mitchell, H. S., Rynbergen, H. J., Anderson, L., et al.: Nutrition in Health and Disease. Sixteenth edition. Philadelphia, J. B. Lippincott Company, 1976.

PHS publications: Height and weight of United States youths 12 through 17 years of age. Am. J. Clin. Nutr., 26:1031-1032, 1973.

Torre, C. T.: Nutritional needs of adolescents. M.C.N., 2:118-127, 1977.

FEEDING OF INFANTS OF LOW BIRTH WEIGHT

All infants of low birth weight (less than 2,500 g) are not alike. Those who are normally grown but premature differ from those who are malnourished in utero and gestationally more mature. The dietary intake and nutritional requirements of the two groups vary considerably. In the lower range of birth weights, however, these two groups can be considered together. In the birth weights of about 1,000 g, there is little difference in early feeding. Between 1,000 and 1,750 g, the mature infant who is small for gestational age usually feeds more vigorously and actively than the gestationally immature infant and requires less special support. At weights of more than 1,750 g, the infant who is small for gestational age usually can be fed as a term infant, whereas the gestationally immature infant still requires special feeding techniques and care. Between 1,750 and 2,500 g, the premature infant without disease requires only experience and care in feeding techniques.

Whenever possible, all mothers of low-birth-weight infants should be encouraged to breast feed. Breast milk may have to be supplemented with synthetic formulas or medium-chain triglycerides, or both, to enrich its caloric concentration. Fresh milk from breast milk donors may be used for infants who cannot tolerate synthetic formulas.

If the low-birth-weight infant is well and free of respiratory distress, the first feedings are begun within 4 to 6 hours of birth. As a general rule, distilled water or, if available, maternal colostrum is used. After a first successful feeding, a half-strength formula or full-strength colostrum and, still later, milk are given. The goal of feeding low-birth-weight infants should be the gradual achievement of between 120 and 150 kcal/kg of body weight per day by the second week of life. In sick and distressed infants, these levels are rarely achieved, but caloric intakes of even half the stated goal may spare tissue catabolism and meet some of the energy needs.

The water and electrolyte requirements of the low-birth-weight infant in the first several days of life depend on the environment in which the infant is kept. If the infant is placed in a radiant warmer, the excess loss of water must be anticipated in providing for daily requirements. For the low-birth-weight infant in a radiant warmer, the goal of the first 2 days is 60 to 80 ml/kg of body weight per day. Amounts are gradually increased until 150 ml/kg of body weight per day is achieved. The feedings are carefully monitored, and the variables indicating hydration are closely followed. If full oral intake cannot achieve proper levels, fluids are given intravenously with glucose and electrolytes to supplement oral feedings.

The means by which these goals are achieved depend entirely on the clinical state of the infant. At the upper scale of low birth weight—between 1,750 and 2,500 g—many infants are vigorous and suck and swallow with skill. Some infants, however, are not. Some larger infants may feed well for a short time but gradually become fatigued in the first several days of life and require other means of calorie provision. For infants of lower weight, a simple technique of continuous orogastric or nasogastric gavage should be used. The volume of intake is gradually increased until the desired caloric goal is achieved. Most infants tolerate these techniques and rapidly thrive to a point at which oral feedings can be started. As oral intake is tolerated, the gavage feeding cycles are gradually reduced until the infant is tolerating all oral intake. In some distressed infants, additional calories must be provided through parenteral alimentation with amino acids and high concentrations of glucose.

SELECTED BIBLIOGRAPHY

Babson, S. G.: Feeding the low-birth-weight infant. J. Pediatr., 79:694-701, 1971.

Committee on Nutrition: Nutritional needs of low-birth-weight infants. Pediatrics, 60:519-530, 1977.

Davidson, M., Levine, S. Z., Bauer, C. H., et al.: Feeding studies in low-birth-weight infants. I. Relationships of dietary protein, fat, and electrolyte to rates of weight gain, clinical courses, and serum chemical concentrations. J. Pediatr., 70:695-713, 1967.

Fomon, S. J., Ziegler, E. E., and Vázquez, H. D.: Human milk and the small premature infant. Am. J. Dis. Child., 131:463-467, 1977.

Liebhaber, M., Lewiston, N. J., Asquith, M. T., et al.: Alterations of lymphocytes and of antibody content of human milk after processing. J. Pediatr., 91:897-900, 1977.

Räihä, N. C. R., Heinonen, K., Rassin, D. K., et al.: Milk protein quantity and quality in low-birthweight infants: I. Metabolic responses and effects on growth. Pediatrics, 57:659-674, 1976.

MODIFICATIONS OF GENERAL DIETS FOR CHILDREN

Therapeutic diets for adults can be modified to meet the nutritional requirements of children. Such diets are individualized according to the child's age, appetite, and activity. See the adult section of this manual for general principles of the diets for protein control, gastrointestinal disorders, sodium control, hyperlipidemia, and anorexia nervosa.

WEIGHT CONTROL FOR CHILDREN

Obesity is a serious national health problem. Although less common and a less serious health threat in the young than in adults, it deserves careful consideration. Obese parents beget obese children. Obesity that begins during childhood is likely to persist into adulthood. If a child enters adolescence obese, the chances are one to four against achievement of normal body weight. If a child is still obese at the end of adolescence, the chances increase to about 28 to one against normality (Stunkard and Burt, 1967). Since programs for the successful control of weight among adults are at best only partially satisfactory, management of the diet during the formative years of childhood may prove to be the most effective single approach to the problem of obesity among adults.

Ideally, the primary goal of weight control in the child is to prevent rather than correct obesity. In the young child, efforts are directed toward education of the family, particularly the mother. Physicians who care for the young must be alerted to the importance of developing or impending obesity and be willing to devote time to the patient and give support to the dietitian in the education of the family. Although there may be a familial type of obesity, most obese children are likely to be obese because of excessive caloric intake based on errors or misunderstandings.

In older children, the success of weight reduction or weight control depends on motivation of the child. Efforts to bring about rapid weight reduction by strenuous diets are rarely justified and even more rarely successful. Instead, a program of gradual caloric reduction accompanied by an increase in activities and augmented by growth is a better approach.

The dietitian begins by taking a dietary history and reviewing the child's schedule of activities. The calorie level established for the child's diet depends on the child's age, degree of overweight, present dietary intake, and present activity level.

A reasonable calorie level for the moderately overweight child might be basal calories for present height, weight, age, and sex, whereas the substantially overweight child may need a restriction equal to basal calories for ideal weight. A program of activity is then discussed. The goal is to increase daily activity from the present level. Emphasis is placed on activities that can be participated in throughout life, such as biking, swimming, walking, and tennis.

Once the calorie and activity goals are established, the dietitian and the child work out a modest but realistic program suited to the child's particular needs. Nutrient requirements for growth and development as well as food sources of essential nutrients are outlined for the child. The interrelationship of energy required by the body, ingested energy, and energy expenditure is explained. The dietitian must reflect confidence in the child's ability to control weight while realistically and honestly discussing the problems that weight control entails. The child is then given an opportunity to ask questions about the program and is assured of continuing support and interest when the program is undertaken. Primary emphasis throughout the program is placed not on the amount of weight lost but on determining if the child is becoming more aware of foods, has a more realistic idea of requirements, and is engaging in activity on a more regular basis.

Parental participation in the program is generally discouraged beyond that of making available the foods included in the dietary program. (See the food exchange list beginning on page 36.)

Successful programs to control weight must be major reeducation efforts in both diet and exercise.

SELECTED BIBLIOGRAPHY

Huse, D. M., Palumbo, P. J., Nelson, R. A., et al.: Grammar school: Site for identifying and treating obese children (abstract). Second International Congress on Obesity, Washington, D.C., October 23-26, 1977.
Stunkard, A., and Burt, V.: Obesity and the body image. II. Age at onset of disturbances in the body image. Am. J. Psychiatry, 123:1443-1447, 1967.

DIETARY MANAGEMENT OF DIABETES

GENERAL CONSIDERATIONS

The nutrient needs of the child with diabetes are the same as those of the child who does not have diabetes (see page 185). Greater attention, however, must be given to the timing of the meals and snacks and the consistency of intake from day to day. Meals should be at regular times each day. The diet for the preadolescent diabetic is planned with midmorning, midafternoon, and bedtime feedings. Diets for older children are planned with a midafternoon and a bedtime feeding. A midmorning feeding may be included if needed. A protein food should be included with each feeding. Meals and snacks are calculated to distribute calories, carbohydrate, and protein in a consistent manner. See page 36 for the food exchange list.

The diet is reevaluated periodically to accommodate the child's changing nutritional needs during growth. Careful attention to helping the child understand the principles of the diabetic diet allows proper lifelong eating habits to be established.

METHODS OF DETERMINING NUTRITIONAL NEEDS

Calorie needs of the child are determined primarily from present dietary intake obtained by a thorough dietary history. Recommended Dietary Allowances and calorie requirements determined by the nomogram and estimated level of activity serve as supportive data for calorie needs. The protein level of the diet should meet the Recommended Dietary Allowances. The dietary history aids in planning the distribution of nutrients among meals and snacks. The diet is prepared to modify existing food habits as little as possible and to ensure adequate nutrition for normal growth and development.

EATING AWAY FROM HOME

The diabetic child may choose to eat a school lunch or a bag lunch brought from home. If the school lunch is chosen, the child can be taught to select the right foods from the cafeteria menu.

School Lunch*

Food Group	Food Item	Serving
Meat and meat alternate†	Lean meat, poultry, or fish	2 oz (edible portion as served)
	or	
	Cheese	2 oz
	or	
	Egg	1
	or	
	Cooked dry beans or dry peas	1/2 cup
	or	
	Peanut butter	4 tbsp
	or	
	An equivalent of any combination of the foods listed above	
Vegetables and fruits	Two or more vegetables or fruits, or both	3/4 cup
Bread	Whole-grain or enriched bread	1 slice
	or	
	Other bread, such as corn bread, biscuits, rolls, and muffins, made of whole-grain or enriched flour	1 serving
Butter or margarine	Butter or fortified margarine	1 tsp
Milk	Fluid milk as beverage	1/2 pt

*Data from Robinson, C. H., and Lawler, M. R.: Normal and Therapeutic Nutrition. Fifteenth edition. New York, Macmillan Publishing Company, 1977, p. 323.

†To meet the requirement, the foods in the meat group must be served in a main dish or in a main dish with one other menu item.

School lunch menus often are published in local newspapers, or the menus can be obtained from the school. Supplements from home may be necessary for lunch and for snacks to meet the needs of the diet.

Nutritional and Exchange Values For Fast Foods*

Exchange values for fast-food restaurants are useful when the child eats away from home. A revised food exchange list should be obtained periodically from the restaurant.

	Nutritional Values				Exchange Values		
	Total Calories	Carbohydrate g	Protein g	Fat g	Medium-fat Meat	Fat	Starch
Arby's							
Roast Beef Sandwich	434		Not available		3	1	2
Super Roast Beef Sandwich	691		Not available		3	5	3
Junior Roast Beef Sandwich	250		Not available		2	…	1
Ham 'N Cheese	457		Not available		4	…	2
Turkey Sandwich (with dressing)	433		Not available		3	1 1/2	2
Arthur Treacher's (fish, chips, coleslaw)							
3-piece Dinner	1,100	91	38	65	4	9	6
2-piece Dinner	905	83	28	51	2 1/2	8	3 1/2
Burger Chef							
Hamburger	250	23	12	12	1	1 1/2	1 1/2
Double Hamburger	325	28	20	15	2 1/2	1	2
Super Chef	530	36	30	29	3 1/2	2	2 1/2
Big Chef	535	41	25	30	3	3	3
French Fries	240	30	3	12	…	2	2
Burger King							
Hamburger	240	25	13	10	2	…	1 1/2
Double Hamburger	370	25	25	20	3	1	1 1/2

Nutritional and Exchange values For Fast Foods (continued)

	Nutritional Values				Exchange Values		
	Total Calories	Carbohydrate g	Protein g	Fat g	Medium-fat Meat	Fat	Starch
Burger King (continued)							
Cheeseburger	310	26	17	15	2	1	1 1/2
Double Cheeseburger	420	26	26	23	3	2	1 1/2
Whopper Junior	300	26	13	16	1 1/2	1 1/2	1 1/2
Whopper Junior with Cheese	350	26	17	20	2	2	1 1/2
Whopper	650	50	27	38	3	4	3
Whopper with Cheese	760	51	34	47	4	5	3
Hot Dog	290	24	11	17	1	2 1/2	1 1/2
French Fries: Small	200	28	3	10	...	2	2
Large	320	42	5	15	...	3	3
Onion Rings: Small	150	20	2	7	...	1	1 1/2
Large	220	31	2	10	...	2	2
Dairy Queen							
Hamburger	260	29	14	10	1 1/2	...	2
Cheeseburger	320	30	18	14	2	1	2
Big Brazier	460	36	26	23	3	1	2 1/2
Big Brazier with Cheese	550	38	31	30	4	1	2 1/2
Super Brazier	780	35	53	48	6	2	2 1/2
Hot Dog	270	23	11	15	1	2	1 1/2
Hot Dog with Chili or Cheese	330	25	14	19	2	1	1 1/2
Fish Sandwich	400	41	20	17	2	1	3

French Fries: Regular	200	25	2	10	...	2	1 1/2
Large	320	40	3	16	...	3	3
Onion Rings	300	33	6	17	...	3	2
Cone: Small	110	18	3	3	...	1	1
Regular	230	35	6	7	...	1 1/2	2 1/2
Large	340	52	10	10	...	2	3 1/2
Kentucky Fried Chicken (fried chicken, mashed potato, coleslaw, rolls)							
3-piece Dinner: Original	830	61	50	43	6	2 1/2	4
Crispy	1,070	74	54	62	6	6 1/2	5
2-piece Dinner: Original	595	51	35	28	2	1 1/2	3 1/2
Crispy	665	40	37	40	4 1/2	3 1/2	3
Long John Silver's (fish, chips, coleslaw)							
3-piece Dinner	1,190	100	55	63	6	7	7
2-piece Dinner	955	89	38	50	4	6	6
McDonald's							
Hamburger	260	30	13	10	1 1/2	...	2
Cheeseburger	300	31	16	13	2	...	2
Quarter-Pounder	420	33	26	21	3	1	2
Quarter-Pounder with Cheese	520	34	31	29	4	2	2
Big Mac	540	39	26	31	3	3	2 1/2
Filet-O-Fish	400	34	14	23	1 1/2	3	2
French Fries	210	26	3	11	...	2	1 1/2
Egg McMuffin	350	26	18	20	2	2	1 1/2

Nutritional and Exchange Values For Fast Foods (continued)

	Nutritional Values				Exchange Values		
	Total Calories	Carbohydrate g	Protein g	Fat g	Medium-fat Meat	Fat	Starch
Pizza Hut (cheese pizza)							
Individual: Thick Crust	1,030	143	71	19	7 1/2	...	9 1/2
Thin Crust	1,005	128	61	28	6	...	8 1/2
1/2 of 13-inch: Thick Crust	900	113	65	21	7	...	7 1/2
Thin Crust	850	103	50	26	5	...	7
1/2 of 15-inch: Thick Crust	1,200	148	83	31	9	...	10
Thin Crust	1,150	144	66	35	7	...	9 1/2
Wendy's							
Hamburger: Single	440	33	25	24	3	2	2
Double	630	34	47	34	6	1	2
Triple	780	27	66	45	9	...	2
Cheeseburger: Single	520	32	31	30	4	2	2
Triple	940	28	73	59	10	2	2
Chili	250	23	22	7	3	...	1 1/2
French Fries	340	42	4	17	...	3	3

*Modified from Nutritional and exchange values for fast foods. Diabetes Forecast, 29:10-11, May-June 1976, and Exchange values for fast food restaurants. Minneapolis, Minnesota, Diabetes Education Center, 1978.

EATING FOR EXTRA ACTIVITY

When the diabetic engages in activities more strenuous than those in the normal daily routine, diet must be readjusted. The following guidelines* will be helpful.

Type of Activity	Examples of Activities	Amount of Food to Be Eaten	
		For Activity Not Directly after a Meal or Snack	*For Activity Directly after a Meal or Snack*
Light	Leisure walking Leisure cycling Vacuuming Golfing	1 fruit exchange before each hour of activity	1 fruit exchange added to meal or snack for 1 hour of activity
Heavy	Strenuous exercise Strenuous cycling Strenuous running Swimming Football Hockey Basketball Shoveling heavy snow	1 bread exchange, 1 meat exchange, 1 fat exchange, and 1 fruit exchange before each hour of activity	1 meat exchange or 1 milk exchange plus 1 fruit exchange added to meal or snack for 1 hour of activity
	Avoid strenuous physical activity directly before a meal.		

*Modified from Methodist Hospital Nutrition Staff: Bone up on exercise and diet. ADAM in Action. March 1977. By permission of American Diabetes Association.

Because of individual tolerances and needs, the child may have to try different amounts of food for a given amount of exercise: Too much will result in excessive glycosuria, while too little may permit an insulin reaction to occur. The parent should be sure the child carries a readily available source of carbohydrate (sugar cubes, sugar candy) to be used in the event of an insulin reaction.

KETOGENIC DIET FOR CHILDREN

GENERAL DESCRIPTION

The ketogenic diet is a weighted diet used in the prophylactic treatment of some types of epilepsy in children. The diet is planned to produce ketosis by reversing the usual ratio of dietary carbohydrate and fat.

NUTRITIONAL ADEQUACY

The physician should prescribe a multivitamin and calcium and iron supplements, since this diet does not meet the Recommended Dietary Allowances for children.

INDICATIONS AND RATIONALE

High in fat and low in carbohydrate, the diet is designed to produce ketone bodies as a result of the incomplete oxidation of fat. Ketone bodies (acetone, acetoacetic acid, and β-hydroxybutyric acid) are thought to have an anticonvulsant action.

The diet is planned to provide adequate calories for normal growth, development, and activity. The amount of fat in the diet is gradually increased, and the carbohydrate content is decreased. The amount of protein stays at the level required by the individual.

This dietary program is used when drug therapy is not fully effective in controlling seizures (Keith, 1963). Although several new and useful anticonvulsant drugs have become available in recent years, some patients have incomplete control of seizures or have unpleasant side effects with drug therapy but obtain a useful therapeutic effect from the diet. The use of drugs is ordinarily continued with the diet, but the dose can often be reduced and sometimes the use of drugs can be discontinued.

To produce ketosis of sufficient degree to have a beneficial effect on seizures, one must achieve a 3:1 ratio of ketogenic to antiketogenic materials.* The time usually required to reverse the usual ratio (1:3) to the 3:1 ratio is 4 days. If this diet does not produce ketosis, a further increase in the amount of fat and a decrease in the amount of carbohydrate may be necessary.

Tests of the urine should show the presence of ketones consistently and definitely when the desired state of ketosis has been achieved. Children on a ketogenic diet tend to excrete ketones at a maximal rate in the midafternoon and at a minimal rate in the early morning hours. Hence, it is usually sufficient to test the urine only on arising.

An abrupt change in a ketogenic diet may cause nausea or even vomiting. The practice is to alter the ratio of ketogenic to antiketogenic substances over a 4-day period to avoid these symptoms. If nausea or vomiting occurs, one or two meals should be omitted and small amounts of fruit juice should be given before the ketogenic diet is resumed.

Instead of the standard ketogenic diet, a diet containing medium-chain triglycerides oil can be used to produce ketosis. Medium-chain triglycerides are said to be more ketogenic than other dietary fats. This diet, however, is usually not as well accepted by the patient and family.

---

*For the purpose of calculating this ratio, it is assumed that glucose is antiketogenic and fatty acids are ketogenic and that 100 g of dietary carbohydrate yields 100 g of glucose, 100 g of dietary fat yields 10 g of glucose and 90 g of fatty acids, and 100 g of dietary protein produces 58 g of glucose and 46 g of fatty acids. Then the ketogenic to antiketogenic ratio may be calculated by dividing the sum of 90% of dietary fat and 46% of dietary protein by the sum of 100% of dietary carbohydrate, 10% of fat, and 58% of protein. All terms in this calculation are in grams of carbohydrate, protein, or fat.

DIETARY REQUIREMENTS

Ratio of Ketogenesis to Antiketogenesis (K:AK). Reversing the ratio of protein and carbohydrate to fat can be achieved in 4 days. The ratio of ketogenic to antiketogenic materials can be altered as suggested in the following table. The physician may indicate a different rate of progression and ratio if desired.

Day	K:AK
First	1.1:1
Second	1.6:1
Third	2.2:1
Fourth	2.8:1

Protein. For a patient 3 years of age or younger, 1.5 g of protein per kilogram of ideal body weight is necessary. For a patient older than 3 years, the amount is 1 g/kg of ideal body weight.

Carbohydrate. The carbohydrate content is determined by subtracting grams of protein from the total value allowed for carbohydrate and protein. See the ketogenic calculation table on page 202 or note the procedure described on page 198. The carbohydrate level should not be reduced below 10 g. For some patients, it may be necessary to decrease carbohydrate content at a slower rate if intolerance to fat is exhibited.

Fat. Note the procedure described on page 198 or see the ketogenic calculation table on page 202.

Calories. The caloric needs of the child are determined primarily from current dietary intake obtained by a thorough dietary history. Recommended Dietary Allowances and calorie requirements determined by the nomogram and the estimated level of activity are additional sources of data for calorie needs.

CALCULATION OF THE KETOGENIC DIET

The 4-day dietary regimen of fat (F) and of protein and carbohydrate (P + C) can be calculated as follows:

Day	K:AK Ratio	Calculation
First	1.1:1	1 g F = 9 kcal × 1.1 = 9.9 kcal 1 g P + C = 4 kcal × 1.0 = 4.0 kcal 13.9 kcal per unit
Second	1.6:1	1 g F = 9 kcal × 1.6 = 14.4 kcal 1 g P + C = 4 kcal × 1.0 = 4.0 kcal 18.4 kcal per unit
Third	2.2:1	1 g F = 9 kcal × 2.2 = 19.8 kcal 1 g P + C = 4 kcal × 1.0 = 4.0 kcal 23.8 kcal per unit
Fourth	2.8:1	1 g F = 9 kcal × 2.8 = 25.2 kcal 1 g P + C = 4 kcal × 1.0 = 4.0 kcal 29.2 kcal per unit

Protein, Fat, and Carbohydrate. Protein, fat, and carbohydrate can be calculated as follows:
1. Determine the total calorie requirement of the child
2. Divide total calories by calories per unit:

$$\frac{\text{Total calories}}{\text{Calories per unit}} = \text{Total units per day}$$

3. For grams of fat, multiply the number of units by the K value in the ratio of ketogenesis to antiketogenesis:

$$\text{Number of units} \times K = \text{grams of fat}$$

4. For grams of protein and carbohydrate, multiply the number of units by the AK value (1) in the ratio of ketogenesis to antiketogenesis:

$$\text{Number of units} \times \text{AK}(1) = \text{grams of protein plus carbohydrate}$$

5. For grams of protein, determine the number of grams needed according to age and kilograms of body weight
6. For grams of carbohydrate, subtract the grams of protein in the diet from the total units per day:

$$\text{Total units per day} - \text{grams of protein} = \text{grams of carbohydrate}$$

SAMPLE DETERMINATION OF THE KETOGENIC DIET

Calculation of the diet, composition of the diet, sample daily food exchanges, and a sample menu pattern are given for the following child.

Patient: 8-year-old boy
Height: 4 feet 1 inch
Weight: 25 kg
Calories: 1,375 (25 kg × 55 kcal)

The values for the 4-day dietary regimen are calculated as follows:

First day			Second day		
1,375 kcal ÷ 13.9 kcal	=	99 units	1,375 kcal ÷ 18.4 kcal	=	75 units
F 99 × 1.1	=	109 g	F 75 × 1.6	=	120 g
P + C = 99 × 1.0	=	99 g	P + C = 75 × 1.0	=	75 g
P (1 g/kg)	=	25 g	P (1 g/kg)	=	25 g
C (99 – 25)	=	74 g	C (75 – 25)	=	50 g

Third day			Fourth day		
1,375 kcal ÷ 23.8 kcal	=	58 units	1,375 kcal ÷ 29.2 kcal	=	47 units
F 58 × 2.2	=	128 g	F 47 × 2.8	=	132 g
P + C = 58 × 1.0	=	58 g	P + C = 47 × 1.0	=	47 g
P (1 g/kg)	=	25 g	P (1 g/kg)	=	25 g
C (58 – 25)	=	33 g	C (47 – 25)	=	22 g

Calculated Values of the Dietary Program

Day	Protein g	Fat g	Carbohydrate g	Calories	K:AK Ratio	Calories per Unit*
First	25	109	74	1,377	1.1:1	13.9
Second	25	120	50	1,380	1.6:1	18.4
Third	25	128	33	1,384	2.2:1	23.8
Fourth	25	132	22	1,376	2.8:1	29.2

*The procedure for calculation is on page 198.

Approximate Composition

The composition will vary slightly from the calculated values according to the foods included in the diet.

Day	Protein g	Fat g	Carbohydrate g	Calories	K:AK Ratio
First	28	110	75	1,406	1.1:1
Second	25	121	50	1,389	1.6:1
Third	24	130	31	1,390	2.2:1
Fourth	24	134	20	1,382	2.8:1

Sample Daily Food Exchanges

Day	Meat	Fat	Whipping Cream	Bread	Bread Product	Vegetable	Fruit
First	2	10	3	3	...	2	4
Second	2	13	3	1 1/2	...	2	3
Third	2	11	4	...	3	2	2
Fourth and following	2	12	4	...	2	2	1/2

Sample Menu Pattern

	Number of Servings*			
	First Day	Second Day	Third Day	Fourth Day
Breakfast				
Fruit	1	1	1	1/2
Bread	1	1	. . .	. . .
Bread product	. . .	. . .	1	1
Fat	2	3	3	3
Whipping cream	1	1	2	2
Noon Meal				
Meat	1	1	1	1
Bread	1	. . .	. . .	. . .
Bread product	. . .	. . .	1	1
Vegetable	1	1	1	1
Fat	4	5	4	4
Whipping cream	1	1	1	1
Fruit	2	1	1/2	. . .
Evening Meal				
Meat	1	1	1	1
Bread	1	1/2	. . .	. . .
Bread product	. . .	. . .	1	. . .
Vegetable	1	1	1	1
Fat	4	5	4	5
Whipping cream	1	1	1	1
Fruit	1	1	1/2	. . .

*All food is weighed.

ALTERNATIVE METHOD OF CALCULATION

Instead of calculating each diet individually, you may use the following ketogenic calculation table. Proceed as follows:

1. Determine the calorie requirement
2. Check the ratio to be used
3. Grams of fat are given in column F
4. Grams of carbohydrate and protein are given in column C + P
5. Subtract the number of grams of protein (page 197) required by the patient from the total number of C + P. The remaining number equals the number of grams of carbohydrate.

Ketogenic Calculation Table

	Ratio of Ketogenesis to Antiketogenesis							
	1.1:1		1.6:1		2.2:1		2.8:1	
Calories	F g	C + P g	F g	C + P g	F g	C + P g	F g	C + P g
800	64	58	69	43	73	33	76	27
900	72	65	78	49	84	38	87	31
1,000	79	72	87	54	92	42	96	32
1,100	87	79	96	60	102	46	105	38
1,200	95	86	104	65	111	50	115	41
1,300	103	94	113	71	120	55	125	45
1,400	111	101	122	76	129	59	134	48
1,500	119	108	130	82	139	63	144	51
1,600	127	115	139	87	148	67	153	55
1,700	135	122	148	92	158	71	163	58
1,800	143	130	157	98	167	76	173	62
1,900	151	137	165	103	176	80	182	65
2,000	159	144	174	109	185	84	192	68
2,100	166	151	183	114	194	88	201	72
2,200	174	159	191	120	203	92	211	75

F = fat; C + P = carbohydrate plus protein.

FOODS TO AVOID

The following foods contain a substantial amount of carbohydrate and should be avoided.

Cake	Molasses
Candy	Pastries
Carbonated beverages	Pies
Chewing gum	Pudding
Cookies	Sherbet
Cough drops or syrups that contain sugar	Sugar
Honey	Sweet rolls
Ice cream	Sweetened condensed milk
Jam	Syrup
Jelly	All breads, bread products, and cereals, unless
Marmalade	they are calculated into the meal plan

FOODS TO USE AS DESIRED

The following foods contain negligible amounts of protein, fat, and carbohydrate and may be used as desired without calculation into the meal plan.

Bouillon, broth, or consommé	Herbs
Chives	Horseradish, without sugar
Cocoa (limit to 1 teaspoon)	Mustard, dry
Coffee	Parsley
Decaffeinated coffee	Pepper
Flavoring extracts	Salt
Gelatin, unsweetened	Tea
(limit to 1 serving per day)	Vinegar

Food Exchange List for the Ketogenic Diet

This exchange list differs from the other food exchange lists in the manual. Only this exchange list should be used in planning menus for a ketogenic diet. Accuracy in portion sizes is important; foods should be weighed.

AVERAGE VALUES

	Weight *g*	Calories	Protein *g*	Fat *g*	Carbohydrate *g*
Meat	30	73	7	5	. . .
Fat	5	36	. . .	4	. . .
Whipping cream	60	187	2	19	2
Bread	varies	68	2	. . .	15
Bread products	2	7	. . .	. . .	1.6
Fruit	varies	24	. . .	. . .	6
Vegetable					
Group 1	100	16	1	. . .	3
Group 2	50	16	1	. . .	3

MEAT EXCHANGE

One meat exchange is equivalent to the weight listed and contains 7 g of protein, 5 g of fat, and 73 kcal.

Grams	
	Medium-fat meat
30	Beef, lamb, pork, veal
30	Liver (add 1 fat exchange and omit 50 g of group 1 vegetable)
40	Pork sausage (omit 2 fat exchanges)
20	Dried beef (add 1 fat exchange)
45	Cold cuts: bologna, luncheon meat, minced ham, liverwurst (all meat, no cereal)
30	Salami (omit 1 fat exchange)
50	Frankfurters or wieners (all meat, no cereal) (omit 1 fat exchange)
	Fowl
30	Chicken, duck, goose, turkey
	Egg (one)
	Fish
30	Salmon or tuna, canned
35	Sardines
50	Clams (add 1 fat exchange and omit 100 g of group 1 vegetable)
40	Lobster (add 1 fat exchange)
70	Oysters (add 1 fat exchange and omit 100 g of group 1 vegetable)
50	Scallops (add 1 fat exchange)
30	Shrimp (add 1 fat exchange)
	Cheese
30	American, brick, cheddar, Roquefort, Swiss, or processed cheese (omit 1 fat exchange)
50	Cottage cheese, creamed (add 1 fat exchange and omit 50 g of group 1 vegetable)

FAT EXCHANGE

One fat exchange is equivalent to the weight listed and contains 4 g of fat and 36 kcal.

Grams	
5	Almonds, slivered
30	Avocado (omit 50 g of group 1 vegetable)
5	Bacon
5	Butter or margarine
5	Cooking fats
5	Mayonnaise
30	Olives, green or ripe
5	Pecans, shelled
5	Salad oils
5	Walnuts, shelled

WHIPPING CREAM EXCHANGE

One whipping cream exchange is 60 g and contains 2 g of protein, 19 g of fat, 2 g of carbohydrate and 187 kcal. Whipping cream that is at least 32% fat should be used. Sixty grams of whipping cream may be exchanged for 65 g of group 1 vegetable and 5 fat exchanges.

BREAD EXCHANGE

One bread exchange is equivalent to the weight listed and contains 2 g of protein, 15 g of carbohydrate and 68 kcal.

Grams	
25	Bread
20	Melba toast
20	Saltines
100	White potato

BREAD PRODUCTS

One bread product contains 1.6 g of carbohydrate and 7 kcal.

Grams	
2	Low-calorie rice wafer

FRUIT EXCHANGE

One fruit exchange is equivalent to the weight listed and contains 6 g of carbohydrate and 24 kcal.

Grams		Grams	
	Apple		*Grapefruit*
40	Fresh	60	Fresh
60	Juice	60	Juice
60	Sauce	40	Nectar
	Apricots	75	Sections, canned
60	Canned		*Grapes*
10	Dried	40	Canned
60	Fresh	40	Fresh
40	Nectar		Juice
	Banana	30	Bottled
30	Whole	40	Frozen
	Berries, fresh	75	*Lemon juice*
50	Blackberries	65	*Lime juice*
40	Blueberries		*Mandarin orange*
60	Boysenberries	100	Canned
50	Cranberries		*Mango*
60	Gooseberries	35	Fresh
50	Loganberries		*Melon*
50	Raspberries	100	Cantaloupe
75	Strawberries	100	Honeydew
	Cherries	100	Watermelon
60	Canned		*Nectarine*
40	Fresh	40	Fresh
	Dates		*Orange*
8	Pitted	50	Fresh, whole
	Figs	60	Juice
60	Canned	50	Sections, fresh or canned
8	Dried		*Papaya*
30	Fresh	60	Fresh
	Fruit cocktail		
60	Canned		

FRUIT EXCHANGE (continued)

Grams		Grams	
	Peach		*Plums*
60	Canned	60	Canned
10	Dried	40	Fresh
60	Fresh		*Prunes*
60	Nectar	30	Juice
	Pear	8	Whole
60	Canned	8	*Raisins*
10	Dried		*Rhubarb*
40	Fresh	160	Raw
	Pineapple		*Tangerine*
60	Canned	50	Fresh, whole
40	Fresh	60	Juice
40	Juice	50	Sections

VEGETABLE EXCHANGE

One serving of group 1 vegetable or group 2 vegetable contains 1 g of protein, 3 g of carbohydrate and 16 kcal.

Group 1 Vegetable, 100 g

Asparagus	Chinese cabbage	Peppers, green or red
Bean sprouts	Collards	Radishes
Beans, green or wax	Cucumber	Sauerkraut
Beet greens	Dill pickle	Spinach
Broccoli	Eggplant	Summer squash
Cabbage	Endive	Tomato juice
Cauliflower	Garden cress	Tomatoes
Celery	Lettuce	Turnip greens
Chard, Swiss	Mushrooms	Turnips
	Mustard greens	Watercress

Group 2 Vegetable, 50 g

Artichokes	Dandelion greens	Okra
Beets	Kale	Onions
Brussels sprouts	Kohlrabi	Pumpkin
Carrots	Leeks	Rutabaga
		Winter squash

SELECTED BIBLIOGRAPHY

Keith, H. M.: Convulsive Disorders in Children With Reference to Treatment With Ketogenic Diet. Boston, Little, Brown & Company, 1963.
Lasser, J. L., and Brush, M. K.: An improved ketogenic diet for treatment of epilepsy. J. Am. Diet. Assoc., 62:281-285, 1973.
Mike, E. M.: Practical guide and dietary management of children with seizures using the ketogenic diet. Am. J. Clin. Nutr., 17: 399-409, 1965.
Signore, J. M.: Ketogenic diet containing medium-chain triglycerides. J. Am. Diet. Assoc., 62:285-290, 1973.

DIETARY GUIDELINES FOR CYSTIC FIBROSIS

Optimal nutrition should be maintained by careful attention to the diet of the patient with cystic fibrosis. Calorie and protein allowances must be sufficient to enable the individual to achieve desirable weight. To achieve desirable weight, the patient may have to increase calorie intake by 50 to 100% of the normal requirement for age and protein intake by 2 or 2 1/2 times normal; maintenance of desirable weight may require somewhat less. Weight gain and linear growth are important criteria of improvement in the evaluation of a patient's response to management.

Dysfunction of pancreatic enzyme secretion results in impaired digestion, particularly of fat. Administration of pancreatic enzymes (pancreatin) with each meal and snack often restores digestion only partially. Therefore, modification of fat intake usually is needed. Some patients should be advised to exert a moderate control of fat intake and limitation of highly fatty foods. The amount of dietary control required depends on the patient's degree of maldigestion and malabsorption. Our experience suggests that no more than 30% of the calories should come from fat. High-fat foods that may be poorly tolerated include whole milk; ice cream; cream; cheese; whole milk yogurt; luncheon meats; wieners; sausage; bacon; fatty and fried meats; peanut butter; rich candy and desserts made with chocolate, nuts, or cream; pies; pastries; doughnuts; salad dressing or oil; creamed foods; and gravy. Fatty snack foods, such as potato chips, corn chips, and French fries, also may cause problems. Moderate amounts of butter or margarine, if tolerated, may be used.

Abdominal distress may occur after ingestion of some vegetables, including corn and those from the cabbage and onion families, and condiments such as horseradish, chili sauce, mustard, catsup, and pickles.

Individual tolerances vary greatly among cystic fibrosis patients. It is recommended that new foods be introduced to the patient gradually and that signs of distress from these foods be noted. Any food that persistently causes distress should be omitted from the diet.

The diet should be reevaluated periodically, since growth and the disease process change the child's needs.

Supplemental vitamins should be prescribed for all cystic fibrosis patients. A multivitamin capsule or tablet containing B complex and C should be given daily in addition to water-soluble forms of vitamins A, D, E, and K. If needed, iron should be given.

VITAMIN PREPARATIONS

Vitamin	Brand Name	Manufacturer	How Supplied	Recommended Doses
Multivitamin supplement containing A, B complex, C, D, and E	Poly-Vi-Sol	Mead Johnson & Company	Drops Tablets	Recommended Dietary Allowance for age
A (water-soluble)	Aquasol A	USV Laboratories	Drops Capsules	Recommended Dietary Allowance for age
E (water-soluble)	Aquasol E	USV Laboratories	Drops Capsules	Infants, 25 to 50 IU Children, 100 to 200 IU
D (water-soluble)	Drisdol	Winthrop Laboratories	Drops Capsules	400 IU
K (water-soluble)	Synkayvite	Roche Laboratories	Tablets	Advisable intake, 15 μg

Characteristically, the cystic fibrosis patient loses abnormally large amounts of salt with sweating. It is, therefore, advisable to give extra salt. The daily dose varies from patient to patient and depends on the amount of sweating, the type of exercise, and the environmental temperature.

Medium-chain triglycerides have been recommended for use in this disorder to help decrease steatorrhea and to provide additional calories. Recent observations, however, suggest that administration of pancreatic enzymes may be needed for their absorption. Thus, medium-chain triglycerides may not provide the nutritional advantage over conventional sources of dietary fat usually attributed to them. See page 147 for a discussion of the manner of use of medium-chain triglycerides and the Pediatric Appendix, page 228, for a listing of a proprietary formula containing these fats. Our experience suggests that 3 tablespoons of medium-chain triglycerides oil per day is tolerated without adverse symptoms by most children.

SELECTED BIBLIOGRAPHY

Ad Hoc Nutrition Committee, Cystic Fibrosis Foundation: Present status of nutrition in cystic fibrosis. Atlanta, Georgia, March 1978.

Allan, J. D., Mason, A., and Moss, A. D.: Nutritional supplementation in treatment of cystic fibrosis of the pancreas. Am. J. Dis. Child., 126:22-26, 1973.

Berry, H. K., Kellogg, F. W., Hunt, M. M., et al.: Dietary supplement and nutrition in children with cystic fibrosis. Am. J. Dis. Child., 129:165-171, 1975.

Durie, P. R., Newth, C. J., Forstner, G. G., et al.: Malabsorption of medium-chain triglycerides in infants with cystic fibrosis: Correction of pancreatic enzyme supplements. J. Pediatr., 96:862-864, 1980.

Kuo, P. T., and Huang, N. N.: The effect of medium chain triglyceride upon fat absorption and plasma lipid and depot fat of children with cystic fibrosis of the pancreas. J. Clin. Invest., 44:1924-1933, 1965.

FOOD ALLERGIES

Food allergies are allergic reactions that can provoke a variety of clinical manifestations. Consistent occurrence of unusual symptoms, such as urticaria, rhinitis, diarrhea, vomiting, and dermatitis, after ingestion of food is an allergic reaction. The causative food is an allergen. The allergic reaction may be immediate or delayed.

There is no standard procedure for dealing with suspected food allergies in children. Offending foods can often be discovered by taking a diet history and having the patient keep a diet diary. For some patients, it is effective to remove all suspected foods from the diet and to add foods one at a time at 2- to 3-day intervals as improvement is shown. One can then work up to a diet that does not contain the offending foods and yet ensures the intake of foods to provide good nutrition.

A child who is allergic to one food is usually allergic to related foods. Peanuts, for example, belong to the pea family, and persons who cannot eat peanuts usually cannot eat beans and peas. They are not necessarily allergic to botanically true nuts. These relationships are shown in the following list.

RELATED FOODS

Family	Food
Apple	Apple, pear, quince
Aster	Lettuce, chicory, endive, escarole, artichoke, dandelion, sunflower seeds, tarragon
Beef	Cow's milk
Beet	Beet, spinach, chard, lamb's-quarters
Bird	All fowl and game birds, including chicken, turkey, duck, goose, guinea fowl, pigeon, quail, and pheasant; eggs
Blueberry	Blueberry, huckleberry, cranberry
Buckwheat	Buckwheat, rhubarb, garden sorrel
Cashew	Cashew, pistachio, mango
Chocolate	Both white and regular chocolate, cocoa, and cola
Citrus	Orange, lemon, grapefruit, lime, tangerine, kumquat, citron
Crustacean	Crab, lobster, shrimp
Fish	All true fish, either freshwater or saltwater, including tuna, sardine, catfish, trout, and crappie
Fungus	Mushroom, yeast, molds, antibiotics
Ginger	Ginger, cardamom, turmeric
Gooseberry	Currant, gooseberry
Grape	Raisin
Grass	Wheat, corn, rice, oats, barley, rye, wild rice, cane, millet, sorghum, bamboo sprouts
Laurel	Avocado, cinnamon, bay leaves, sassafras
Mallow	Cottonseed, okra

RELATED FOODS (continued)

Family	Food
Melon (gourd)	Watermelon, cucumber, cantaloupe, pumpkin, squash, other melons
Mollusk	Oyster, clam, abalone, mussel
Mustard	Mustard, turnip, radish, horseradish, watercress, cabbage, kraut, Chinese cabbage, broccoli, cauliflower, Brussels sprouts, collards, kale, kohlrabi, rutabaga
Myrtle	Allspice, guava, clove, pimento
Onion	Onion, garlic, asparagus, chives, leeks, sarsaparilla
Palm	Coconut, date
Parsley	Carrot, parsnip, celery, parsley, celeriac, anise, dill, fennel, angelica, celery seed, cumin, coriander, caraway
Pea	Peanuts, peas (green, field, black-eyed), beans (navy, lima, pinto, string, soybeans, etc.), licorice, acacia, tragacanth
Plum	Plum, cherry, peach, apricot, nectarine, wild cherry, almond
Potato	Potato, tomato, eggplant, peppers (including green pepper, red pepper, chili pepper, paprika, cayenne, and capsicum, but not black and white peppers)
Reptile	Turtle, rattlesnake, frog
Rose	Strawberry, raspberry, blackberry, dewberry, loganberry, youngberry, boysenberry
Walnut	English walnut, black walnut, pecan, hickory nut, butternut

SELECTED BIBLIOGRAPHY

Rapaport, H. G., and Linde, S. M.: The Complete Allergy Guide. New York, Simon & Schuster, 1970.

SPECIAL DIETS FOR INFANTS WITH INBORN ERRORS
OF AMINO ACID METABOLISM

Management of a hereditary aminoacidopathy may require the restriction of dietary intake of one or more amino acids to the level of minimal requirement.

The amount of the restricted amino acid provided by the diet must be sufficient to meet the metabolic requirements dependent on it, including the requirement for growth; yet its intake must not permit an excess accumulation in body fluids of the amino acid or its derivatives. The nutrient requirements can be met by a semisynthetic diet derived either from a modified protein hydrolysate or from a mixture of L-amino acids, so that the diet either contains an extremely low amount of the implicated amino acid or is free of it. Other dietary sources of protein can furnish the implicated amino acid or acids in an amount sufficient to sustain normal metabolism but low enough to avoid toxicity. Requirements for other nutrients—calories, fat (including essential fatty acids), carbohydrates, minerals, and vitamins—are met either by special dietary formulations added to the amino acid product or by further supplementation with natural foods of known composition.

Careful monitoring of treatment and its effect is essential throughout the period of dietary management. Total nutritional intake, including the micronutrient composition, should be known and monitored to be certain the child is receiving a nutritionally adequate diet. The concentration of appropriate amino acids in the blood should be determined often enough to assure that the level is adequate to sustain normal protein metabolism but is not high enough to be harmful. The child must be observed frequently to be certain that nutritional deficiencies do not develop.

The principles of therapy call for development of a precise diet appropriate to the problem, nutritional surveillance to assure that the diet is adequate, mechanisms for follow-up of the child for symptoms or signs of toxicity of nutritional deficiency, and provision of general support for the child.*

Metabolic centers that are accumulating experience and have good laboratory support may be the most efficient providers of adequate treatment for patients with inborn errors of metabolism. The American Academy of Pediatrics maintains and periodically publishes a list of these metabolic centers.

---

*Committee on Nutrition: Special diets for infants with inborn errors of amino acid metabolism. Pediatrics, 57:783-791, 1976.

PEDIATRIC APPENDIX

GROWTH PERCENTILES

Graphs

**BOYS: BIRTH TO 36 MONTHS
PHYSICAL GROWTH
NCHS PERCENTILES**

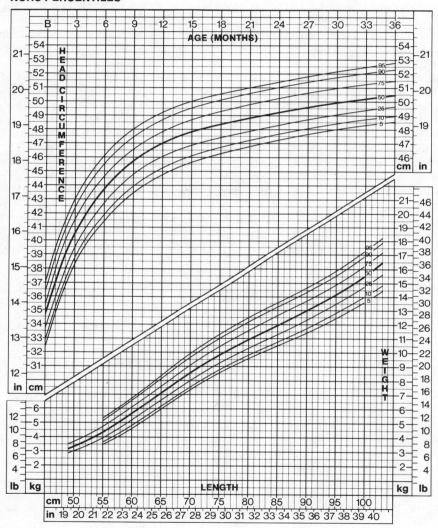

Adapted from: Hamill PVV, Drizd TA, Johnson CL, Reed RB, Roche AF, Moore
WM: Physical growth: National Center for Health Statistics percentiles. AM J
CLIN NUTR 32:607-629,1979. Data from the Fels Research Institute, Wright
State University School of Medicine, Yellow Springs, Ohio.

© 1980 ROSS LABORATORIES

BOYS: BIRTH TO 36 MONTHS
PHYSICAL GROWTH
NCHS PERCENTILES

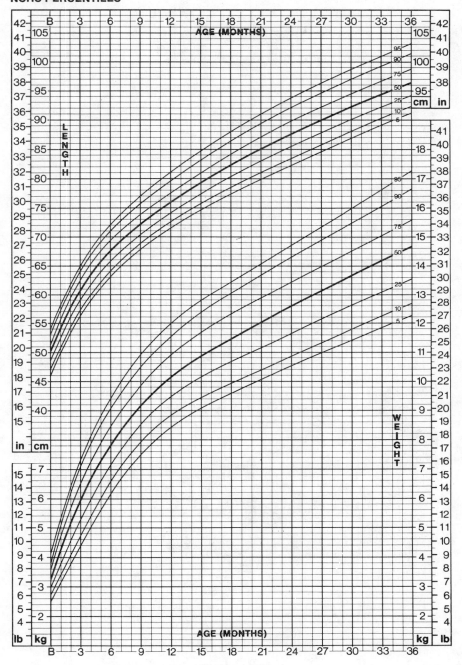

Adapted from: Hamill PVV, Drizd TA, Johnson CL, Reed RB, Roche AF, Moore
WM: Physical growth: National Center for Health Statistics percentiles. AM J
CLIN NUTR 32:607-629,1979. Data from the Fels Research Institute, Wright
State University School of Medicine, Yellow Springs, Ohio.

© 1980 ROSS LABORATORIES

GIRLS: BIRTH TO 36 MONTHS
PHYSICAL GROWTH
NCHS PERCENTILES

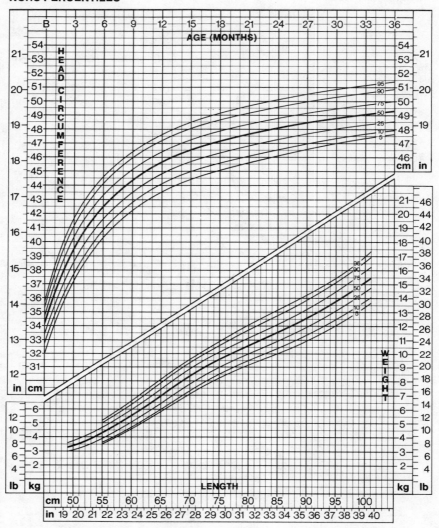

Adapted from: Hamill PVV, Drizd TA, Johnson CL, Reed RB, Roche AF, Moore
WM: Physical growth: National Center for Health Statistics percentiles. AM J
CLIN NUTR 32:607-629,1979. Data from the Fels Research Institute, Wright
State University School of Medicine, Yellow Springs. Ohio.

© 1980 ROSS LABORATORIES

**GIRLS: BIRTH TO 36 MONTHS
PHYSICAL GROWTH
NCHS PERCENTILES**

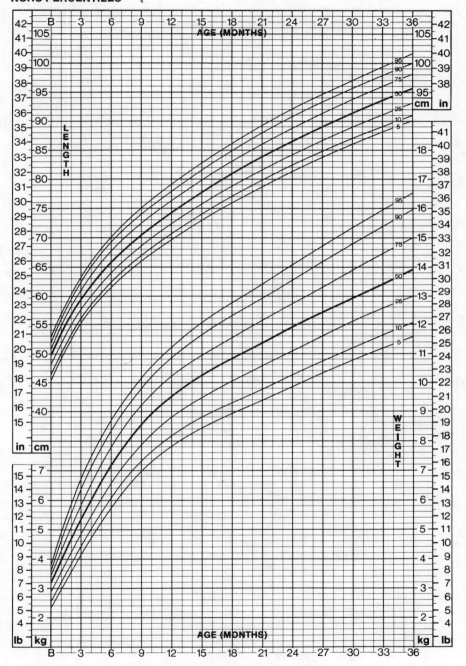

Adapted from: Hamill PVV, Drizd TA, Johnson CL, Reed RB, Roche AF, Moore
WM: Physical growth: National Center for Health Statistics percentiles. AM J
CLIN NUTR 32:607-629,1979. Data from the Fels Research Institute, Wright
State University School of Medicine, Yellow Springs, Ohio.

**BOYS: 2 TO 18 YEARS
PHYSICAL GROWTH
NCHS PERCENTILES**

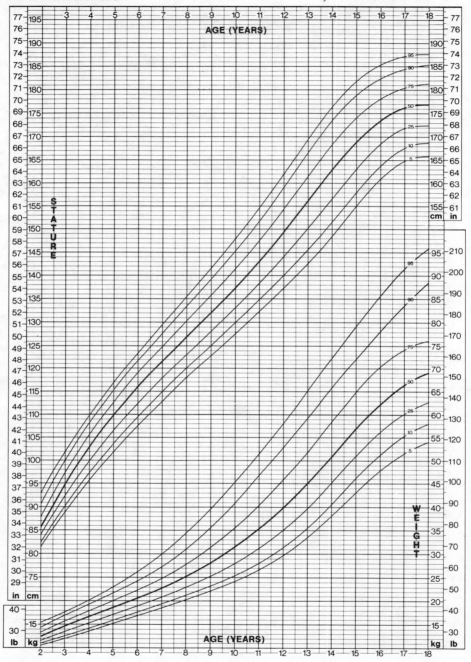

Adapted from: Hamill PVV, Drizd TA, Johnson CL, Reed RB, Roche AF, Moore
WM: Physical growth: National Center for Health Statistics percentiles. AM J
CLIN NUTR 32:607-629,1979. Data from the National Center for Health
Statistics (NCHS) Hyattsville, Maryland.

© 1980 ROSS LABORATORIES

**BOYS: PREPUBESCENT
PHYSICAL GROWTH
NCHS PERCENTILES**

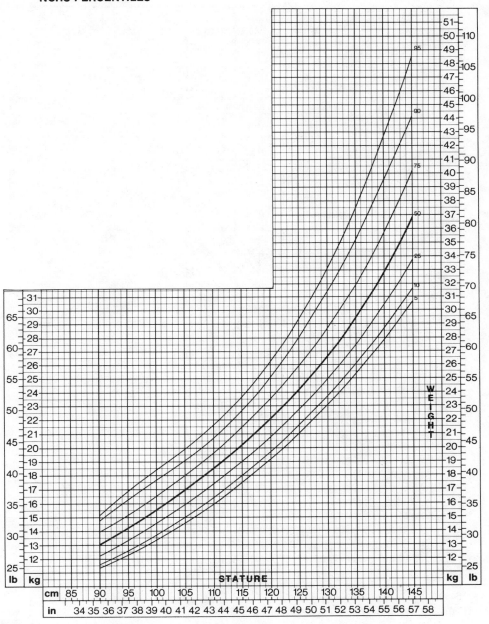

Adapted from: Hamill PVV, Drizd TA, Johnson CL, Reed RB, Roche AF, Moore
WM: Physical growth: National Center for Health Statistics percentiles. AM J
CLIN NUTR 32:607-629,1979. Data from the National Center for Health
Statistics (NCHS) Hyattsville, Maryland.

© 1980 ROSS LABORATORIES

GIRLS: 2 TO 18 YEARS
PHYSICAL GROWTH
NCHS PERCENTILES

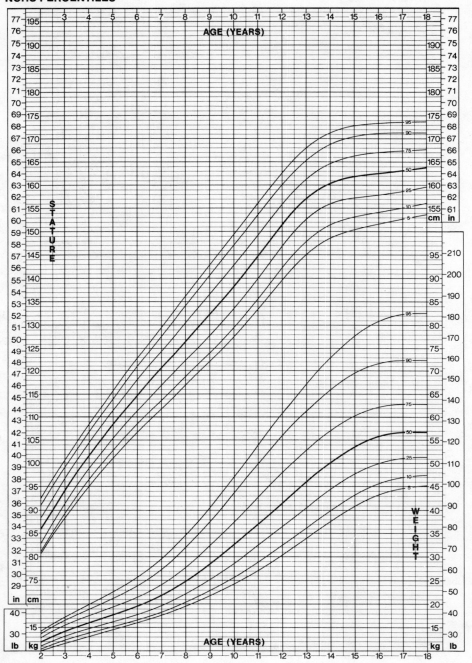

Adapted from: Hamill PVV, Drizd TA, Johnson CL, Reed RB, Roche AF, Moore
WM: Physical growth: National Center for Health Statistics percentiles. AM J
CLIN NUTR 32:607-629,1979. Data from the National Center for Health
Statistics (NCHS) Hyattsville, Maryland.

© 1980 ROSS LABORATORIES

GIRLS: PREPUBESCENT
PHYSICAL GROWTH
NCHS PERCENTILES

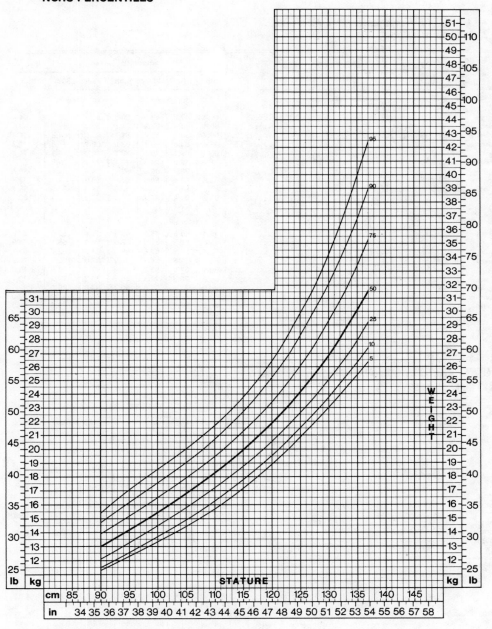

STATURE

Adapted from: Hamill PVV, Drizd TA, Johnson CL, Reed RB, Roche AF, Moore
WM: Physical growth: National Center for Health Statistics percentiles. AM J
CLIN NUTR 32:607-629,1979. Data from the National Center for Health
Statistics (NCHS) Hyattsville, Maryland.

Tables*

PERCENTILES OF RECUMBENT LENGTH BY SEX AND AGE, BIRTH TO 36 MONTHS

Sex and age	Smoothed percentile						
	5th	10th	25th	50th	75th	90th	95th
Male	Recumbent length in centimeters						
Birth	46.4	47.5	49.0	50.5	51.8	53.5	54.4
1 month	50.4	51.3	53.0	54.6	56.2	57.7	58.6
3 months	56.7	57.7	59.4	61.1	63.0	64.5	65.4
6 months	63.4	64.4	66.1	67.8	69.7	71.3	72.3
9 months	68.0	69.1	70.6	72.3	74.0	75.9	77.1
12 months	71.7	72.8	74.3	76.1	77.7	79.8	81.2
18 months	77.5	78.7	80.5	82.4	84.3	86.6	88.1
24 months	82.3	83.5	85.6	87.6	89.9	92.2	93.8
30 months	87.0	88.2	90.1	92.3	94.6	97.0	98.7
36 months	91.2	92.4	94.2	96.5	98.9	101.4	103.1
Female							
Birth	45.4	46.5	48.2	49.9	51.0	52.0	52.9
1 month	49.2	50.2	51.9	53.5	54.9	56.1	56.9
3 months	55.4	56.2	57.8	59.5	61.2	62.7	63.4
6 months	61.8	62.6	64.2	65.9	67.8	69.4	70.2
9 months	66.1	67.0	68.7	70.4	72.4	74.0	75.0
12 months	69.8	70.8	72.4	74.3	76.3	78.0	79.1
18 months	76.0	77.2	78.8	80.9	83.0	85.0	86.1
24 months	81.3	82.5	84.2	86.5	88.7	90.8	92.0
30 months	86.0	87.0	88.9	91.3	93.7	95.6	96.9
36 months	90.0	91.0	93.1	95.6	98.1	100.0	101.5

PERCENTILES OF WEIGHT BY SEX AND AGE, BIRTH TO 36 MONTHS

Sex and age	Smoothed percentile						
	5th	10th	25th	50th	75th	90th	95th
Male	Weight in kilograms						
Birth	2.54	2.78	3.00	3.27	3.64	3.82	4.15
1 month	3.16	3.43	3.82	4.29	4.75	5.14	5.38
3 months	4.43	4.78	5.32	5.98	6.56	7.14	7.37
6 months	6.20	6.61	7.20	7.85	8.49	9.10	9.46
9 months	7.52	7.95	8.56	9.18	9.88	10.49	10.93
12 months	8.43	8.84	9.49	10.15	10.91	11.54	11.99
18 months	9.59	9.92	10.67	11.47	12.31	13.05	13.44
24 months	10.54	10.85	11.65	12.59	13.44	14.29	14.70
30 months	11.44	11.80	12.63	13.67	14.51	15.47	15.97
36 months	12.26	12.69	13.58	14.69	15.59	16.66	17.28
Female							
Birth	2.36	2.58	2.93	3.23	3.52	3.64	3.81
1 month	2.97	3.22	3.59	3.98	4.36	4.65	4.92
3 months	4.18	4.47	4.88	5.40	5.90	6.39	6.74
6 months	5.79	6.12	6.60	7.21	7.83	8.38	8.73
9 months	7.00	7.34	7.89	8.56	9.24	9.83	10.17
12 months	7.84	8.19	8.81	9.53	10.23	10.87	11.24
18 months	8.92	9.30	10.04	10.82	11.55	12.30	12.76
24 months	9.87	10.26	11.10	11.90	12.74	13.57	14.08
30 months	10.78	11.21	12.11	12.93	13.93	14.81	15.35
36 months	11.60	12.07	12.99	13.93	15.03	15.97	16.54

*From Hamill, P. V. V., Drizd, T. A., Johnson, C. L., et al.: NCHS growth curves for children birth–18 years. Vital Health Stat. [11], No. 165: 1–74, November 1977.

PERCENTILES OF STATURE BY SEX AND AGE, 2 THROUGH 24 YEARS

Sex and age	N	Observed percentile						
		5th	10th	25th	50th	75th	90th	95th
Male		Stature in centimeters						
2.00-2.25 years	419	82.6	83.5	86.1	87.8	90.3	91.9	97.3
2.25-2.75 years	945	86.1	87.0	89.0	91.2	93.8	97.3	98.3
2.75-3.25 years	785	88.9	90.5	92.4	95.1	97.2	100.1	101.2
3.25-3.75 years	857	92.1	93.3	95.7	98.2	101.1	102.8	104.4
3.75-4.25 years	856	96.2	97.3	100.0	102.6	105.3	107.5	110.8
4.25-4.75 years	937	98.0	100.2	103.4	105.8	108.6	111.8	113.2
4.75-5.25 years	874	100.7	103.2	105.5	108.8	112.4	115.4	116.5
5.25-5.75 years	878	106.2	107.7	110.1	113.5	116.1	118.2	119.5
5.75-6.25 years	908	108.5	110.1	112.8	117.0	119.4	122.2	123.1
6.25-6.75 years	1,033	108.9	110.0	114.8	118.2	121.9	125.0	127.1
6.75-7.25 years	988	114.1	115.6	118.5	122.3	125.9	128.3	129.8
7.25-7.75 years	1,120	115.6	118.3	120.8	124.5	127.9	131.4	133.4
7.75-8.25 years	1,014	119.3	121.0	123.8	127.9	131.7	134.9	138.0
8.25-8.75 years	902	121.2	123.4	126.2	129.6	133.2	136.4	138.8
8.75-9.25 years	943	121.1	124.5	127.5	132.8	136.3	139.4	141.9
9.25-9.75 years	958	125.2	127.7	131.2	135.0	138.7	142.7	144.7
9.75-10.25 years	1,030	127.3	130.0	133.7	138.6	142.1	145.9	149.0
10.25-10.75 years	1,070	130.5	132.5	135.8	139.4	144.1	148.4	151.4
10.75-11.25 years	1,052	132.5	135.3	138.7	143.5	147.9	151.4	154.0
11.25-11.75 years	952	135.1	138.0	141.4	145.8	150.8	154.5	156.1
11.75-12.25 years	1,010	138.5	140.1	144.1	148.6	153.7	159.4	162.6
12.25-12.75 years	1,092	139.3	141.8	146.4	152.1	157.2	162.6	165.5
12.75-13.25 years	1,155	142.2	144.8	149.7	154.8	159.6	165.3	167.8
13.25-13.75 years	1,056	145.6	148.6	153.6	160.0	166.5	172.2	175.5
13.75-14.25 years	954	149.2	153.0	157.7	164.4	169.9	175.1	177.6
14.25-14.75 years	1,019	152.9	156.4	161.1	167.6	173.1	177.8	179.4
14.75-15.25 years	1,112	155.0	157.6	163.0	169.4	173.8	178.2	181.8
15.25-15.75 years	914	158.8	161.4	166.6	171.6	175.4	180.4	183.4
15.75-16.25 years	1,051	160.5	164.3	169.0	173.5	177.8	181.5	185.8
16.25-16.75 years	876	163.8	165.5	170.6	174.9	179.5	183.3	186.4
16.75-17.25 years	1,054	164.4	166.2	170.7	176.8	181.8	184.6	187.3
17.25-17.75 years	935	163.3	167.7	172.1	176.4	181.0	185.0	187.8
17.75-18.25 years	866	166.5	170.1	173.1	176.0	180.2	186.1	187.3
18.25-19.00 years	1,067	166.8	169.3	172.0	175.8	180.1	185.9	186.8
19.00-20.00 years	1,770	162.8	166.9	171.6	177.2	180.8	185.0	186.2
20.00-21.00 years	1,668	159.4	168.4	172.2	177.4	181.2	183.6	185.8
21.00-22.00 years	1,703	166.2	168.3	172.5	177.3	181.1	184.8	190.0
22.00-23.00 years	1,662	167.2	167.7	171.3	177.1	180.6	187.1	192.0
23.00-24.00 years	1,589	161.3	165.3	172.3	176.8	183.0	188.5	189.2
24.00-25.00 years	1,595	165.4	168.5	172.9	178.1	183.0	186.7	189.5

PERCENTILES OF STATURE BY SEX AND AGE, 2 THROUGH 24 YEARS *(Continued)*

Sex and age	N	Observed percentile						
		5th	10th	25th	50th	75th	90th	95th
Female		Stature in centimeters						
2.00-2.25 years	440	81.3	82.5	84.6	86.8	89.9	93.6	94.6
2.25-2.75 years	972	84.2	85.3	87.1	90.3	93.4	94.8	96.4
2.75-3.25 years	622	90.2	90.7	92.7	95.3	96.7	99.1	100.6
3.25-3.75 years	887	91.8	92.8	95.0	97.4	99.8	102.1	103.6
3.75-4.25 years	775	94.8	96.2	97.9	100.5	103.8	106.0	108.2
4.25-4.75 years	848	96.8	97.6	100.5	103.8	106.2	109.4	112.0
4.75-5.25 years	876	99.1	101.1	105.2	108.1	111.6	113.7	114.7
5.25-5.75 years	890	103.8	106.1	108.4	111.8	115.5	118.7	121.3
5.75-6.25 years	866	107.1	109.0	111.9	115.4	118.8	122.1	124.6
6.25-6.75 years	1,025	109.3	111.6	114.3	117.7	121.7	125.2	126.9
6.75-7.25 years	945	111.7	113.2	117.4	120.8	124.3	126.8	128.6
7.25-7.75 years	952	115.8	117.2	120.0	123.7	127.9	131.7	134.2
7.75-8.25 years	1,004	117.8	119.5	122.8	127.5	130.6	132.9	134.6
8.25-8.75 years	968	118.9	121.4	124.4	129.2	133.4	135.8	138.0
8.75-9.25 years	988	122.2	124.8	128.4	132.7	137.7	141.0	142.3
9.25-9.75 years	885	126.6	127.6	131.1	135.1	139.8	144.4	147.6
9.75-10.25 years	1,092	129.0	130.3	134.4	138.5	143.0	147.0	149.8
10.25-10.75 years	1,086	129.4	131.1	135.2	140.6	144.7	149.8	152.4
10.75-11.25 years	870	132.1	134.8	139.5	143.9	148.8	153.7	157.0
11.25-11.75 years	862	134.5	135.8	141.7	147.3	152.6	157.1	158.8
11.75-12.25 years	1,082	139.4	142.2	146.7	151.8	156.4	161.4	165.9
12.25-12.75 years	1,019	141.7	145.9	150.8	154.8	159.7	164.0	165.7
12.75-13.25 years	1,058	143.7	147.7	163.0	157.5	161.4	165.5	167.4
13.25-13.75 years	1,120	149.4	151.6	155.4	159.6	163.8	165.9	169.2
13.75-14.25 years	1,080	149.8	151.6	155.7	160.0	163.4	167.1	168.7
14.25-14.75 years	951	150.3	153.2	157.4	161.6	165.4	169.5	171.1
14.75-15.25 years	1,012	151.5	153.3	157.2	161.2	166.3	171.2	174.9
15.25-15.75 years	980	152.6	154.8	157.9	162.9	167.6	172.1	176.2
15.75-16.25 years	959	152.5	154.8	158.2	163.6	167.7	170.7	172.3
16.25-16.75 years	836	150.7	153.3	157.6	162.1	166.5	171.5	172.6
16.75-17.25 years	1,108	151.8	154.6	158.0	161.8	166.5	171.6	173.8
17.25-17.75 years	810	150.7	154.3	158.0	162.6	166.6	170.0	172.5
17.75-18.25 years	826	152.2	155.5	159.8	163.9	168.0	171.0	171.8
18.25-19.00 years	1,420	154.9	157.8	161.2	165.3	167.2	172.4	174.2
19.00-20.00 years	1,384	155.0	155.9	159.9	163.0	166.8	170.6	173.1
20.00-21.00 years	1,771	152.3	155.1	159.0	163.2	168.8	172.4	175.3
21.00-22.00 years	1,818	152.0	154.6	158.5	162.5	167.0	170.8	173.0
22.00-23.00 years	1,734	150.4	153.0	156.9	162.8	167.2	171.2	174.5
23.00-24.00 years	1,800	154.2	156.0	158.6	163.1	166.8	170.5	172.6
24.00-25.00 years	1,796	152.3	155.4	158.3	162.3	167.4	170.4	171.6

PERCENTILES OF WEIGHT BY SEX AND AGE, 2 THROUGH 24 YEARS

Sex and age	N	Observed percentile						
		5th	10th	25th	50th	75th	90th	95th
Male		Weight in kilograms						
2.00-2.25 years	419	9.97	11.10	11.63	12.67	14.05	14.85	15.47
2.25-2.75 years	945	11.31	11.89	12.63	13.53	14.57	15.69	16.80
2.75-3.25 years	785	12.28	12.84	13.55	14.43	15.34	16.39	17.37
3.25-3.75 years	857	12.70	13.34	14.33	15.39	16.46	17.77	18.63
3.75-4.25 years	856	13.83	14.70	15.46	16.64	17.85	18.87	20.62
4.25-4.75 years	937	14.42	15.09	16.02	17.71	19.17	20.45	21.51
4.75-5.25 years	874	14.99	15.52	16.91	18.47	20.22	21.02	22.59
5.25-5.75 years	878	17.01	17.31	18.33	19.88	21.39	23.21	25.32
5.75-6.25 years	908	16.87	17.80	19.53	21.21	22.85	24.98	26.40
6.25-6.75 years	1,033	17.21	17.82	19.70	21.59	23.41	26.21	28.18
6.75-7.25 years	992	18.59	19.39	21.37	22.93	25.22	28.74	30.72
7.25-7.75 years	1,120	18.76	20.07	22.04	24.33	26.48	29.08	32.31
7.75-8.25 years	1,014	20.20	21.47	23.47	25.65	28.70	31.36	35.15
8.25-8.75 years	902	21.71	22.63	24.35	26.31	29.27	33.08	34.96
8.75-9.25 years	943	22.01	22.98	25.13	27.89	31.75	36.62	40.23
9.25-9.75 years	958	23.11	24.30	26.40	29.65	33.63	38.58	45.67
9.75-10.25 years	1,030	24.40	25.63	27.98	31.83	36.09	41.08	43.69
10.25-10.75 years	1,070	26.09	27.73	29.49	32.57	36.39	40.75	45.66
10.75-11.25 years	1,052	27.98	28.79	31.23	35.86	39.68	44.71	51.83
11.25-11.75 years	952	28.17	30.14	34.07	37.48	41.94	47.16	52.45
11.75-12.25 years	1,010	30.10	31.18	34.21	38.75	46.43	55.24	62.43
12.25-12.75 years	1,092	31.72	32.98	36.18	41.98	47.30	54.05	58.45
12.75-13.25 years	1,155	32.17	34.61	38.43	43.62	50.17	59.22	64.29
13.25-13.75 years	1,056	36.24	37.80	42.92	49.23	58.38	63.44	68.39
13.75-14.25 years	954	38.25	41.47	46.98	51.65	60.77	67.04	76.61
14.25-14.75 years	1,019	40.52	43.64	49.70	55.32	62.62	72.69	77.03
14.75-15.25 years	1,112	42.14	44.93	50.35	56.35	63.63	71.27	76.91
15.25-15.75 years	914	46.26	49.12	54.29	58.92	66.68	75.40	81.81
15.75-16.25 years	1,051	46.83	51.29	55.79	61.74	69.33	76.78	86.07
16.25-16.75 years	876	50.46	53.22	56.77	64.71	72.28	81.62	87.57
16.75-17.25 years	1,054	52.15	55.42	60.65	65.90	73.76	81.72	91.23
17.25-17.75 years	935	51.80	55.53	60.81	66.64	75.36	83.35	92.16
17.75-18.25 years	866	54.76	58.18	62.04	68.96	75.49	88.36	94.71
18.25-19.00 years	1,067	54.96	60.35	63.62	69.88	78.67	92.66	99.60
19.00-20.00 years	1,770	55.40	57.38	65.91	70.66	76.43	87.01	96.48
20.00-21.00 years	1,668	55.86	57.71	65.04	71.89	78.44	88.86	94.84
21.00-22.00 years	1,703	52.66	58.17	65.29	72.12	80.96	89.04	96.13
22.00-23.00 years	1,662	55.02	59.14	65.09	71.77	79.66	90.57	96.93
23.00-24.00 years	1,589	59.16	60.69	65.54	74.71	82.44	94.05	105.35
24.00-25.00 years	1,595	60.87	63.96	67.96	79.37	85.69	97.60	103.19

PERCENTILES OF WEIGHT BY SEX AND AGE, 2 THROUGH 24 YEARS (Continued)

Sex and age	N	Observed percentile						
		5th	10th	25th	50th	75th	90th	95th
Female		Weight in kilograms						
2.00-2.25 years	440	10.06	10.66	11.41	12.21	12.86	13.84	14.57
2.25-2.75 years	972	10.77	11.20	11.98	12.76	13.94	14.74	15.09
2.75-3.25 years	622	12.14	12.40	13.12	13.93	15.61	16.84	17.74
3.25-3.75 years	887	12.29	13.03	13.58	14.60	15.93	17.54	18.28
3.75-4.25 years	775	13.13	13.63	14.51	15.68	17.15	18.22	18.94
4.25-4.75 years	848	13.45	14.05	15.04	16.57	17.78	19.35	20.26
4.75-5.25 years	876	14.33	15.21	16.48	17.73	19.66	21.23	22.10
5.25-5.75 years	890	15.18	16.20	17.47	18.92	20.96	23.44	25.01
5.75-6.25 years	866	15.99	17.09	18.21	20.19	22.39	24.88	28.71
6.25-6.75 years	1,025	17.02	17.71	19.24	21.06	23.55	26.17	27.89
6.75-7.25 years	945	17.86	18.74	20.20	22.13	23.98	26.91	29.58
7.25-7.75 years	952	18.84	19.60	21.33	23.72	26.54	29.61	31.55
7.75-8.25 years	1,004	20.11	20.79	22.49	24.89	27.73	32.63	35.20
8.25-8.75 years	968	20.47	21.50	23.30	26.39	29.69	33.65	36.45
8.75-9.25 years	988	22.20	23.17	25.27	28.79	33.40	39.66	42.69
9.25-9.75 years	885	23.29	24.72	26.92	30.26	34.54	39.87	43.62
9.75-10.25 years	1,092	24.34	25.25	28.03	31.68	36.38	43.16	45.92
10.25-10.75 years	1,086	25.28	26.69	29.42	33.00	37.63	45.90	48.37
10.75-11.25 years	870	26.73	28.32	32.09	36.13	42.27	47.72	54.49
11.25-11.75 years	862	27.44	29.45	32.88	37.97	44.38	50.77	58.09
11.75-12.25 years	1,082	29.72	32.74	36.42	41.70	48.78	57.77	64.79
12.25-12.75 years	1,019	32.59	34.97	39.46	45.37	51.40	58.10	63.21
12.75-13.25 years	1,058	34.21	37.17	41.44	47.06	54.79	62.20	66.61
13.25-13.75 years	1,120	37.72	39.45	45.00	50.30	56.81	67.05	75.78
13.75-14.25 years	1,080	37.74	39.86	44.86	50.22	56.44	66.44	74.70
14.25-14.75 years	951	40.77	42.96	47.21	53.03	60.95	68.88	78.43
14.75-15.25 years	1,012	41.14	43.65	47.48	53.29	59.72	71.57	75.36
15.25-15.75 years	980	42.99	46.11	48.98	55.25	60.80	71.45	77.78
15.75-16.25 years	959	43.64	45.74	49.22	54.92	61.58	67.70	78.03
16.25-16.75 years	836	43.86	45.69	49.46	54.97	62.64	72.37	83.10
16.75-17.25 years	1,108	43.87	45.57	50.76	56.49	62.22	72.45	84.19
17.25-17.75 years	810	42.90	45.36	50.56	55.23	61.59	70.62	84.82
17.75-18.25 years	826	45.05	47.89	52.68	57.68	62.32	69.62	75.86
18.25-19.00 years	1,420	44.83	45.89	51.03	56.97	63.16	72.62	78.70
19.00-20.00 years	1,384	48.65	48.83	51.62	57.24	63.48	76.33	83.48
20.00-21.00 years	1,771	44.40	47.23	51.70	57.22	63.94	72.15	75.89
21.00-22.00 years	1,818	46.08	48.54	52.15	58.36	64.64	72.88	81.76
22.00-23.00 years	1,734	42.86	46.18	51.35	58.82	67.38	75.54	85.35
23.00-24.00 years	1,800	45.59	47.77	52.16	59.87	64.64	72.80	84.62
24.00-25.00 years	1,796	46.65	48.13	52.06	58.88	66.33	77.17	86.04

PERCENTILES OF WEIGHT BY SEX AND STATURE

Sex and stature	N	Observed percentile						
		5th	10th	25th	50th	75th	90th	95th
Male, 2-11.5 years		Weight in kilograms						
90-92 centimeters	330	12.02	12.22	12.81	13.80	14.90	15.56	15.79
92-94 centimeters	451	12.06	12.22	12.71	13.51	14.61	15.51	15.81
94-96 centimeters	451	12.31	12.66	13.68	14.66	15.46	15.94	16.61
96-98 centimeters	555	12.31	13.08	14.28	15.04	15.80	17.12	17.77
98-100 centimeters	359	13.70	14.05	14.50	15.26	16.10	18.04	19.06
100-102 centimeters	557	13.92	14.20	14.82	15.87	17.12	17.88	18.96
102-104 centimeters	414	14.31	14.64	15.63	16.66	17.51	18.19	19.30
104-106 centimeters	561	14.45	14.91	16.14	17.16	18.30	19.33	19.67
106-108 centimeters	553	15.51	15.83	16.56	17.70	18.98	19.76	20.53
108-110 centimeters	702	16.20	16.43	17.10	18.31	19.77	22.13	23.16
110-112 centimeters	641	16.15	16.50	17.57	18.83	19.91	21.50	22.37
112-114 centimeters	706	16.94	17.78	18.66	19.85	21.27	22.63	23.85
114-116 centimeters	912	18.04	18.32	19.16	20.41	21.39	21.98	23.22
116-118 centimeters	1,013	18.36	18.80	20.06	21.03	22.01	23.41	23.88
118-120 centimeters	1,284	18.43	19.01	20.29	21.43	22.81	23.76	24.64
120-122 centimeters	1,194	19.49	20.23	21.31	22.85	24.40	25.76	26.85
122-124 centimeters	1,430	20.42	21.12	22.42	23.62	25.19	26.78	27.95
124-126 centimeters	647	21.50	22.19	22.95	24.33	26.15	27.80	30.14
126-128 centimeters	1,565	22.30	22.92	24.31	25.55	27.31	29.91	31.05
128-130 centimeters	1,277	22.84	23.91	24.79	26.22	28.32	31.31	34.33
130-132 centimeters	1,524	23.96	24.35	25.41	27.29	29.35	31.17	31.96
132-134 centimeters	1,443	24.45	25.33	26.74	28.54	31.33	34.75	35.82
134-136 centimeters	1,554	24.65	25.46	27.45	29.55	32.18	37.22	39.83
136-138 centimeters	1,281	26.47	27.21	28.68	30.52	33.40	36.53	37.73
138-140 centimeters	1,184	28.11	28.48	29.59	31.91	33.85	37.25	39.62
140-142 centimeters	1,356	28.65	29.46	31.19	33.87	36.81	40.96	48.32
142-144 centimeters	1,043	29.82	31.10	32.82	35.24	38.80	42.37	44.39
144-146 centimeters	709	30.45	31.47	34.24	37.28	40.89	44.51	48.88
Female, 2-10 years								
90-92 centimeters	332	11.73	12.08	12.46	13.08	13.70	14.71	15.84
92-94 centimeters	429	12.04	12.19	12.66	13.45	14.51	15.51	15.85
94-96 centimeters	566	12.08	12.30	12.97	14.09	15.25	15.94	16.49
96-98 centimeters	608	13.08	13.22	13.66	14.53	15.49	16.35	17.21
98-100 centimeters	522	12.49	12.99	14.20	15.17	16.33	17.57	17.99
100-102 centimeters	421	14.03	14.26	14.95	16.12	17.36	18.79	22.16
102-104 centimeters	425	14.14	14.38	15.09	16.32	17.62	18.92	19.50
104-106 centimeters	524	14.38	14.95	16.19	17.00	17.81	19.08	19.66
106-108 centimeters	522	14.81	15.73	16.47	17.34	18.46	19.51	19.86
108-110 centimeters	533	14.55	15.40	16.42	17.33	18.55	19.78	20.87
110-112 centimeters	651	16.09	16.36	17.16	18.42	19.51	20.64	21.45
112-114 centimeters	793	16.28	16.92	18.30	19.41	20.89	22.04	23.14
114-116 centimeters	909	17.35	18.13	18.81	19.95	21.34	22.70	23.79
116-118 centimeters	1,099	18.09	18.37	19.23	20.63	21.93	23.65	25.07
118-120 centimeters	1,162	18.39	18.86	20.15	21.40	23.18	25.02	25.90
120-122 centimeters	1,277	19.43	20.16	21.09	22.56	23.90	25.65	27.36
122-124 centimeters	1,246	19.96	20.39	21.59	23.02	24.61	26.58	28.67
124-126 centimeters	1,319	20.47	21.47	22.59	23.77	25.72	27.74	29.72
126-128 centimeters	1,219	21.53	22.25	23.28	25.35	27.42	29.51	31.19
128-130 centimeters	1,327	22.52	23.28	24.62	26.21	28.73	31.21	33.04
130-132 centimeters	1,102	23.66	24.30	25.39	27.20	29.73	33.45	35.21
132-134 centimeters	1,088	24.47	25.30	26.67	28.42	32.47	35.43	38.82
134-136 centimeters	969	25.25	26.30	28.18	30.51	33.03	36.17	39.20
136-138 centimeters	667	26.05	26.75	28.47	30.70	34.32	37.65	42.36
138-140 centimeters	...	...	...	...	...	...	...	...
140-142 centimeters	...	...	...	...	...	...	...	...
142-144 centimeters	...	...	...	...	...	...	...	...
144-146 centimeters	...	...	...	...	...	...	...	...

INFANT FORMULAS

Name	Company	Classifi-cation	Food Source	Use	Normal Dilution with Water	Kcal/fl oz, Normal Dilution	Pro-tein g	Fat g	Carbo-hydrate g
Casec	Mead Johnson	Infant food modifier	Dried calcium caseinate derived from skim milk curd and limewater	To increase protein and calcium intake	Varies	370	88	2˙	0
Cho-Free	Syntex	Formula base without added carbohy-drate	Soy protein isolate (soy oil)	For intolerance to disaccharides, other carbohy-drates, or milk	Diluted with an equal volume of 12.8% carbohy-drate solution	20	1.8	3.5	6.4
Enfamil	Mead Johnson	Infant formula	Nonfat milk, lactose, soy and coconut oils, soy lecithin	Infant feeding; may be used for infants with poor tolerance of milk fat	Liquid, 1:1 Powder, 1:6	20	1.5	3.7	7
Enfamil with Iron	Mead Johnson	Infant formula	Nonfat milk, lactose, soy and coconut oils, soy lecithin	Infant feeding	Liquid, 1:1 Powder, 1:6	20	1.5	3.7	7
Enfamil Premature Formula	Mead Johnson	Infant formula	Nonfat milk, lactose, sucrose, medium-chain triglycerides, corn and coconut oils	To provide nutrients in a readily absorbable form for low-birth-weight infants	None	24	2.2	4.1	9.2
Evaporated milk	Several brands	Infant formula	Cow's milk	Infant feeding	1:2	13	2.3	2.6	3.2
Lofenalac	Mead Johnson	Modified infant formula	Casein hydrolysate low in phenylala-nine, corn oil, corn syrup solids, modified tapioca starch	For children with phenylketonuria	1:6	20	2.2	2.7	8.8
Lytren	Mead Johnson	Oral electro-lyte mixture		To supply water and electrolytes for maintenance; to replace mild to moderate fluid losses	Powder, 80 g:1 qt Liquid, none	9	0	0	8.4
MBF (Meat Base Formula)	Gerber	Modified infant formula	Beef heart, sugar, modified tapioca starch, sesame oil	May be used in galactosemia or milk allergies	13:19.5	15	2.1	2.5	4.7
Milk, cow's		Infant formula	Cow's milk	Infant feeding	Varies	20	3.5	3.7	4.9
Milk, human		Natural food	Human milk	Infant feeding	None	23	1.1	4.5	6.8

AND FEEDINGS*

					Composition per 100 ml, Normal Dilution†							
Calcium mg	Phosphorus mg	Iron mg	Sodium mg	Potassium mg	Vitamin A IU	Vitamin D IU	Thiamin mg	Riboflavin mg	Niacin mg	Ascorbic acid mg	Other	Miscellaneous Information
1600	800	3	150	30	0	0	0	0	0	0		Powder mixes easily with cereals, milk drinks, and mixed vegetable and meat dishes
85	64	0.88	37	90	220	44	0.055	0.110	0.77	5.7	Other vitamins and minerals	
57.5	48.7	0.16	29	73	177	44.2	0.055	0.066	0.89	5.8	Other vitamins and minerals	
57.5	48.7	1.33	29	73	177	44.2	0.055	0.066	0.89	5.8	Other vitamins and minerals	
133	66	0.19	33	90	212.4	53.1	0.066	0.077	1.06	6.9	Other vitamins and minerals	Available for hospital use only
84	67	Tr	40	102	107.2	27.6	0.013	0.11	0.59	Tr	Vitamin and mineral addition varies from brand to brand	Values are for normal dilution with no added sugar; generally requires added carbohydrates
66.4	49.8	1.33	33	71.9	177	44.2	0.055	0.066	0.89	5.8	Other vitamins and minerals	Should be used only for children with PKU‡
9.9	8.2	0	71.2	104	0	0	0	0	0	0		
74	48	1.03	14	29	130.5	34.5	0.045	0.075	0.54	4.4	Other vitamins and minerals	Nonsoy, milk-free formula; additional carbohydrate is normally added before feeding
117	92	0.05	51	137	102.5	1.4	0.044	0.175	0.094	1.1	Other vitamins and minerals	Composition is only approximate because of seasonal variations, differences in breeds and manufacturing, and so forth
34	14	0.05	16	51	189.8	2.2	0.016	0.036	0.147	4.3	Other vitamins and minerals	Composition is only approximate because of individual differences, varying degrees of maturity, diet of mother, and so forth

Table continued on the following page

Name	Company	Classifi-cation	Food Source	Use	Normal Dilution with Water	kcal/fl oz, Normal Dilution	Pro-tein g	Fat g	Carbo-hydrate g
Milk, goat's		Infant formula	Goat's milk	Infant feeding	Varies	20	3.2	4	4.6
Dale Dehy-drated Goat Milk	Cutter	Infant formula	Goat's milk	Infant feeding	Liquid, 1:1 Powder, 1:8	20	3.3	4.1	4.7
Miracle Goat Milk	Milk Foods	Infant formula	Evaporated goat's milk		1:1				
Neo-Mull-Soy	Syntex	Infant formula	Soy protein isolate, sucrose, soybean oil	Hypoallergenic formula for infants sensitive to cow's milk	1:1	20	1.8	3.5	6.4
Nursoy	Wyeth	Infant formula	Sucrose; soy protein isolate; oleo, safflower, soybean, and coconut oils	Hypoallergenic formula for infants sensitive to cow's milk	1:1	20	2.3	3.6	6.8
Nutramigen	Mead Johnson	Modified infant formula	Protein hydrol-ysate: casein enzymatically hydrolyzed, sucrose, modified tapioca starch, corn oil	For infants sensitive to milk proteins or who have galactosemia	1:6	20	2.2	2.6	8.8
Pedialyte	Ross	Oral electro-lyte mixture		To supply water and electrolytes for maintenance; to replace mild to moderate fluid losses	None needed	6	0	0	5
Portagen	Mead Johnson	Modified infant formula	Sodium caseinate, MCT§ and corn oils, corn syrup solids, sucrose	For infants and adults who do not efficiently digest and absorb conven-tional long-chain food fats	1:6 (infant)	20	2.5	3.4	8.1
Pregestimil	Mead Johnson	Modified infant formula	Protein hydrol-ysate, MCT§ and corn oils, corn syrup solids, dextrose, modified tapioca starch	For infants with malabsorption disorders	1:6	20	2.2	2.8	8.8

AND FEEDINGS* *(Continued)*

					Composition per 100 ml, Normal Dilution†							
Calcium mg	Phosphorus mg	Iron mg	Sodium mg	Potassium mg	Vitamin A IU	Vitamin D IU	Thiamin mg	Riboflavin mg	Niacin mg	Ascorbic acid mg	Other	Miscellaneous Information
129	106	0.1	35	180	207.4	2.4	0.040	0.184	0.19	1.5	Other vitamins and minerals	Goat's milk is a relatively poor source of folic acid; therefore, a supplement of 50 µg/day is recommended
130	106	0.05	41	179			0.0480	0.1140	0.27	1.4		Fat from goat's milk may be more readily digested than that from cow's milk because of having more essential fatty acids, a greater percentage of medium-chain and short-chain fatty acids, and fewer long-chain fatty acids
85	64	0.88	37	90	220	44	0.055	0.110	0.77	5.7	Other vitamins and minerals	
66	46	1.32	21	77	275	44	0.080	0.011	1.04	6	Other vitamins and minerals	
66	49.8	1.33	33	72	177	44.2	0.055	0.066	0.89	5.8	Other vitamins and minerals	Nonsoy milk-free formula
16	0	0	69	78	0	0	0	0	0	0	0.4 meq of magnesium; 3 meq of chloride; 2.8 meq of lactate	Contraindications: intractable vomiting, adynamic ileus, intestinal obstruction of perforated bowel, severe dehydration secondary to diarrhea; use with caution in decreased renal function
66.4	49.8	1.33	33.2	88.5	553	55.3	0.111	0.133	1.44	5.5	Other vitamins and minerals	
66.4	49.8	1.33	33.2	71.9	177	44.2	0.055	0.066	0.88	5.8	Other vitamins and minerals	

Table continued on the following page

INFANT FORMULAS

Name	Company	Classifi-cation	Food Source	Use	Normal Dilution with Water	kcal/fl oz, Normal Dilution	Pro-tein g	Fat g	Carbo-hydrate g
Probana	Mead Johnson	Modified infant formula	Whole and nonfat cow's milk, banana powder, casein hydrol-ysate, dextrose, corn oil	For use in celiac conditions and diarrhea	1:6	20	4.2	2.2	7.9
ProSobee	Mead Johnson	Infant formula	Soy protein isolate with added L-methionine, soy oil, sucrose, corn syrup solids	Hypoallergenic formula for infants sensitive to cow's milk	1:1	20	2.5	3.4	6.8
SMA	Wyeth	Infant formula	Nonfat cow's milk, partially demin-eralized whey; lactose; coconut, oleo, soybean, and safflower oils	Infant feeding	Liquid, 1:1 Powder, 1:8	20	1.5	3.6	7.2
Similac	Ross	Infant formula	Nonfat cow's milk, lactose, coconut and soy oils	Infant feeding	Liquid, 1:1	20	1.55	3.6	7.2
Similac with Iron	Ross	Infant formula	Nonfat cow's milk, lactose, coconut and soy oils	Infant feeding	Liquid, 1:1	20	1.55	3.6	7.2
Similac Advance	Ross	Infant formula	Nonfat cow's milk, soy protein isolate, corn syrup, soy and corn oils	Infant feeding	1:1	16	2.8	2	6.2
Similac Isomil	Ross	Infant formula	Soy protein isolate, sucrose, corn syrup, soy and coconut oils	Hypoallergenic formula for infants sensitive to cow's milk	1:1	20	2	3.6	6.8
Similac PM 60/40	Ross	Infant formula	Partially demin-eralized nonfat cow's milk, partially demin-eralized whey, lactose, corn and coconut oils	For infants whose renal system might be taxed by a solute load greater than that of human milk	1:8	20	1.6	3.5	7.6
Soyalac	Loma Linda	Infant formula	Soybean and corn syrup solids, sugar, soybean oil	Hypoallergenic formula for infants sensitive to cow's milk	Liquid, 1:1	20	2.1	4	5.9

*Modified from Dietary Department, University of Iowa Hospitals and Clinics: Recent Advances in Therapeutic Diets. Third edition. Ames, Iowa, Iowa State University Press, 1979, pp. 128–131. By permission.

†For Casec, composition per 100 g of powder.

‡Precautions: Intake of phenylalanine must be carefully controlled to prevent excessive blood levels and urinary excretion and still provide enough for growth. Phenylalanine blood levels and weight and growth curves should be determined. Symptoms of phenylalanine deprivation may include lethargy, nausea, vomiting, and fever.

§Medium-chain triglycerides.

AND FEEDINGS* *(Continued)*

| | | | | | Composition per 100 ml, Normal Dilution† | | | | | | | |
Cal-cium mg	Phos-phorus mg	Iron mg	Sodium mg	Potas-sium mg	Vitamin A IU	Vitamin D IU	Thia-min mg	Ribo-flavin mg	Nia-cin mg	Ascorbic acid mg	Other	Miscellaneous Information
121.7	94	0.15	64.2	127	553	110.6	0.066	0.111	0.885	5.8	Other vitamins and minerals	
83	55	1.33	44.3	77.4	177	44.2	0.055	0.066	0.89	5.5	Other vitamins and minerals	
45	33	1.27	16	53	265	42.3	0.071	0.106	0.7	5.8	60:40 lactal-bumin:casein ratio; other vitamins and minerals	Demineralized whey is used to produce a formu-la based on cow's milk but similar in mineral compo-sition to human milk
51	39	Tr	22	70	250	40	0.065	0.1	0.7	5.5	Other vitamins and minerals	
51	0.39	1.2	22	70	250	40	0.065	0.1	0.7	5.5	Other vitamins and minerals	
80	60	1.8	45	110	240	40	0.075	0.090	1	5	Other vitamins and minerals	Recommended for babies 4 months of age and older
70	50	1.2	30	71	250	40	0.04	0.06	0.9	5.5	Other vitamins and iron	
40	20	0.26	16	58	250	40	0.065	0.10	0.73	5.5	60:40 lactal-bumin:casein ratio; other vitamins and minerals	Demineralized whey is used to produce a for-mula based on cow's milk but similar in min-eral composition to human milk
42	33	1	32	90	158.4	42.3	0.042	0.063	0.600	3.2	Other vitamins and minerals	

CALCULATION OF BASAL CALORIC REQUIREMENT
FOR INFANTS AND CHILDREN

For a child less than 5 years of age, the basal caloric requirement for 24 hours is computed by multiplying the standard weight for the measured height by the basal requirement for calories per pound per 24 hours for the appropriate age (see table of "Basal Requirement for Calories per Pound per 24 Hours" below). The height is that of the child measured without shoes. The weight to be used is an estimate of a desirable weight based on evaluation of the child's muscular development and body fat with the additional aid of the tables on pages 222 through 227. The age to be used is that of the child to the nearest year or half year. Depending on activity, actual calorie expenditure of a child is generally 50 to 80% greater than basal expenditure.

BASAL REQUIREMENT FOR CALORIES PER POUND PER 24 HOURS

	Calories	
Age	*Boys*	*Girls*
6 months	25.0	25.0
1 year	25.5	25.5
2 years	25.0	24.5
3 years	23.5	23.5
4 years	23.0	22.0

SELECTED BIBLIOGRAPHY

Benedict, F. G., and Talbot, F. B.: Metabolism and Growth from Birth to Puberty. Washington, D.C., The Carnegie Institution of Washington, 1921, 213 pp.

Lewis, R. G., Kinsman, G. M., and Iliff, A.: The basal metabolism of normal boys and girls from two to twelve years old, inclusive. Am. J. Dis. Child., 53:348–428, 1937.

SECTION 6

FORMULAS,
FOOD SUPPLEMENTS,
AND TOTAL PARENTERAL
NUTRITION

FORMULAS FOR TUBE FEEDING AND ORAL FEEDING

GENERAL DESCRIPTION

Commercial formulas that provide feedings with standardized nutrient composition and uniform viscosity may be administered either orally or by tube to provide nutritional support for persons unable or unwilling to ingest or tolerate conventional foods.

INDICATIONS AND RATIONALE

Commercial formulas are generally preferable to blenderized food because of convenience, bacteriologic safety, lower cost, and fewer problems of delivery through a tube. Standard feeding formulas cost about $5 per day for amounts required to maintain the average patient; chemically defined diets may cost two to four times this amount. Formulas can be selected to be lactose-free or restricted in fat if required by the clinical situation. Chemically defined formulas provide protein in the form of mixtures of amino acids or small peptide units, carbohydrates as simple sugars or oligosaccharides, and fat as polyunsaturated fat in amounts only large enough to provide the necessary essential fatty acids and, in some preparations, as medium-chain triglycerides in ·addition. Thus, chemically defined formulas tend to be higher in osmolality, less pleasant in taste, and more expensive than standard formulas but are appropriate for use in states of maldigestion, malabsorption, partial intestinal obstruction, and enterocutaneous fistulas. Diets to identify food allergies may be begun with chemically defined formulas, which presumably are nearly or completely free of allergens.

ORAL FEEDINGS

Persons with dysphagia, inadequate food intake, or wired jaw may require liquid feedings. Conventional hospital clear liquid and full liquid diets in quantities usually consumed by patients are inadequate in several nutrients and should not be used as the sole nutritional support for more than 2 or 3 days. Formulas can be used to provide palatable feedings, which alone or in addition to the conventional hospital liquid diets will satisfy the nutritional needs of these patients.

TUBE FEEDINGS

Tube feeding techniques are used when the person is unable to swallow readily or safely, such as in neurologic disorders or after extensive surgical procedures of the head or neck. Patients with maldigestion, malabsorption, partial intestinal obstruction, or fistulas may require chemically defined diets (elemental diets) to satisfy their nutritional needs.

HAZARDS

Tube feeding preparations are excellent media for growth of bacteria. This fact should be kept in mind in handling and administration. Diarrhea may occur as a consequence of bacterial growth in the preparation, lactase deficiency, high osmolality of the formula, inappropriate positioning of the tube, or excessively rapid administration of the formula. Long-term disuse of the intestinal tract may lead to malabsorption; thus, feedings are often tolerated better if small amounts (perhaps one-fourth or less of the estimated caloric needs) are given initially and the volume of the feeding is gradually increased over the space of several days. It is often desirable to maintain parenteral nutrition during this transitional period until the patient's gastrointestinal tract can tolerate enough of the formula to maintain a satisfactory nutritional state. Dilution of formulas to half strength may also be necessary to prevent diarrhea when feedings are resumed after a week or more without oral or tube feeding. Dehydration, hypernatremia, hyperglycemia, and hyperosmolar coma are all potential hazards, particularly if the patient has diabetes or if too little water is given with the formula. Insulin-taking diabetics may require increased doses of insulin during tube feeding. In the patient with impaired renal function, plasma urea concentration better reflects the degree of retained protein catabolic products than does the creatinine level. Risks of vomiting and aspiration may be lessened if the precautions listed under ordering information are observed.

MONITORING TECHNIQUES

Serum sodium, potassium, and chloride and plasma urea and glucose concentrations should be measured at intervals of 2 or 3 days during the first 2 weeks of tube feedings and at less frequent intervals thereafter when the condition of the patient seems stable. Frequent weighing reflects short-term changes in water and sodium balance and provides a long-term measure of correction of malnutrition. An increase in serum sodium concentration may indicate water depletion and the need to add enough water beyond that supplied by the formula to correct the imbalance. The introduction of tube feeding may result in so-called starvation edema if the person has been substantially protein- and calorie-depleted; congestive failure is rare but has occurred.

A decreased serum albumin level is commonly regarded as an indication of protein malnutrition, but changes in hydration may influence this measurement and thus limit its usefulness in identifying protein-depleted states and in monitoring the response to treatment. Changes in protein status can be assessed by calculating nitrogen balance (nitrogen intake minus nitrogen loss). Total nitrogen loss can be estimated by measuring and adding stool and urine nitrogen and the nitrogen content of the exudate, if any. Total nitrogen intake can be estimated by dividing the total protein content of the formula and intravenous infusions by 6.25. If the nitrogen balance is positive, the protein deficit is being corrected. If the nitrogen balance is negative, the deficit is increasing.

ORDERING INFORMATION

Specify the *product*. Order "standard feeding formula" for oral or tube feeding of patients who have intact gastrointestinal tracts but who are unable to take adequate amounts of food in other forms. Specify "chemically defined diet" for patients who have maldigestion or malabsorption, need minimal residue, or require a test diet for indication of food allergies. Specific products can be ordered by name as well.

Specify *total volume* of formula for 24 hours. If the caloric density of the formula prepared at standard dilutions is about 1 kcal per milliliter, the volume in milliliters will be about equal to the calories desired. Calorie requirements can be estimated by use of the following guide.

Weight maintenance for adults with	kcal/kg of ideal body weight
Normal metabolic needs	25
Hypermetabolic states	40 to 50

The amount of protein that would be included in a standard formula with these calorie levels should be adequate for most circumstances. In general, only one-half the expected full amounts of feedings should be ordered for the first day or two to allow the intestinal tract to accommodate itself to the new manner of feeding.

Indicate the *allowance of water*. The recommended intake of water is usually 1 ml per 1 kcal of feeding. Generally, water requirements can be met by giving an additional amount of water equal to one-fourth to one-third the volume of the tube feeding. The amount of water needed in addition to that in the formula can be determined more closely if the moisture content of the formula is known. To determine water supplied by the formula, multiply the percentage of moisture content by the total volume of the feeding. (The moisture content of most formulas is 75 to 80% of weight/volume.) The difference between the total volume and the calculated water content of the formula is the amount of free water that must be given in addition to the formula to meet recommendations.

Specify *rate and timing* of administration. Formulas given by tube preferably should be administered continuously, either throughout the 24 hours or during the waking hours, for example, from 6 a.m. to 10 p.m. or from 7 a.m. to 9 p.m. If feedings are given intermittently, the formula should be administered at a drip rate not exceeding 240 ml per 20 minutes. Too rapid a rate of administration may produce cramping or diarrhea.

NURSING PRECAUTIONS

A 6F or 8F feeding tube is generally acceptable to most patients, but a 10F tube may be used if problems are encountered maintaining the flow of the formula. It is useful to administer the needed amount of water in amounts of 50 to 100 ml several times daily to flush the tubing and gavage feeding bag. The feeding may be interrupted 30 to 60 minutes before and during any physically stressful activity, such as physiotherapy or intermittent positive pressure breathing. The head of the bed should be elevated as much as the patient can tolerate to reduce the chance of vomiting and aspiration.

Bottled formulas may be stored at room temperature until opened. An open bottle should have the time and date of opening marked on it and should be stored in the refrigerator—but no longer than 24 hours. Prepared formulas should be placed in the refrigerator. Any unused formula should be discarded when the 24 hours has expired. The formula should be kept refrigerated, and portions sufficient for no more than 4 to 5 hours may be added to the gavage feeding bags; the formula will then warm to nearly room temperature as it passes slowly through the plastic tubing. Formulas should be thoroughly mixed before administration. The gavage bags should either be replaced daily or be cleansed thoroughly in water and detergent and be carefully rinsed daily. The physician should judge when the nasogastric tube needs to be replaced.

During the first 3 days, the possibility of gastric retention should be determined by aspirating the stomach contents every 6 to 8 hours. If more than 200 ml of gastric content is obtained, the feeding should be interrupted for 2 or more hours and the stomach contents should be aspirated again. Feedings may be resumed if the physician judges the residual volume of the stomach contents to be small enough (usually 100 ml or less) that risk of regurgitation and aspiration is acceptably small. If no evidence of gastric retention is found in the first 3 days, the residual volume need be determined only once daily at a time the formula has been administered for at least 3 to 4 hours. The time intervals and volumes are likely to be appropriate for many patients but must be individualized for each patient's needs. Nurses should notify the physician if diarrhea occurs. If the patient has emesis or complains of abdominal distress or nausea, the nurse should discontinue the feeding immediately and report this to the physician.

PHYSICIANS: HOW TO ORDER DIETS

Requests for formulas for tube feeding or oral feeding should supply the following information.

Product.

Standard feeding formula—For oral or tube feeding of patients who have intact gastrointestinal tracts but who are unable to take adequate amounts of food in other forms; *or*

Chemically defined diet—For patients who have maldigestion or malabsorption, need minimal residue, or require a test diet for identification of food allergies; *or*

Specific products may be ordered by name.

Volume. Twenty-five milliliters of formula per kilogram of ideal body weight provides sufficient calories and protein for most patients. Up to 50 ml/kg may be needed for hypermetabolic states.

Supplemental water. Generally, supplemental water equal to 20% or more of the volume of full-strength feeding formulas is needed.

Rate of administration. The rate usually should be specified as "continuously" or "continuously during waking hours." If feedings are given intermittently, one should specify no more than 240 ml in 20 minutes.

COMPOSITION OF

Product and Manufacturer	Caloric Density kcal/ml	How Supplied	kcal	Protein	Fat
Intact Protein and Protein Isolates: Low-Lactose, Low-Residue					
Ensure Ross	1.06	240-ml bottles and cans	106	3.7 g; 14% of kcal Sodium and calcium caseinates Soy protein isolate	3.7 g; 31.5% of kcal Corn oil
Ensure Osmolite Ross	1.06	240-ml bottles and cans; 960-ml cans	106	3.6 g; 13.6% of kcal Sodium and calcium caseinates Soy protein isolate	3.8 g; 32.3% of kcal MCT‡ oil Corn oil Soy oil
Ensure Plus Ross	1.50	240-ml cans	150	5.5 g; 14.7% of kcal Sodium and calcium caseinates Soy protein isolate	5.3 g; 32% of kcal Corn oil
Isocal Mead Johnson	1.04	240-ml bottles and cans; 360-ml and 960-ml cans	104	3.4 g; 12.9% of kcal Sodium and calcium caseinates Soy protein isolate	4.4 g; 38.5% of kcal Soy oil MCT‡ oil
Precision High Nitrogen Diet Doyle	1.05	82-g packet; mix with 240 ml of water to yield 285 ml	105	4.4 g; 17% of kcal Egg albumin	0.05 g; 0.4% of kcal Soybean oil
Precision Isotonic Diet Doyle	0.96	58-g packet; mix with 240 ml of water to yield 260 ml	96	2.9 g; 11.8% of kcal Egg albumin	3 g; 28.2% of kcal Vegetable oil
Precision LR Diet Doyle	1.11	84-g packet; mix with 240 ml of water to yield 285 ml	111	2.6 g; 9.5% of kcal Egg albumin	0.08 g; 0.6% of kcal Soybean oil
Precision Moderate Nitrogen Diet Doyle	1.21	77-g packet; mix with 240 ml of water to yield 275 ml	121	3.9 g; 13% of kcal Egg albumin	3.8 g; 28% of kcal Soybean oil
Hydrolyzed Protein and Amino Acids: Low-Lactose, Low-Residue, Chemically Defined Formula					
Flexical Mead Johnson	1	56-g packet; mix with 207 ml of water to yield 250 ml	100	2.2 g; 9% of kcal Hydrolyzed casein Crystalline amino acids	3.4 g; 30% of kcal Soy oil MCT‡ oil
Vital Ross	1	78-g packet; mix with 255 ml of water to yield 300 ml	100	4.2 g; 16.7% of kcal Hydrolyzed whey, soy, and meat proteins Free essential amino acids	1 g; 9.3% of kcal Sunflower oil

SELECTED FORMULAS*

Composition per 100 ml

Carbohydrate	Lactose g	Sodium meq	Potassium meq	Chloride meq	Calcium mg	Phosphorus mg	Osmolality† mOsm/kg of Water	Moisture % wt/vol
14.5 g; 54.5% of kcal Corn syrup solids Sucrose	0	3.2	3.25	2.9	52.8	52.8	450	84
14.3 g; 54% of kcal Corn syrup solids Glucose polymers (Polycose)	0	2.3	2.3	2.3	54.2	54.2	300	83
19.7 g; 53.3% of kcal Corn syrup solids Sucrose	0	4.6	4.9	4.5	63	63	600	§
13 g; 49.6% of kcal Corn syrup solids	0	2.3	3.3	2.9	62.5	52.1	350	78
21.8 g; 83% of kcal Maltodextrin Sucrose	0	4.3	2.3	3.4	35.1	35.1	557	§
14.4 g; 60% of kcal Glucose oligosaccharides Sucrose	0	3.3	2.5	2.9	65.4	65.4	300	§
24.9 g; 89.9% of kcal Maltodextrin Sucrose	0	3.0	2.2	3.1	58.4	58.4	500-545	§
18.2 g; 59% of kcal Maltodextrin Sucrose	0	4.5	2.3	3.1	60.6	60.6	395	§
15.4 g; 61% of kcal Sucrose Dextrin Citrate	0	1.5	3.2	3.5	60.0	50.0	723	§
18.5 g; 74% of kcal Glucose oligosaccharides and polysaccharides Sucrose Cornstarch	0	1.7	3.0	1.9	66.6	66.6	450	86

Table continued on following page

COMPOSITION OF SELECTED FORMULAS* (Continued)

Product and Manufacturer	Caloric Density kcal/ml	How Supplied	kcal	Protein	Fat
Vivonex Eaton	1	80-g packet; dilute to 300 ml	100	2.1 g; 8.5% of kcal Crystalline amino acids	0.1 g; 1.3% of kcal Safflower oil
Vivonex HN Eaton	1	80-g packet; dilute to 300 ml	100	4.2 g; 18.26% of kcal Crystalline amino acids	0.1 g; 0.78% of kcal Safflower oil
Intact Protein Containing Milk: Moderate- and Low-Residue					
Compleat-B Doyle	1	250-ml bottles and 400-ml cans	100	4 g; 16% of kcal Intact meat, beef, and wheat protein	4 g; 36% of kcal Corn oil Beef fat
Carnation Instant Breakfast**†† Carnation	1.22	34-35 g packets; mix with 240 ml of whole milk to yield 260 ml	122	5.8 g; 22.1% of kcal Whole milk Nonfat milk Sodium caseinate Soy protein isolate	3.1 g; 28% of kcal Milk fat
Meritene liquid** Doyle	1	240-ml and 300-ml cans	100	6.1 g; 24% of kcal Concentrated skim milk Sodium caseinate	3.4 g; 30% of kcal Vegetable oil Monoglycerides and diglycerides
Meritene powder** and milk†† Doyle	1.06	Mix 32 g of powder with 240 ml of whole milk to yield 260 ml	106	6.9 g; 25.8% of kcal Whole milk Nonfat milk	3.5 g; 31.3% of kcal Milk fat
Sustacal liquid** Mead Johnson	1	240-ml, 360-ml, and 960-ml cans	100	6 g; 24.4% of kcal Concentrated skim milk Sodium and calcium caseinates Soy protein isolate	2.3 g; 20.1% of kcal Soy oil
Sustacal powder** and milk†† Mead Johnson	1.33	53-g packet; mix with 240 ml of whole milk to yield 270 ml	133	8 g; 24% of kcal Nonfat milk Whole milk	3.3 g; 22% of kcal Milk fat
Sustagen powder** and water Mead Johnson	1.66	Mix 100 g of powder with 160 ml of water to yield 240 ml	166	10 g; 24% of kcal Nonfat milk Whole milk Calcium caseinate	1.4 g; 7.5% of kcal Milk fat

*Not all these formulas are currently available at the Mayo Clinic and its associated institutions. Data are based on information available from the manufacturer at the time this manual was being prepared for publication. Formulations may be altered periodically. These data are intended to be used for comparison. If additional information is needed, the manufacturer should be written.

†Unflavored; the osmolality of the product varies with the flavor packet used. If the product is mixed with a soft drink or a juice rather than water, the osmolality of the mixing product should be included when the osmolality of the solution is determined.

‡MCT = medium-chain triglycerides.

§Information not available.

**Values for vanilla flavor.

††Whole milk added.

Composition per 100 ml

Carbohydrate	Lactose g	Sodium meq	Potassium meq	Chloride meq	Calcium mg	Phosphorus mg	Osmolality† mOsm/kg of Water	Moisture % wt/vol
22.6 g; 90.2% of kcal Glucose oligosaccharides	0	3.7	3.0	5.1	44.3	44.3	500-1,180	85
21.0 g; 80.96% of kcal Glucose oligosaccharides	0	3.3	1.8	5.2	26.7	26.7	810-1,150	85
12 g; 48% of kcal Maltodextrin Lactose	2.4	6.8	3.4	2.3	62.5	168.7	490	80
13.5 g; 49.9% of kcal Sucrose Corn syrup solids Lactose	9.5	4.2	7.2	§	137.1	110.5	§	§
11.7 g; 46% of kcal Sucrose Lactose Corn syrup solids	5.7	4.0	4.3	4.7	125.0	125.0	700-750	§
11.9 g; 42.9% of kcal Lactose Corn syrup solids	9.8	4.0	7.1	6.5	217.9	181.6	690	§
13.8 g; 55.2% of kcal Sucrose Lactose Corn syrup solids	1.7	4.0	5.3	4.4	100.0	91.7	625	§
17.9 g; 54% of kcal Sucrose Lactose Corn syrup solids	11.4	5.3	8.6	5.0	214.8	177.8	756	§
28.6 g; 68.5% of kcal Corn syrup solids Glucose	9.5	5.0	8.5	§	304.8	228.6	1,334	§

DIETARY SUPPLEMENTS

Dietary supplements are a concentrated source of nutrients prescribed to increase intake of a specific nutrient. Dietary supplements are used in addition to the individual's diet. The supplement should be chosen according to the specific needs of the patient. For example, nonfat dry milk could be incorporated into foods to increase the protein and calorie content of the diet.

PHYSICIANS: HOW TO ORDER DIETS

Generally, the dietitian will incorporate dietary supplements or other supplementary oral feedings into the diet as the situation indicates and notify the physician. If the physician chooses to request a specific supplement, the diet order should indicate the **kind of supplement** and the **amount**.

COMPOSITION OF SELECTED SUPPLEMENTS

Product and Manufacturer	Type	How Supplied	Amount to Give 100 kcal	Composition per 100 kcal				
				Protein g	Fat g	Carbohydrate g	Sodium meq	Potassium meq
Cal-Power General Mills	Carbohydrate source	Liquid: 1 carton = 8 fl oz (300 g)	55 g, liquid	0.06	0	27.2	0.24	0.07
Citrotein Doyle	Calorie supplement	Powder: 1/4 cup = 33 g	26.3 g, dry wt	6.05	0.26	18.42	4.58	2.68
Controlyte Doyle	Calorie supplement: low-electrolyte, low-protein	Powder	19.8 g, dry wt	Trace	4.80	14.3	0.13	0.02
Hycal Beecham	Carbohydrate source	Liquid	40.7 ml, liquid	0.01	0.01	24.41	0.24	0.01
Lipomul-Oral Upjohn	Fat source	Liquid	16.7 ml, liquid	0.01	11.11	0.11	0.29	0.01
MCT Oil Mead Johnson	Fat source: medium-chain triglycerides	Liquid: 1 tbsp = 14 g	12.05 g, liquid	0	12.05	0	0	0
Nonfat dry milk	Protein, calorie supplement	Powder: 1 tbsp = 7 g	28 g; 4 tbsp	10	0.2	14.6	6.5	12.6
Polycose Ross	Carbohydrate source: oligosaccharides	Powder: 1 tbsp = 8 g; Liquid: 1 bottle = 120 ml	25 g, dry wt; 50 ml, liquid	0	0	25	1.23	0.03

SELECTED BIBLIOGRAPHY
(Formulas for Tube Feeding and
Oral Feeding, Dietary Supplements)

Shils, M. E., ed.: Defined-Formula Diets for Medical Purposes. Chicago, American Medical Association, 1977.
Shils, M. E., Bloch, A. S. and Chernoff, R.: Liquid formulas for oral and tube feeding. Clin. Bull., 6:151-158, 1976.

TOTAL PARENTERAL NUTRITION

Total parenteral nutrition is commonly used to meet the full nutritional needs of the patient who is unable to take food orally or by tube feeding for a substantial period. Patients undergoing surgery ordinarily have sufficient nutritional reserves to sustain them for a few days to a week if needs for water and electrolytes are met by peripheral vein infusions of glucose and electrolyte solutions. If the patient is already malnourished, if inability to eat is likely to be prolonged, or if, as in inflammatory bowel disease, there is a need to "rest the bowel," solutions of glucose, amino acids, electrolytes, and vitamins are given by way of a catheter into a large vein near the heart. These concentrated solutions are irritating to the vein walls unless given into a large vein, where the large volume of blood flow results in prompt dilution.

Although total parenteral nutrition is not the immediate responsibility of the dietitian, one must be aware of the need to protect the nutritional gains achieved by a period of parenteral feeding. This is done by providing oral feedings in increasing amounts as the parenteral feedings are gradually reduced over a period of days. During this transitional period, the dietitian and physician should see that no substantial calorie deficits occur.

SELECTED BIBLIOGRAPHY

Feliciano, D. V., and Telander, R. L.: Total parenteral nutrition in infants and children. Mayo Clin. Proc., 51:647-654, 1976.
Fleming, C. R., McGill, D. B., Hoffman, H. N., II, et al.: Total parenteral nutrition. Mayo Clin. Proc., 51:187-199, 1976.

SECTION 7

OTHER DIETARY
PROGRAMS

SPECIAL DIETARY PRECAUTIONS

DIETARY PRECAUTIONS FOR CARDIAC SURGERY PATIENTS

GENERAL DESCRIPTION

The dietary progression for postoperative cardiac surgery patients is similar to that for other types of surgery. The diet is also controlled in sodium.

INDICATIONS AND RATIONALE

Sodium is controlled as a precaution against congestive heart failure. The degree and duration of sodium restriction vary with the type of surgery and the response of the patient. The patient follows the diet postoperatively until dismissal from the hospital or for several weeks after dismissal. Then the diet is advanced to a lesser degree of sodium restriction, which is followed for several weeks or longer. Most patients may then resume their usual dietary practices. The following chart summarizes the general types of heart surgery and the level of sodium restriction usually prescribed.

Condition	Sodium Level and Progression
Repair of complex forms of congenital heart defects Prosthetic valve replacement	Begin with 20 meq of sodium; advance to 90 meq of sodium or no-extra-salt diet
Repair of simpler forms of congenital heart defects (for example, atrial septal defect, isolated pulmonary stenosis) Coronary artery bypass grafting	Begin with 90 meq of sodium; advance to usual diet

It may be appropriate for persons who have had surgery related to coronary artery disease to follow a diet intended for weight control or to lower serum lipids.

SODIUM RESTRICTION FOR ADULTS

See page 65 for calculation of sodium-controlled diets.

SODIUM RESTRICTION FOR CHILDREN

There are two levels of sodium restriction: strict (1 meq of sodium per 100 calories) and mild (4 meq of sodium per 100 calories). These levels correspond to the 20 meq and 90 meq of sodium diets for adults.

The diet is based on the total number of calories necessary for the child to maintain normal weight. Generally, the hospitalized child does not require the same number of calories that a healthy, more active child does. The following guide may be used to estimate calorie needs.

Body Weight (kg)	Suggested Calorie Intake (kcal)
<10	100/kg
10 to 20	1,000 + 50 for each kg over 10
>20	1,500 + 20 for each kg over 20

The following guide may be used for sodium intake.

Suggested Calorie Intake (kcal)	Control of Sodium (meq)	
	Strict	Mild
<1,000	<10	<40
1,000 to 1,500	10 to 15	40 to 60
>1,500	15 to 25	60 to 90

The diet should not exceed the upper limit of sodium allowed in each group. The food exchange list for sodium control (see page 67) may be used.

PHYSICIANS: HOW TO ORDER DIETS

The diet order should specify the **initial level of sodium**. This is automatically continued through each stage of the postoperative series (clear liquid, full liquid, and soft diets). Requests for instruction in home diet should also indicate the level of sodium restriction:

For adults—
**20 meq of sodium, advance to 90 meq of sodium
or no extra salt;** *or*
90 meq of sodium, advance to usual diet.

For children—
**Strict sodium restriction, advance to mild sodium
restriction;** *or*
Mild sodium restriction, advance to usual diet.

The physician should discuss the duration of diet modifications with the patient.

SELECTED BIBLIOGRAPHY

Peterson, C. R.: Dietary counseling for patients admitted for coronary artery bypass graft. J. Am. Diet. Assoc., 68:158-159, 1976.

DIETARY PRECAUTIONS FOR CARDIAC MEDICAL PATIENTS

GENERAL DESCRIPTION

The dietary program for patients in the coronary care unit routinely consists of control of sodium, cholesterol, and calories and restriction of caffeine-containing beverages.

INDICATIONS AND RATIONALE

The diet is modified primarily as a precautionary measure, rather than as therapy, for patients who have sustained a myocardial infarction.

During the first several days or weeks after a myocardial infarction, the patient may have congestive heart failure. Control of sodium in the diet lessens the cardiac work load, is a precaution against congestive failure, and favors control of hypertension if it is a factor. Cardiac arrhythmia, a particular hazard during this time, may possibly be provoked by caffeine.

Large meals may stress the circulation, interfere with breathing by distending the stomach, increase the metabolic rate (postprandial thermogenesis), and thus increase the cardiac work load. Generally, several small meals are well tolerated. If the patient is obese and the diet to be followed after dismissal is expected to be limited to a certain calorie level (for example, 1,000 or 1,200 calories), the diets served in the coronary care unit should not exceed this figure. This policy facilitates instruction of the patient at dismissal and emphasizes the importance of long-term weight control.

The patient usually knows that the infarction was the consequence of atherosclerosis of the coronary arteries and may be fearful of foods high in cholesterol or saturated fats during the several days or weeks of the postinfarction period, even though the atherosclerotic process had evolved only after many years of interaction between genetic and dietary factors. Control of cholesterol and saturated fats (see page 58) is reasonable to allay the apprehensions of the patient and relatives and to initiate dietary modifications that may help to avoid further atherogenesis and an infarction months or years later. Control of dietary fats and cholesterol is thought to be less necessary for patients beyond the seventh decade and is often not done.

GENERAL DIETARY RECOMMENDATIONS

The dietary recommendations vary according to the recovery phase of the patient, which is organized into three stages. The length of each stage varies according to the type of infarct and the protocol of the unit.

Stage 1. The diet is low in sodium ($\leqslant$90 meq) and cholesterol and consists of soft or liquid foods (see "Soft Diet," page 12, or "Full Liquid Diet," page 10). The meals are small. Caffeine-containing beverages, such as coffee and tea, are not permitted. Decaffeinated coffee may be served.

Stage 2 (Days 6-10). The diet is low in sodium ($\leqslant$90 meq) and cholesterol. Calorie needs are assessed with a view toward the dismissal diet.

Stage 3 (Days 11-15). The diet is individualized according to the need for long-term control of sodium, cholesterol, and saturated fats.

PHYSICIANS: HOW TO ORDER DIETS

The diet order should indicate **dietary precautions for coronary care unit patient** and any additional dietary modifications necessary.

SELECTED BIBLIOGRAPHY

Christakis, G., and Winston, M.: Nutritional therapy in acute myocardial infarction. J. Am. Diet. Assoc., 63: 233-238, 1973.
Hemzacek, K. I.: Dietary protocol for the patient who has suffered a myocardial infarction. J. Am. Diet. Assoc., 72:182-185, 1978.
Jones, R. J.: Dietary management in the coronary care unit (questions and answers). J.A.M.A., 237:2645, 1977.

TYRAMINE CONTROL

GENERAL DESCRIPTION

The diet restricts foods that contain large amounts of tyramine either naturally or through aging, a process that increases tyramine content by protein breakdown. Foods that have high levels of other pressor amines and foods that have been implicated in hypertensive reactions during monoamine oxidase therapy are also restricted.

INDICATIONS AND RATIONALE

The diet should be used as a precautionary measure for all patients takine monoamine oxidase inhibitors. These drugs, such as tranylcypromine (Parnate) and pargyline, either alone (Eutonyl) or in combination with a thiazide diuretic (Eutron), are basically safe for treating depression or hypertension. The concomitant ingestion of foods having a high concentration of tyramine or other pressor amines may precipitate a hypertensive crisis characterized by headaches and nausea. Tyramine and other pressor amines are normally degraded in the body by the enzyme monoamine oxidase. Monoamine oxidase inhibitors interfere with this process, and the result is the accumulation of a variety of amine substances in the adrenergic nerve terminals. The ingestion of tyramine may trigger the sudden release of large quantities of these pressor amines from their nerve terminal storage sites. Some of the released catecholamines are strongly active vasopressor materials; therefore, a hypertensive crisis may occur.

In patients taking monoamine oxidase inhibitors, it has been reported that as little as 6 mg of tyramine may cause increased blood pressure and that 25 mg may induce a hypertensive crisis.

FOODS TO ALLOW AND FOODS TO AVOID*

Food Groups	Allow	Avoid
Beverage	Decaffeinated coffee; cereal beverage; artificially flavored fruit drink	Limit coffee, tea, and carbonated beverages to a total of 3 cups/day
Meat	Cottage cheese; soft or semidry sausage; cured meat; all others except those in "Avoid" column	Aged and processed cheese; pickled herring; dried herring; liver; peanuts and peanut butter; aged meats, including dry sausage, hard salami, pepperoni, and summer sausage; any prepared with meat tenderizers or soy sauce
Fat	Cream cheese; all others except sour cream and avocado	Sour cream; avocado
Milk	All except chocolate milk and yogurt	Chocolate milk; yogurt
Starch	All beans, including Italian broad beans, string beans, wax beans, and kidney beans, except broad (fava) beans; all other starches	Broad (or fava) beans†
Vegetable	All except sauerkraut	Sauerkraut
Fruit	All except those in "Avoid" column	Canned figs; raisins; raspberries
Soup	All except those in "Avoid" column	Commercial canned soup; any made with soup cubes or meat extracts
Dessert	All except those with chocolate	Any with chocolate
Sweets	All except those with chocolate	Any with chocolate
Miscellaneous	All products, including bakers' yeast (as a leavening agent in bakery products), except those listed in "Avoid" column	Meat tenderizers; meat extracts; yeast extracts: therefore, canned soup, soup cubes, and brewers' yeast; soy sauce; chocolate Beer; wine; other alcoholic beverages

*Data available on the content of tyramine and other pressor amines show a great deal of variation. The tyramine content is likely to vary among different brands of a particular food, since several factors related to the preparation, processing, and storing of foods may contribute to their tyramine content. The tyramine content may also vary with the time the food is left unrefrigerated: the longer the time, the greater the protein degradation. For practical purposes, the diet is intended to prohibit or limit foods that tend to be high in tyramine or other pressor amines and foods that have been implicated in the development of a hypertensive crisis in patients taking monoamine oxidase inhibitors.

†Broad (or fava) beans resemble lima beans but are rounder and have a larger and thicker pod.

MEDICATIONS

Many drugs are likely to interact with monoamine oxidase inhibitors (Lipman, 1978). The patient should be cautioned to avoid all other drugs, whether over-the-counter or previously prescribed by a physician, unless the current physician considers them to be acceptable.

PHYSICIANS: HOW TO ORDER DIETS

The diet order should indicate **tyramine control** *or* request **dietary precautions during use of monoamine oxidase inhibitors.**

SELECTED BIBLIOGRAPHY

Headache, tyramine, serotonin, and migraine. Nutr. Rev., 26:40-44, 1968.

Lipman, A. G.: Potential interactions between monoamine oxidase inhibitors and nonprescription drugs. Mod. Med., 46:45-46, Feb. 28, 1978.

Marley, E., and Blackwell, B.: Interactions of monoamine oxidase inhibitors, amines, and foodstuffs. Adv. Pharmacol. Chemother., 8:185-239, 1970.

TEST DIETS

TEST DIET FOR STEATORRHEA

GENERAL DESCRIPTION

Fat intake is estimated during the test period. The diet is generally planned to provide 100 g of fat. Estimates of actual fat intake are made, since many patients may not be able to consume this amount of fat and since test results can be interpreted according to the fat intake. This diet was formerly called the "100-gram fat test diet."

INDICATIONS AND RATIONALE

The test diet is used to determine if steatorrhea is present. Steatorrhea is an indication of gastrointestinal maldigestion or malabsorption.

Stools are collected during a 3-day period in which the patient follows the test diet. Ordinarily, the test is done in the hospital or in a facility for serving accurately measured diets to outpatients.

Food intake is monitored and fat intake is estimated. An average daily intake of 100 ± 10 g of fat is usually considered acceptable. The physician should be notified if intake is outside this range.

Some patients may find it especially difficult to eat a diet containing 100 g of fat. If the patient's actual fat intake can be estimated, this information can be used to interpret results of the stool fat collection.

Ordinarily, stool fat for normal adult subjects consuming this diet is 4 to 5 g per day. A value greater than 7 g per day is considered to indicate steatorrhea.* Because of the large variation in total fecal solids, fat excretion expressed as a percentage of the dry weight of the stool is not a satisfactory measure of steatorrhea. Average stool fat increases with increased dietary fat. The formula

$$(0.021 \times \text{grams of dietary fat per 24 hours}) + 2.93$$
$$= \text{grams of fecal fat per 24 hours}\dagger$$

describes this relationship and may permit interpretation of fecal fat analysis even when fat intake differs considerably from that in the standard test diet. In addition to reporting the amount of fat actually consumed, the dietitian can determine the expected amount of stool fat for this level of intake.

Stool nitrogen remains remarkably constant over a wide range of protein intake, although a high-fiber diet tends to increase stool nitrogen somewhat. Mean stool nitrogen on the standard 100-gram fat test diet was 1.7 g/24 hours (range, 0.8 to 2.5 g). Other studies suggest a somewhat lower range, with means of 1.2 to 1.3 g of nitrogen per 24 hours (Reifenstein et al., 1945; Wollaeger et al., 1946). Stool nitrogen, like stool fat, is increased in malabsorption and maldigestion and can be used to confirm stool fat data.

Stool fat and nitrogen data should be viewed not only as numbers to confirm or disprove a diagnosis but also as a means of assessing the nutritional consequences of an intestinal disorder. Stool fat in excess of 7 g per day can be multiplied by the factor of 9 kcal/g to obtain calories wasted by steatorrhea. Stool nitrogen in excess of 2 g per day multiplied by the factor of 6.25 g of protein per gram of nitrogen gives the equivalent amount of protein wasted. This figure multiplied by the factor of 4 kcal/g yields protein calories wasted by malabsorption or maldigestion.

PHYSICIANS: HOW TO ORDER DIETS

The diet order should indicate **test diet for steatorrhea** or **100-gram fat test diet** and the date the diet is to begin. The dietitian will notify the physician if fat intake is outside the range of 100 ± 10 g.

---

*In children, steatorrhea is defined as fecal fat excretion of 5 or more grams per day with a diet containing 40 to 65 g of fat. If the child is an outpatient, having the mother keep an accurate diet diary during the test period helps in the determination of steatorrhea.

†According to this formula, a stool fat of 5.03 g would be expected after a dietary fat intake of 100 g, and a stool fat of 3.98 g would be expected after a dietary fat intake of 50 g. Example: (0.021 × 50 g of dietary fat) + 2.93 = 3.98 g of stool fat.

SUGGESTED DAILY FOOD EXCHANGES

In a structured food service setting, such as a hospital, any foods may be served as long as their fat content can be reliably determined. A general hospital diet or modified diet may be served if the fat content of the foods is known.

In an outpatient setting, the diet will be more accurate if fat-free and low-fat foods are used and measured amounts of fat are added. See page 149 for foods to allow and to avoid. The following guide may be used to plan a diet containing 100 g of fat.

Whole Milk	Skim Milk	Vegetable	Fruit	Bread	Meat*	Fat	Low-fat Dessert	Low-fat Sweets
2	...	Ad lib	Ad lib	Ad lib	6	10	Ad lib	Ad lib
...	2	Ad lib	Ad lib	Ad lib	6	14	Ad lib	Ad lib
...	...	Ad lib	Ad lib	Ad lib	8	12	Ad lib	Ad lib

*Calculations are based on values for medium-fat meats.

SELECTED BIBLIOGRAPHY

Reifenstein, E. C., Jr., Albright, F., and Wells, S. L.: The accumulation, interpretation, and presentation of data pertaining to metabolic balances, notably those of calcium, phosphorus, and nitrogen. J. Clin. Endocrinol., 5:367-395, 1945.

Wollaeger, E. E., Comfort, M. W., and Osterberg, A. E.: Total solids, fat and nitrogen in the feces: III. A study of normal persons taking a test diet containing a moderate amount of fat; comparison with results obtained with normal persons taking a test diet containing a large amount of fat. Gastroenterology, 9:272-283, 1947.

Wollaeger, E. E., Comfort, M. W., Weir, J. F., et al.: The total solids, fat and nitrogen in the feces: I. A study of normal persons and of patients with duodenal ulcer on a test diet containing large amounts of fat. Gastroenterology, 6:83-92, 1946.

RENIN TEST DIET

GENERAL DESCRIPTION

The renin test diet contains no more than 20 meq of sodium and approximately 90 meq of potassium* daily. The patient follows the diet for 3 days and is weighed just before and after completion of the diet. On the fourth day, a plasma sample is drawn for renin determination.

---

*Potassium content of the diet does not need to be calculated closely. Although a precise level of potassium is not mandatory, it is important that the diet not be deficient in potassium. If the suggested daily food exchanges are followed, the diet will contain adequate potassium.

INDICATIONS AND RATIONALE

The diet is used to evaluate renin activity in some patients with hypertension. The purpose of the test diet is to stimulate renin production by restricting sodium intake.

Renin, a substance formed by the kidney, is part of a complex mechanism for maintaining blood pressure within normal limits. The amount of renin in the blood normally increases when the body must conserve sodium to maintain a normal volume of extracellular fluid and, hence, normal blood volume. A low-sodium diet, the use of diuretics, or maintaining an upright posture for several hours increases renin secretion. Since depletion of body potassium may impair this relationship, potassium content of the diet is also controlled. Conversely, a high intake of sodium may result in a decrease in secretion and low or undetectable levels of circulating renin.

If the low-sodium diet does not elevate renin production in a hypertensive patient, the patient may have an aldosterone-producing tumor.

A more common use of this test diet is to prepare the patient with suspected renal arterial vascular disease for bilateral renal vein catheterization. The level of renin in venous blood from an ischemic kidney is higher than that in blood from a normal kidney. Stimulating the renin-releasing mechanism by restricting sodium increases the difference between the response of an ischemic kidney and that of a normal kidney and thus improves the reliability of the interpretation of renal venous renin measurements.

PHYSICIANS: HOW TO ORDER DIETS

The diet order should indicate **renin test diet** *and* the date the test diet is to begin.

SUGGESTED DAILY FOOD EXCHANGES

See page 67 for sodium exchange list.

Milk	Salt-free Vegetable	Fruit	Salt-free Bread	Salt-free Meat	Salt-free Fat	Salt-free Sweets
1	3 or 4	3 or 4	6 or 7	6 or 7	Ad lib	Ad lib

DIETS IN PREPARATION FOR DIAGNOSTIC PROCEDURES

DIET IN PREPARATION FOR TREADMILL TESTS

INDICATIONS AND RATIONALE

Exercise stress testing is performed primarily to diagnose and determine the severity of coronary artery disease. A common form of exercise testing is the treadmill test; the patient walks at a known speed on a known grade while electrocardiographic recordings are made. One source of abnormal response to the treadmill test is recent ingestion of food. It is recommended that the meal preceding treadmill testing be small and light and be served 3 to 4 hours before the test.

GENERAL DIETARY RECOMMENDATIONS

Hospitalized patients are generally served a light breakfast or lunch. Although the items can vary according to the preferences of the patient, suggested menus are:

Light Breakfast	Light Lunch
Juice	Juice
Toast, 1 or 2 slices	Sandwich
Margarine, 1 or 2 tsp	Gelatin
Beverage	Beverage

PHYSICIANS: HOW TO ORDER DIETS

This diet order should indicate **breakfast [or lunch] for treadmill test.**

SELECTED BIBLIOGRAPHY

Riley, C. P., Oberman, A., and Sheffield, L. T.: Electrocardiographic effects of glucose ingestion. Arch. Intern. Med., 130:703-707, 1972.
Simonson, E.: Electrocardiographic stress tolerance tests. Prog. Cardiovasc. Dis., 13:269-292, 1970.

DIET IN PREPARATION FOR TESTS OF CARBOHYDRATE METABOLISM

INDICATIONS AND RATIONALE

Patients scheduled for glucose tolerance testing (oral and intravenous) or tolbutamide response testing should receive a diet with ample carbohydrate for at least 3 days before the test is performed. The diet should contain adequate protein (at least the Recommended Dietary Allowance), adequate calories (at least maintenance level), and at least 150 g of carbohydrate.*

The purpose of the diet is to condition the insulin-releasing mechanism and the glucose-disposing enzyme systems to respond fully to a glucose or tolbutamide challenge. This diet also helps assure adequate stores of hepatic glycogen to provide a source of glucose for restoration of plasma glucose levels after the initial hypoglycemic response to tolbutamide. In normal persons who have fasted, missed meals during the several days before testing, or followed a diet very low in carbohydrate, the response to challenge by a glucose load or tolbutamide may be abnormal. Results of glucose tolerance tests in hospitalized patients are commonly invalid because of the stress of current or recent illness, inactivity, drugs, or the supine position during the test.

GENERAL DIETARY RECOMMENDATIONS

Hospitalized patients are served a general diet (which contains about 250 g of carbohydrate). The physician should be notified if the patient's intake is inadequate.

Outpatients should be advised to eat their usual diet and some additional sweets and desserts. If the patient has been following a weight reduction diet, a diet very low in carbohydrate, or other unusual dietary practices, a dietitian should discuss an appropriate diet with the patient at least 3 days before the test.

PHYSICIANS: HOW TO ORDER DIETS

The diet order should indicate ⩾**150-gram carbohydrate diet** *or* **diet in preparation for glucose tolerance test.**

SELECTED BIBLIOGRAPHY

Marble, A.: Laboratory procedures useful in diagnosis and treatment. *In* Marble, A., White, P., Bradley, R. F., et al., eds.: Joslin's Diabetes Mellitus. Eleventh edition. Philadelphia, Lea & Febiger, 1971, pp. 191–208.

Seltzer, H. S.: Oral glucose tolerance tests. *In* Fajans, S. S., and Sussman, K. E., eds.: Diabetes Mellitus: Diagnosis and Treatment. Vol. 3. New York, American Diabetes Association, 1971, pp. 101–106.

Wilkerson, H. L. C., Hyman, H., Kaufman, M., et al.: Diagnostic evaluation of oral glucose tolerance tests in nondiabetic subjects after various levels of carbohydrate intake. N. Engl. J. Med., 262:1047–1053, 1960.

---

*Although 300-gram carbohydrate diets have traditionally been used in preparation for tests of carbohydrate metabolism, valid testing results have been reported with intakes of 150 to 200 g (Wilkerson et al., 1960).

DIET IN PREPARATION FOR 5–HIAA TESTING

INDICATIONS AND RATIONALE

The presence of 5–HIAA (5-hydroxyindoleacetic acid) in the urine is an indication of serotonin metabolism. An excess of 5–HIAA may indicate that the patient has a carcinoid tumor. For 24 hours before urine collection, patients scheduled for 5–HIAA testing should avoid ingesting exogenous sources of 5–HIAA and compounds that interfere with the test.

FOODS TO AVOID

Avocado	Plums
Bananas	Walnuts
Eggplant	Alcohol
Pineapple	

MEDICATIONS TO AVOID

Cough syrup containing glyceryl guaiacolate

Acetaminophen (Tylenol)

Phenacetin

PHYSICIANS: HOW TO ORDER DIETS

This diet may be ordered as **diet in preparation for 5–HIAA testing.**

SELECTED BIBLIOGRAPHY

5 Hydroxyindoleacetic acid—patient instructions. Lab. Med. Bull. (Mayo Clinic), 2 No. 11:3, 1977.

APPENDIX

FOOD AND NUTRITION BOARD, NATIONAL ACADEMY OF SCIENCES–NATIONAL RESEARCH COUNCIL RECOMMENDED DAILY DIETARY ALLOWANCES,* Revised 1974

Designed for the maintenance of good nutrition of practically all healthy people in the USA

	Age	Weight		Height		Energy	Protein	Fat-Soluble Vitamins			
								Vitamin A Activity		Vitamin D	Vitamin E Activity∥
	yr	kg	lb	cm	in.	kcal†	g	RE‡	IU	IU	IU
Infants	0.0–0.5	6	14	60	24	kg × 117	kg × 2.2	420§	1,400	400	4
	0.5–1.0	9	20	71	28	kg × 108	kg × 2.0	400	2,000	400	5
Children	1–3	13	28	86	34	1,300	23	400	2,000	400	7
	4–6	20	44	110	44	1,800	30	500	2,500	400	9
	7–10	30	66	135	54	2,400	36	700	3,300	400	10
Males	11–14	44	97	158	63	2,800	44	1,000	5,000	400	12
	15–18	61	134	172	69	3,000	54	1,000	5,000	400	15
	19–22	67	147	172	69	3,000	54	1,000	5,000	400	15
	23–50	70	154	172	69	2,700	56	1,000	5,000		15
	51+	70	154	172	69	2,400	56	1,000	5,000		15
Females	11–14	44	97	155	62	2,400	44	800	4,000	400	12
	15–18	54	119	162	65	2,100	48	800	4,000	400	12
	19–22	58	128	162	65	2,100	46	800	4,000	400	12
	23–50	58	128	162	65	2,000	46	800	4,000		12
	51+	58	128	162	65	1,800	46	800	4,000		12
Pregnant						+300	+30	1,000	5,000	400	15
Lactating						+500	+20	1,200	6,000	400	15

*Modified from National Research Council: Recommended Dietary Allowances. Eighth edition. Washington, D.C., National Academy of Sciences, 1974.

The allowances are intended to provide for individual variations among most normal persons as they live in the United States under usual environmental stresses. Diets should be based on a variety of common foods in order to provide other nutrients for which human requirements have been less well defined.

†Kilojoules (kJ) = 4.2 × kcal.

‡Retinol equivalents.

§Assumed to be all as retinol in milk during the first six months of life. All subsequent intakes are assumed to be half as retinol and half β-carotene when calculated from international units. As retinol equivalents, three-fourths are as retinol and one-fourth as β-carotene.

Water-Soluble Vitamins							Minerals					
Ascorbic acid	Fola- cin¶	Nia- cin#	Ribo- flavin	Thia- mine	Vitamin B$_6$	Vitamin B$_{12}$	Cal- cium	Phos- phorus	Iodine	Iron	Mag- nesium	Zinc
mg	µg	mg	mg	mg	mg	µg	mg	mg	µg	mg	mg	mg
35	50	5	0.4	0.3	0.3	0.3	360	240	35	10	60	3
35	50	8	0.6	0.5	0.4	0.3	540	400	45	15	70	5
40	100	9	0.8	0.7	0.6	1.0	800	800	60	15	150	10
40	200	12	1.1	0.9	0.9	1.5	800	800	80	10	200	10
40	300	16	1.2	1.2	1.2	2.0	800	800	110	10	250	10
45	400	18	1.5	1.4	1.6	3.0	1,200	1,200	130	18	350	15
45	400	20	1.8	1.5	2.0	3.0	1,200	1,200	150	18	400	15
45	400	20	1.8	1.5	2.0	3.0	800	800	140	10	350	15
45	400	18	1.6	1.4	2.0	3.0	800	800	130	10	350	15
45	400	16	1.5	1.2	2.0	3.0	800	800	110	10	350	15
45	400	16	1.3	1.2	1.6	3.0	1,200	1,200	115	18	300	15
45	400	14	1.4	1.1	2.0	3.0	1,200	1,200	115	18	300	15
45	400	14	1.4	1.1	2.0	3.0	800	800	100	18	300	15
45	400	13	1.2	1.0	2.0	3.0	800	800	100	18	300	15
45	400	12	1.1	1.0	2.0	3.0	800	800	80	10	300	15
60	800	+2	+0.3	+0.3	2.5	4.0	1,200	1,200	125	18+**	450	20
80	600	+4	+0.5	+0.3	2.5	4.0	1,200	1,200	150	18	450	25

∥Total vitamin E activity, estimated to be 80% as α-tocopherol and 20% as other tocopherols.

¶ The folacin allowances refer to dietary sources as determined by *Lactobacillus casei* assay. Pure forms of folacin may be effective in doses less than one-fourth of the Recommended Dietary Allowance.

#Although allowances are expressed as niacin, it is recognized that on the average 1 mg of niacin is derived from each 60 mg of dietary tryptophan.

**This increased requirement cannot be met by ordinary diets; therefore, the use of supplemental iron is recommended.

FOOD AND NUTRITION BOARD, NATIONAL ACADEMY OF SCIENCES—NATIONAL RESEARCH COUNCIL RECOMMENDED DAILY DIETARY ALLOWANCES,* Revised 1980

Designed for the maintenance of good nutrition of practically all healthy people in the USA

	Age	Weight		Height		Protein	Fat-Soluble Vitamins			Vitamin C
							Vitamin A	Vitamin D	Vitamin E	
	yr	kg	lb	cm	in.	g	μg RE†	μg‡	mg α-TE§	mg
Infants	0.0–0.5	6	13	60	24	kg × 2.2	420	10	3	35
	0.5–1.0	9	20	71	28	kg × 2.0	400	10	4	35
Children	1–3	13	29	90	35	23	400	10	5	45
	4–6	20	44	112	44	30	500	10	6	45
	7–10	28	62	132	52	34	700	10	7	45
Males	11–14	45	99	157	62	45	1,000	10	8	50
	15–18	66	145	176	69	56	1,000	10	10	60
	19–22	70	154	177	70	56	1,000	7.5	10	60
	23–50	70	154	178	70	56	1,000	5	10	60
	51+	70	154	178	70	56	1,000	5	10	60
Females	11–14	46	101	157	62	46	800	10	8	50
	15–18	55	120	163	64	46	800	10	8	60
	19–22	55	120	163	64	44	800	7.5	8	60
	23–50	55	120	163	64	44	800	5	8	60
	51+	55	120	163	64	44	800	5	8	60
Pregnant						+30	+200	+5	+2	+20
Lactating						+20	+400	+5	+3	+40

*Modified from National Research Council: Recommended Dietary Allowances. Ninth edition. Washington, D.C., National Academy of Sciences, 1980.

The allowances are intended to provide for individual variations among most normal persons as they live in the United States under usual environmental stresses. Diets should be based on a variety of common foods in order to provide other nutrients for which human requirements have been less well defined. See table on page 270 for suggested average energy intakes.

†Retinol equivalents. 1 retinol equivalent = 1 μg retinol or 6 μg β-carotene.

‡As cholecalciferol. 10 μg of cholecalciferol = 400 IU of vitamin D.

§α-Tocopherol equivalents. 1 mg of d-α-tocopherol = 1 α-TE.

∥1 NE (niacin equivalent) is equal to 1 mg of niacin or 60 mg of dietary tryptophan.

Water-Soluble Vitamins						Minerals					
Thia-mine	Ribo-flavin	Niacin	Vitamin B_6	Fola-cin¶	Vitamin B_{12}	Cal-cium	Phos-phorus	Mag-nesium	Iron	Zinc	Iodine
mg	mg	mg NE‖	mg	µg	µg	mg	mg	mg	mg	mg	µg
0.3	0.4	6	0.3	30	0.5#	360	240	50	10	3	40
0.5	0.6	8	0.6	45	1.5	540	360	70	15	5	50
0.7	0.8	9	0.9	100	2.0	800	800	150	15	10	70
0.9	1.0	11	1.3	200	2.5	800	800	200	10	10	90
1.2	1.4	16	1.6	300	3.0	800	800	250	10	10	120
1.4	1.6	18	1.8	400	3.0	1,200	1,200	350	18	15	150
1.4	1.7	18	2.0	400	3.0	1,200	1,200	400	18	15	150
1.5	1.7	19	2.2	400	3.0	800	800	350	10	15	150
1.4	1.6	18	2.2	400	3.0	800	800	350	10	15	150
1.2	1.4	16	2.2	400	3.0	800	800	350	10	15	150
1.1	1.3	15	1.8	400	3.0	1,200	1,200	300	18	15	150
1.1	1.3	14	2.0	400	3.0	1,200	1,200	300	18	15	150
1.1	1.3	14	2.0	400	3.0	800	800	300	18	15	150
1.0	1.2	13	2.0	400	3.0	800	800	300	18	15	150
1.0	1.2	13	2.0	400	3.0	800	800	300	10	15	150
+0.4	+0.3	+2	+0.6	+400	+1.0	+400	+400	+150	**	+5	+25
+0.5	+0.5	+5	+0.5	+100	+1.0	+400	+400	+150	**	+10	+50

¶ The folacin allowances refer to dietary sources as determined by *Lactobacillus casei* assay after treatment with enzymes (conjugases) to make polyglutamyl forms of the vitamin available to the test organism.

#The Recommended Dietary Allowance for vitamin B_{12} in infants is based on average concentration of the vitamin in human milk. The allowances after weaning are based on energy intake (as recommended by the American Academy of Pediatrics) and consideration of other factors, such as intestinal absorption.

**The increased requirement during pregnancy cannot be met by the iron content of habitual American diets nor by the existing iron stores of many women; therefore, the use of 30 to 60 mg of supplemental iron is recommended. Iron needs during lactation are not substantially different from those of nonpregnant women, but continued supplementation of the mother for 2 to 3 months after parturition is advisable to replenish stores depleted by pregnancy.

MEAN HEIGHTS AND WEIGHTS AND RECOMMENDED ENERGY INTAKE*

Category	Age yr	Weight kg	lb	Height cm	in.	Energy Needs (with range) kcal	MJ†
Infants	0.0–0.5	6	13	60	24	kg × 115 (95–145)	kg × 0.48
	0.5–1.0	9	20	71	28	kg × 105 (80–135)	kg × 0.44
Children	1–3	13	29	90	35	1,300 (900–1,800)	5.5
	4–6	20	44	112	44	1,700 (1,300–2,300)	7:1
	7–10	28	62	132	52	2,400 (1,650–3,300)	10.1
Males	11–14	45	99	157	62	2,700 (2,000–3,700)	11.3
	15–18	66	145	176	69	2,800 (2,100–3,900)	11.8
	19–22	70	154	177	70	2,900 (2,500–3,300)	12.2
	23–50	70	154	178	70	2,700 (2,300–3,100)	11.3
	51–75	70	154	178	70	2,400 (2,000–2,800)	10.1
	76+	70	154	178	70	2,050 (1,650–2,450)	8.6
Females	11–14	46	101	157	62	2,200 (1,500–3,000)	9.2
	15–18	55	120	163	64	2,100 (1,200–3,000)	8.8
	19–22	55	120	163	64	2,100 (1,700–2,500)	8.8
	23–50	55	120	163	64	2,000 (1,600–2,400)	8.4
	51–75	55	120	163	64	1,800 (1,400–2,200)	7.6
	76+	55	120	163	64	1,600 (1,200–2,000)	6.7
Pregnancy						+300	
Lactation						+500	

*Modified from National Research Council: Recommended Dietary Allowances. Ninth edition. Washington, D.C., National Academy of Sciences, 1980.

The energy allowances for the young adults are for men and women doing light work. The allowances for the two older age groups represent mean energy needs over these age spans; they allow for a 2% decrease in basal (resting) metabolic rate per decade and a reduction in activity of 200 kcal/day for men and women between 51 and 75 years, 500 kcal for men over 75 years, and 400 kcal for women over 75 years. The customary range of daily energy output is shown in parentheses for adults and is based on a variation in energy needs of ±400 kcal at any one age; the values emphasize the wide range of energy intakes appropriate for any group of people.

Energy allowances for children through age 18 are based on median energy intakes of children of these ages who participated in longitudinal growth studies. The values in parentheses are 10th and 90th percentiles of energy intake; they indicate the range of energy consumption among children of these ages.

†Megajoule.

ESTIMATED SAFE AND ADEQUATE DAILY DIETARY INTAKES OF ADDITIONAL SELECTED VITAMINS AND MINERALS*

	Age	Vitamins			Trace Elements†						Electrolytes		
		Vitamin K	Biotin	Pantothenic acid	Copper	Manganese	Fluoride	Chromium	Selenium	Molybdenum	Sodium	Potassium	Chloride
	yr	µg	µg	mg	mg	mg	mg	mg	mg	mg	mg	mg	mg
Infants	0–0.5	12	35	2	0.5–0.7	0.5–0.7	0.1–0.5	0.01–0.04	0.01–0.04	0.03–0.06	115–350	350–925	275–700
	0.5–1	10–20	50	3	0.7–1.0	0.7–1.0	0.2–1.0	0.02–0.06	0.02–0.06	0.04–0.08	250–750	425–1,275	400–1,200
Children	1–3	15–30	65	3	1.0–1.5	1.0–1.5	0.5–1.5	0.02–0.08	0.02–0.08	0.05–0.1	325–975	550–1,650	500–1,500
and	4–6	20–40	85	3–4	1.5–2.0	1.5–2.0	1.0–2.5	0.03–0.12	0.03–0.12	0.06–0.15	450–1,350	775–2,325	700–2,100
adolescents	7–10	30–60	120	4–5	2.0–2.5	2.0–3.0	1.5–2.5	0.05–0.2	0.05–0.2	0.10–0.3	600–1,800	1,000–3,000	925–2,775
	11+	50–100	100–200	4–7	2.0–3.0	2.5–5.0	1.5–2.5	0.05–0.2	0.05–0.2	0.15–0.5	900–2,700	1,525–4,575	1,400–4,200
Adults		70–140	100–200	4–7	2.0–3.0	2.5–5.0	1.5–4.0	0.05–0.2	0.05–0.2	0.15–0.5	1,100–3,300	1,875–5,625	1,700–5,100

*Modified from National Research Council: Recommended Dietary Allowances. Ninth edition. Washington, D.C., National Academy of Sciences, 1980. Because there is less information on which to base allowances, these figures are not given in the main table of the Recommended Dietary Allowances and are provided here in the form of ranges of recommended intakes.

†Since the toxic levels for many trace elements may be only several times usual intakes, the upper levels for the trace elements given in this table should not be habitually exceeded.

VITAMIN SUPPLEMENTS

Under what circumstances is vitamin supplementation appropriate? There is no simple answer, but a general guide is available in the form of the Recommended Dietary Allowances (RDA). However, the RDA are not intended to apply to conditions of stress and illness. The clinician and dietitian must be guided by textbooks and other such sources concerned with the condition at issue.

RECOMMENDED DIETARY ALLOWANCES

The Food and Nutrition Board of the National Academy of Sciences has prepared recommendations for the amounts of a number of vitamins and minerals that should provide for the needs of nearly all normal people living in the United States under usual environmental stresses. A table of these recommendations is reproduced in the Appendix on pages 268 and 269. These allowances are designed to provide for possible variations in individual needs and in most instances are substantially greater than the minimum amounts needed to prevent symptoms of vitamin deficiency. Thus, a diet supplying less than some of the RDA should not necessarily be considered unsatisfactory or in need of vitamin supplementation.

The RDA should not be confused with the United States Recommended Daily Allowances (USRDA). The latter standards have been derived from the RDA by the Food and Drug Administration as standards for nutrition labeling. These are given in the Appendix on page 273.

For general vitamin supplementation, there is one generic formulation: Decavitamin USP. This formula consists of the following substances, but the quantity of each component is not specified; only the amount of each vitamin is required to appear on the label: vitamin A (retinol), thiamine (B_1), riboflavin (B_2), pyridoxine (B_6), cyanocobalamin (B_{12}), folic acid, niacin, pantothenate, ascorbic acid (vitamin C), vitamin D (calciferol), and vitamin E (tocopherol). The term *hexavitamin* has been applied to the preparations containing vitamin A, thiamine, riboflavin, niacin, ascorbic acid, and vitamin D.

The responsibility of the clinician is to choose the preparation that will provide the amounts and kinds of vitamins needed for a particular situation.

CLINICAL SETTINGS

For restricted calorie diets below 1,000 to 1,200 calories, a multivitamin preparations such as a decavitamin or hexavitamin formula with amounts of individual vitamins approximately equal to the USRDA may be appropriate. Higher potency or "therapeutic" formulas are not necessary for this purpose.

Patients having malabsorption or maldigestion secondary to pancreatic or intestinal disease may benefit from the regular use of supplemental vitamins. Liquid vitamin preparations may be absorbed better than those in capsule form when rapid transit may interfere with dissolution of the capsule. Measurement of prothrombin activity guides the need for additional vitamin K and the response to this agent. Water-soluble forms of vitamin K, such as menadiol sodium diphosphate (available in 5-mg tablets) and vitamin K_5 (available in 4-mg capsules), used regularly may be effective in states characterized by steatorrhea. Measurements of folate and vitamin B_{12} serum levels may be useful in establishing whether and in what quantities these substances should be given. Folic acid (available in 1-mg tablets) may be given orally in doses of 1 to 5 mg daily in malabsorption and, if necessary, may be administered parenterally in doses of 1 mg daily. Vitamin B_{12} is best administered intramuscularly in a dose of 100 to 1,000 μg daily until clinical evidences of B_{12} deficiency are corrected; thereafter, 100 to 1,000 μg is given at intervals of 2 to 4 weeks.

Emotional stress should not increase vitamin needs, but surgical or traumatic stress possibly increases rates of vitamin losses or degradation. Very little objective information exists on which to base recommendations for vitamin administration in stress, however. The previously well-nourished patient probably experiences no harm if supplementary vitamins are not administered in the first several days after injury or surgery. If regular meals containing the usual complement of vitamins cannot be consumed within a few days, it would be reasonable to provide a decavitamin formula with at least one USRDA, parenterally or orally as circumstances demand.

There does not appear to be any special need for vitamins in old age, but disease and social factors often limit the variety and quality of foods eaten by the elderly. Hence, vitamin supplementation may be needed for the older patient. A diet history may warn of possible vitamin deficiency. Special needs for vitamins in such conditions as infancy, pregnancy, and renal disease are explained in those sections of the diet manual.

SELECTED BIBLIOGRAPHY

Hines, C., Jr.: Vitamins: Absorption and malabsorption. Arch. Intern. Med., 138:619-621, 1978.

RECOMMENDED DAILY ALLOWANCES OF VITAMINS, UNITED STATES (USRDA)*

	Infants and Children < 4 yr	Children > 4 yr and Adults
Vitamin A	2,500 IU	5,000 IU
Thiamine (B_1)	0.7 mg	1.5 mg
Riboflavin (B_2)	0.8 mg	1.7 mg
Vitamin B_6	0.7 mg	2 mg
Vitamin B_{12}	3 μg	6 μg
Folacin (B_c)	0.2 mg	0.4 mg
Biotin	0.15 mg	0.3 mg
Niacin	9 mg	20 mg
Pantothenic acid	5 mg	10 mg
Ascorbic acid (C)	40 mg	60 mg
Vitamin D	400 IU	400 IU
Vitamin E	10 IU	30 IU

*From White, P. L.: Vitamin preparations: Proper use in medical practice. Postgrad. Med., 60:204-209, Oct. 1976. By permission of McGraw-Hill, Inc.

TRACE MINERALS

The same considerations governing the use of vitamin supplements apply to trace minerals.

Most of the essential trace minerals are available in adequate amounts in protein-containing foods. Persons who consume adequate amounts of protein are not likely to have trace mineral deficiencies.

Infants and children reared in fluoride-deficient areas and not consuming fluoridated water may require fluoride supplementation. Iodide deficiency is now rare because of the wide use of iodized salt, foods derived from different geographic areas, and some food additives containing iodides. Iron may be needed for iron-deficient states, but these states are usually the result of blood loss rather than restricted dietary intake. Deficiencies of zinc, manganese, copper, and other trace elements may occur in patients receiving only parenterally administered nutrients. Plasma levels of these substances can be a guide to their administration, but because of the way the substances bind to plasma protein, interpretation of plasma levels in states characterized by protein deficiency is difficult.

MAYO CLINIC PHYSIOLOGIC VALUES

(NORMAL RANGES)

BLOOD OR SERUM VALUES

Ascorbic acid (vitamin C)	0.6–2.0 mg/dl
Bleeding time—Ivy	1–6 min
Calcium	8.9–10.1 mg/dl
Carotene	48–200 μg/dl
Chloride	100–108 meq/liter
Copper	0.75–1.45 μg/ml
Erythrocyte count	M, 4.5–$6.2 \times 10^6/\mu$l
	F, 4.2–$5.4 \times 10^6/\mu$l
Ferritin	M, 20–300 ng/ml
	F, 20–120 ng/ml
Folate (serum)	2–20 ng/ml
Glucose, fasting	70–100 mg/dl
Hematocrit	M, 42–54%
	F, 38–46%
Hemoglobin	M, 14–17 g/dl
	F, 12–15 g/dl
Iron	M. 75–175 μg/dl
	F, 65–165 μg/dl
Iron binding capacity, total	240–450 μg/dl
Iron binding capacity, % saturation	18–50%
Lipids	

Lipids, serum — Upper limits, 95%
(mg/dl)

Age	Males		Females	
	Cholesterol	Triglycerides	Cholesterol	Triglycerides
6	200	86	208	97
8	200	96	208	107
10	200	104	208	113
12	200	114	208	116
14	200	122	208	116
16	200	131	208	115
18	202	138	209	112
20	210	143	210	107
—				
—				
55	291	197	291	133
65	296	199	320	145

Lipids, lipoproteins fractions —
Upper limits, 95%
Cholesterol, mg/dl

Age	Males			Females		
	VLDL	LDL	HDL	VLDL	LDL	HDL
6–11	20	140	65	20	150	65
12–14	25	140	65	25	150	65
15–19	30	140	65	25	150	70
20–29	45	175	70	35	160	75
30–39	60	190	70	35	170	80
40–49	60	205	70	35	190	80
> 50	60	220	70	35	200	80

Upper limits, 95%
Triglycerides, mg/dl

Age	Males			Females		
	VLDL	LDL	HDL	VLDL	LDL	HDL
6–7	60	25	15	60	25	15
8–11	60	25	15	85	25	15
12–14	90	25	15	85	25	15
15–19	105	25	15	85	25	15
20–29	155	30	20	90	30	15
30–39	155	40	20	90	40	15
40–49	155	50	20	90	40	15
> 50	155	50	20	90	40	15

MAYO CLINIC PHYSIOLOGIC VALUES

(NORMAL RANGES) *(Continued)*

BLOOD OR SERUM VALUES *(Continued)*

Magnesium	1.7–2.1 mg/dl
Osmolality	275–295 mOsm/kg
Phosphorus	2.5–4.5 mg/dl
Potassium	3.6–4.8 meq/liter
Protein, total	6.6–7.9 g/dl
Protein electrophoresis	
Albumin	3.05–4.30 g/dl
Alpha-1 globulin	0.13–0.32 g/dl
Alpha-2 globulin	0.60–1.04 g/dl
Beta-globulin	0.72–1.25 g/dl
Gamma globulin	0.70–1.60 g/dl
Sodium	135–145 meq/liter
Urea	M, 17–51 mg/dl
	F, 13–45 mg/dl
Uric acid	M, 4.3–8.0 mg/dl
	F, 2.3–6.0 mg/dl
Vitamin A	125–150 IU/dl
Zinc	0.75–1.4 μg/ml

URINE VALUES

Calcium	M, <275 mg/24 h
	F, <250 mg/24 h, normal diet
Creatinine clearance	70–135 ml/min/1.73 m^2 at age 20
	(decreased by 6 ml/min/decade)
	300–800 mOsm/kg; overhydration
Osmolality	<100, dehydration > 800
	20–60 mg/24 h
Oxalate	30–90 meq/24 h
Potassium	<0.27 g/24 h
Protein, total	
Renal clearance — standard	
Glomerular filtration rate (inulin	
or iothalamate ^{125}I)	90–130 ml/min/1.73 m^2 at age 20
	(decreased by 4 ml/min/decade)
Effective renal plasma flow (PAH)	400–700 ml/min/1.73 m^2 at age 20
	(decreased by 17 ml/min/decade)
Filtration fraction	18–22%
Renal clearance — short	
Glomerular filtration rate	
(iothalamate ^{125}I)	90–130 ml/min/1.73 m^2 at age 20
	(decreased by 4 ml/min/decade)
Glomerular filtration rate	
(creatinine)	See creatinine clearance
Sodium	130–200 meq/24 h
Uric acid	<750 mg/24 h

MAYO CLINIC PHYSIOLOGIC VALUES

(NORMAL RANGES) *(Continued)*

MISCELLANEOUS VALUES

Basal metabolism rate	−10 to +10%
Stool examination	
Fat, quantitative	2–7 g/24 h
Nitrogen	1–2 g/24 h
Vitamin B_{12} absorption (Schilling test)	>9% excretion

AVERAGE WEIGHT IN RELATION TO HEIGHT*

HEIGHT		WEIGHT							
		MEN				WOMEN			
		Pounds		Kilograms		Pounds		Kilograms	
Feet	Meters	Average	Range	Average	Range	Average	Range	Average	Range
4'10"	1.47	–	–	–	–	102	92-119	46.3	41.7-54.0
4'11"	1.50	–	–	–	–	104	94-122	47.1	42.6-55.3
5' 0"	1.52	–	–	–	–	107	96-125	48.5	43.5-56.7
5' 1"	1.55	–	–	–	–	110	99-128	50.0	44.9-58.1
5' 2"	1.58	123	112-141	55.8	50.8-63.9	113	102-131	51.3	46.3-59.4
5' 3"	1.60	127	115-144	57.6	52.2-65.3	116	105-134	52.6	47.6-60.8
5' 4"	1.63	130	118-148	58.9	53.5-67.1	120	108-138	54.4	49.0-62.6
5' 5"	1.65	133	121-152	60.3	54.9-68.9	123	111-142	55.8	50.3-64.4
5' 6"	1.68	136	124-156	61.7	56.2-70.8	128	114-146	58.1	51.7-66.2
5' 7"	1.70	140	128-161	63.5	58.1-73.0	132	118-150	59.9	53.5-68.0
5' 8"	1.73	145	132-166	65.8	59.9-75.3	136	122-154	61.7	55.3-69.9
5' 9"	1.75	149	136-170	67.6	61.7-77.1	140	126-158	63.5	57.2-71.7
5'10"	1.78	153	140-174	69.4	63.5-78.9	144	130-163	65.3	59.0-73.9
5'11"	1.80	158	144-179	71.7	65.3-81.2	148	134-168	67.1	60.8-70.2
6' 0"	1.83	162	148-184	73.5	67.1-83.5	152	138-173	68.9	62.6-78.5
6' 1"	1.85	166	152-189	75.3	68.9-85.7	–	–	–	–
6' 2"	1.88	171	156-194	77.6	70.8-88.0	–	–	–	–
6' 3"	1.91	176	160-199	79.8	72.6-90.3	–	–	–	–
6' 4"	1.93	181	164-204	82.1	74.4-92.5	–	–	–	–

*From Bray, G. A.: The obese patient. Major Probl. Intern. Med., 9:1–450, 1976. By permission of W. B. Saunders Company. Subject should be without shoes for height measurement and in light clothing or no clothing for weight measurement.

BODY FAT AND SKINFOLDS*

The equivalent fat content, as a percentage of body weight, for a range of values for the sum of four skinfolds (biceps, triceps, subscapular, and suprailiac) of males and females of different ages.

Skinfolds mm	Age in years							
	Males				Females			
	17-29	30-39	40-49	50+	16-29	30-39	40-49	50+
15	4·8	—	—	—	10·5	—	—	—
20	8·1	12·2	12·2	12·6	14·1	17·0	19·8	21·4
25	10·5	14·2	15·0	15·6	16·8	19·4	22·2	24·0
30	12·9	16·2	17·7	18·6	19·5	21·8	24·5	26·6
35	14·7	17·7	19·6	20·8	21·5	23·7	26·4	28·5
40	16·4	19·2	21·4	22·9	23·4	25·5	28·2	30·3
45	17·7	20·4	23·0	24·7	25·0	26·9	29·6	31·9
50	19·0	21·5	24·6	26·5	26·5	28·2	31·0	33·4
55	20·1	22·5	25·9	27·9	27·8	29·4	32·1	34·6
60	21·2	23·5	27·1	29·2	29·1	30·6	33·2	35·7
65	22·2	24·3	28·2	30·4	30·2	31·6	34·1	36·7
70	23·1	25·1	29·3	31·6	31·2	32·5	35·0	37·7
75	24·0	25·9	30·3	32·7	32·2	33·4	35·9	38·7
80	24·8	26·6	31·2	33·8	33·1	34·3	36·7	39·6
85	25·5	27·2	32·1	34·8	34·0	35·1	37·5	40·4
90	26·2	27·8	33·0	35·8	34·8	35·8	38·3	41·2
95	26·9	28·4	33·7	36·6	35·6	36·5	39·0	41·9
100	27·6	29·0	34·4	37·4	36·4	37·2	39·7	42·6
105	28·2	29·6	35·1	38·2	37·1	37·9	40·4	43·3
110	28·8	30·1	35·8	39·0	37·8	38·6	41·0	43·9
115	29·4	30·6	36·4	39·7	38·4	39·1	41·5	44·5
120	30·0	31·1	37·0	40·4	39·0	39·6	42·0	45·1
125	30·5	31·5	37·6	41·1	39·6	40·1	42·5	45·7
130	31·0	31·9	38·2	41·8	40·2	40·6	43·0	46·2
135	31·5	32·3	38·7	42·4	40·8	41·1	43·5	46·7
140	32·0	32·7	39·2	43·0	41·3	41·6	44·0	47·2
145	32·5	33·1	39·7	43·6	41·8	42·1	44·5	47·7
150	32·9	33·5	40·2	44·1	42·3	42·6	45·0	48·2
155	33·3	33·9	40·7	44·6	42·8	43·1	45·4	48·7
160	33·7	34·3	41·2	45·1	43·3	43·6	45·8	49·2
165	34·1	34·6	41·6	45·6	43·7	44·0	46·2	49·6
170	34·5	34·8	42·0	46·1	44·1	44·4	46·6	50·0
175	34·9	—	—	—	—	44·8	47·0	50·4
180	35·3	—	—	—	—	45·2	47·4	50·8
185	35·6	—	—	—	—	45·6	47·8	51·2
190	35·9	—	—	—	—	45·9	48·2	51·6
195	—	—	—	—	—	46·2	48·5	52·0
200	—	—	—	—	—	46·5	48·8	52·4
205	—	—	—	—	—	—	49·1	52·7
210	—	—	—	—	—	—	49·4	53·0

In two-thirds of the instances, the error was within ± 3·5% of the body-weight as fat for the women and ± 5% for the men.

*Modified from Durnin, J. V. G. A., and Womersley, J.: Body fat assessed from total body density and its estimation from skinfold thickness: Measurements on 481 men and women aged from 16 to 72 years. Br. J. Nutr., 32:77-97, 1974. By permission of the Nutrition Society.

ESTIMATION OF IDEAL WEIGHT OR GOAL WEIGHT

Correction of obesity or even attainment of a distinctly lean weight is of great importance in the treatment of diabetes, orthopedic problems involving weight-bearing structures, and many cardiovascular conditions, such as angina pectoris and hypertension. When use of an oral hypoglycemic agent to treat diabetes in an overweight person is questionable, imposition of a low-calorie diet without use of the drug often achieves satisfactory control of glycemia and glycosuria even before a substantial loss of weight has occurred. Thus, if an appropriate diet is vigorously applied, the controversial issue of whether to use an oral hypoglycemic agent does not often arise.

If one was in good health and considered oneself well proportioned at age 20 to 22, weight at that age may be a useful indication of ideal weight. The use of the weight in young adult life as a measure of one's ideal weight compensates in some measure for variations in body build. Commonly, the 50- or 60-year-old person has gained 10 to 15 kg (22 to 33 lb) since age 20 and yet regards this weight gain as normal. He defends this weight gain, stating that most of his friends and relatives have gained a similar amount. It is often difficult for such a person to understand that his muscle and skeletal masses have diminished somewhat with age and with lessened physical conditioning and that if he returned to the weight he had at age 20, he would still have a greater amount of body fat than he had in his prime. Many patients are unable to conceive of losing enough to return to their age-20 weight, and the physician or dietitian must compromise and agree to a goal of a lesser weight loss. Thus, in discussions with patients, two estimates can be made: an ideal weight and a goal weight. The ideal weight should be physiologically optimum, and for the middle-aged or older individual, this often equals or is less than the weight of that person in early maturity. A goal weight is a weight that is acceptable to the individual and yet represents a loss large enough to be of benefit. If the physician and dietitian accept a weight substantially greater than desirable, they create an obstacle to losing below that weight in the future.

Estimations of what weight a patient should be seeking are somewhat more difficult since the introduction of the less familiar metric measurements of height and weight. A hand calculator is almost a necessity for quick and easy conversion of kilograms and centimeters to pounds and inches. Height-weight tables are useful additional guides for establishing ideal weight. Another method, convenient if a calculator is available, is to square the height in meters and multiply this value by the factor 22. For example, a person 180 cm in height would be assigned an ideal weight of 71 kg by the following computation: $1.8 \times 1.8 \times 22 = 71.28$. This formula is based on the finding by Keys and associates (1972) that of the several proposed formulas for describing degrees of adiposity in terms of height and weight, the body mass index correlates most closely with fatness as determined by body density and skinfold measurements. West (1980) used the Fogarty International Conference on Obesity standards for nude weight without shoes to calculate that the factor should be 22.1 for men and 20.6 for women. For subjects weighed with light clothing and no shoes, the factor would be 22.4 in men and 20.9 in women.

Formal skinfold thickness measurements with the Lange caliper* or a similar device permit calculation of an ideal weight by means of the table of Durnin and Womersley (page 279). One assumes that at ideal weight, either 15% (for men) or 20% (for women) of body weight will be fat and applies the following formula:

$$\frac{\text{Actual weight} - \left(\text{actual weight} \times \begin{array}{c}\% \text{ of body weight} \\ \text{as fat derived} \\ \text{from tables}\end{array}\right)}{100\% - \text{desired \% of body weight as fat}} = \text{ideal weight}$$

*Cambridge Scientific Industries, 101 Virginia Avenue, Cambridge, Maryland 21613.

An example for a 110-kg man whose skinfold measurements indicate that 40% of body weight is fat and whom the physician or dietitian would like to see achieve a weight such that 15% of body weight is fat:

$$\frac{110 \text{ kg} - (110 \times 0.40)}{1 - 0.15} = 77.6 \text{ kg}$$

No formula or calculation can substitute for commonsense clinical evaluation, however. Often, it is well to provide the patient with an agreed-upon intermediate goal weight and reassess the degree of fatness when that level is achieved. Some obese persons have a surprisingly large muscle mass as a consequence of carrying about their excess weight (the "weight-lifter effect"), and they may prove to have a desirable proportion of fat if they can lose to a weight of 5 to 15 kg above that which would be calculated from height-weight tables or the body mass index.

SELECTED BIBLIOGRAPHY

Cork, R. C., and Vaughan, R. W.: Indices of obesity (letter to the editor). J.A.M.A., 242:1140, 1979.
Keys, A., Fidanza, F., Karvonen, M. J., et al.: Indices of relative weight and obesity. J. Chronic Dis., 25:329-343, 1972.
West, K. M.: Computing and expressing degree of fatness (letter to the editor). J.A.M.A., 243:1421-1422, 1980.

FOOD NOMOGRAM*

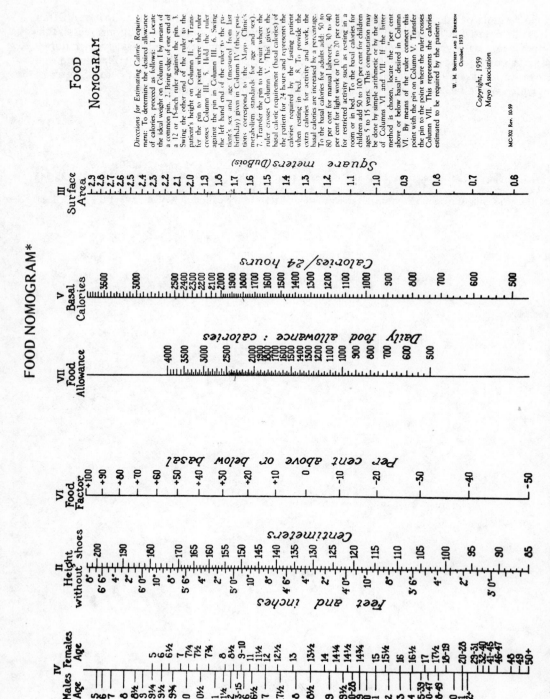

FOOD NOMOGRAM

Directions for Estimating Caloric Requirement: To determine the desired allowance of calories, proceed as follows: 1. Locate the ideal weight on Column I by means of a common pin. 2. Bring edge of one end of a 12 or 15-inch ruler against the pin. 3. Swing the other end of the ruler to the patient's height on Column II. 4. Transfer the pin to the point where the ruler crosses Column III. 5. Hold the ruler against the pin in Column III. 6. Swing the left hand end of the ruler to the patient's sex and age (measured from last birthday) given in Column IV (these positions correspond to the Mayo Clinic's metabolism standards for age and sex). 7. Transfer the pin to the point where the ruler crosses Column V. This gives the basal caloric requirement (basal calories) of the patient for 24 hours and represents the calories required by the fasting patient when resting in bed. 8. To provide the extra calories for activity and work, the basal calories are increased by a percentage. To the basal calories for adults add: 50 to 80 per cent for manual laborers, 30 to 40 per cent for light work or 10 to 20 per cent for restricted activity such as resting in a room or in bed. To the basal calories for children add 50 to 100 per cent for children ages 5 to 15 years. This computation may be done by simple arithmetic or by the use of Columns VI and VII. If the latter method is chosen, locate the "per cent above or below basal" desired in Column VI. By means of the ruler connect this point with the pin on Column V. Transfer the pin to the point where the ruler crosses Column VII. This represents the calories estimated to be required by the patient.

W. M. BOOTHBY AND J. BERKSON
October, 1933

Copyright, 1959
Mayo Association

MC-702 Rev. 10-59

---

*Note: The error in some published versions of the nomogram devised by Boothby and Sandiford for determining body surface area (see Turcotte, G.: Erroneous nomograms for body-surface area a [letter to the editor], N. Engl. J. Med., 300:1339, 1979) does not occur in this food nomogram.

WEIGHT LOSS RECORD*

WEIGHT LOSS RECORD
MAYO CLINIC — ROCHESTER, MINNESOTA

CLINIC NO. _____ NAME _____ CONSULTANT _____ SHEET NO. _____

AGE _____ HEIGHT _____ WEIGHT _____ IDEAL WT. _____ DIETITIAN _____

Weigh and record weight once a week.

Date	Weight	Date	Weight

Diet:

BASAL CALORIES FOR _____ POUNDS =

BASAL + _____ % =

CALORIE INTAKE =

CALORIE DEFICIT =

ESTIMATED WEIGHT LOSS PER WEEK =

ESTIMATED WEIGHT LOSS IN _____ WEEKS =

PLEASE RETURN THIS RECORD ON _____
                                      DATE

TO _____ ROCHESTER, MINNESOTA 55901

THE DIETITIAN WILL REVIEW YOUR PROGRESS WITH YOUR PHYSICIAN.

ANOTHER WEIGHT LOSS RECORD, SHEET NO. _____ WILL BE MAILED TO YOU.

*Format for mailed weight records.

FATTY ACID AND CHOLESTEROL CONTENT OF FOODS

Food	Amount	Total Fat, g	Fatty Acids, g* Saturated	Fatty Acids, g* Polyunsaturated	Cholesterol, mg
Meat, lean (≤ 3 g fat/oz)	1 oz				
Beef		2.6	0.9	0.1	25
Lamb		2.9	1.2	0.1	28
Pork		2.8	0.8	0.3	25
Veal		3.1	1.3	0.2	28
Poultry (without skin)	1 oz				
Chicken					
Light		1	trace	trace	22
Dark		2.7	0.7	0.5	25
Turkey					
Light		0.7	trace	trace	22
Dark		1.5	0.4	0.3	28
Others: duck, goose, pheasant		2.3	0.5	0.2	25
Finfish	1 oz				
≤ 5% fat		0.5	trace	trace	18
Bass, cod, halibut, haddock, skipjack tuna, sole, red snapper, pike perch					
5–10% fat		2	trace	trace	18
Trout; drained anchovy, salmon, albacore, and sardines; mackerel; Atlantic herring					
≥ 12% fat		3.8	0.6	0.6	27
Pacific herring					
Shellfish	1 oz				
< 2% fat		0.5	. . .	0.2	15
Abalone, clams, mussel, oysters, scallops					
Crab, lobster		0.5	. . .	0.2	26
Shrimp		0.4	. . .	0.2	42
Caviar		4.2	. . .	. . .	84
Organ meats	1 oz				
Heart		1.6	0.5	0.2	77
Liver					
Beef, veal		1.1	0.4	0.2	122
Chicken		1.2	0.5	0.3	208
Brains		2.4	0.6	0.3	560
Sweetbreads		6.5	2.7	0.3	130
Kidney		3.4	1.3	0.5	225
Tongue		4.7	1.6	0.6	25
Giblets		0.9	0.3	0.2	60
Gizzard		0.9	0.3	0.2	55
Meat, medium-fat (≤ 5 g fat/oz): cooked, separable lean	1 oz				
Beef		4.3	1.8	0.2	25
Pork		4	1.3	0.4	25

FATTY ACID AND CHOLESTEROL CONTENT OF FOODS (Continued)

Food	Amount	Total Fat, g	Fatty Acids, g*		Cholesterol, mg
			Saturated	Polyunsaturated	
Meat, high-fat (≥ 10 g fat/oz)	1 oz				
Beef		9	3.7	0.3	26
Pork		8.6	3.3	1.0	25
Lamb (untrimmed)		8.2	3.8	0.5	27
Veal (untrimmed)		7	2.6	0.4	28
Cold cuts		7.6	2.7	0.9	25
Sausage		12.4	4.5	1.5	25
Bacon: cooked, 50% fat	1 slice	3.4	1.3	0.4	3
Dairy products					
Milk	1 cup				
Skim (< 1% fat)		0.2	0.1	. . .	4
Buttermilk		0.2	0.1	. . .	4
1%		2.4	1.4	trace	7
2%		4.8	2.9	0.2	14
Whole		8.4	5.3	0.3	32
Chocolate					
Skim		5.5	2.2	0.1	16
Whole		8.2	5.2	0.3	32
Yogurt	1 cup				
Part skim milk		2	1.3	0.1	11
Whole milk		8.2	5.3	2.4	32
Processed milk	1 oz				
Condensed		2.4	1.5	0.1	10
Evaporated		2.4	1.4	trace	9
Cottage cheese	1/4 cup (2 oz)				
1%		0.5	0.3	trace	2
2%		1	0.6	trace	3
Regular		2.3	1.4	0.7	7
Cheese	1 oz				
< 1% fat Dietetic		0.3	0.2	trace	2
< 10% fat Imitation processed cheese spread		2.2	1.4	0.1	9
< 20% fat Farmer, mozzarella (part skim), ricotta		4.6	2.9	0.1	18
< 30% fat Pasteurized processed cheese foods and spreads, Bel Paese, Camembert, Edam, feta, Gouda, Limburger, mozzarella (low-moisture), Neufchâtel, Parmesan, Samsoe, Swiss		7.4	4.7	0.2	27
> 30% fat Blue, brick, cheddar, colby, cream, Muenster, Port du Salut		9.2	5.6	0.3	29
Polyunsaturated cheese		6.4	0.8	3.7	1

FATTY ACID AND CHOLESTEROL CONTENT OF FOODS (Continued)

Food	Amount	Total Fat, g	Fatty Acids, g*		Cholesterol, mg
			Saturated	Polyunsaturated	
Dairy products (Continued)					
Cream	1 oz				
Half-and-half		3.3	2.0	0.9	12
Light (sweet or sour)		5.8	3.6	0.2	18
Heavy		10.6	6.6	0.4	38
Whipped (aerosol)		6.5	4.1	0.3	24
Dairy desserts	3 1/2 oz				
Ice milk		5.1	3.2	0.2	14
Ice cream					
Regular		10.6	6.6	0.4	40
Rich		16	10	0.6	57
Ice cream sandwich		8.2	4.7	0.5	40
Butterfat	1 tsp				
Butter		4	2.5	0.2	12
Butter oil		5	3.1	0.2	14
Eggs					
Whole	1				
Small (≤ 40 g)		4.5	1.4	0.5	192
Medium (≤ 44 g)		5	1.5	0.6	222
Large (≤ 50 g)		5.7	1.7	0.6	252
Extra large (≤ 57 g)		6.4	1.9	0.7	281
Yolk	100 g	33.5	10.1	3.8	1,480
Fats and oils					
Margarine	1 tsp				
Vegetable (P/S ratio†)					
> 3: e.g., soft safflower		4	0.5	2.3	...
2.6–3: e.g., stick safflower		4	0.6	1.7	...
2–2.5: e.g., soft corn		4	0.7	1.8	...
1.6–1.9: e.g., stick corn		4	0.8	1.3	...
1–1.5: e.g., liquid soybean		4	0.9	1.3	...
0.5–0.9: e.g., partially hydrogenated oil		4	0.8	0.5	...
< 0.5: e.g., hydrogenated oil		4	0.8	0.5	...
Vegetable-animal		4	1.7	0.3	4
Animal fats					
Beef	1 tsp				
Tallow		5	2.4	0.2	5
Lard		5	2	0.6	5
Chicken					
Fat	1 tsp	5	1.6	0.8	4
Skin, 35% fat	5 g	1.8	0.5	0.5	6
Salt pork, raw	1 oz	23.8	8.5	2.7	19
Mutton	5 g	5	2.2	0.4	4
Vegetable oils	1 tsp				
Safflower		5	0.5	3.7	...
Sunflower		5	0.5	3.2	...
Soybean					
Nonhydrogenated		5	0.8	2.9	...
Part hydrogenated		5	0.7	2	...

FATTY ACID AND CHOLESTEROL CONTENT OF FOODS *(Continued)*

Food	Amount	Total Fat, g	Fatty Acids, g* Saturated	Fatty Acids, g* Polyunsaturated	Cholesterol, mg
Fats and oils *(Continued)*					
Wheat germ		5	0.9	3	. . .
Corn		5	0.6	2.9	. . .
Sesame		5	0.8	2	. . .
Cottonseed		5	1.3	2.5	. . .
Peanut		5	0.9	1.2	. . .
Olive		5	0.7	0.4	. . .
Palm		5	2.4	0.5	. . .
Cocoa butter		5	3	0.2	. . .
Coconut		5	4.3	0.1	. . .
Soybean lecithin		5	0.8	2.4	. . .
Processed vegetable oils	1 tsp				
Oil blends					
90% sunflower and 10% cottonseed		5	0.6	3.1	. . .
90% soybean and 10% cottonseed		5	0.8	2.8	. . .
50% cottonseed and 50% soybean		5	1.2	2.7	. . .
10% olive and 90% other vegetable		5	0.7	1.8	. . .
Shortenings					
All-vegetable		5	1.6	1	. . .
Vegetable-animal		5	2.1	0.5	3
Dressings					
Mayonnaise		4	0.6	2.3	4
Mayonnaise-type		2.1	0.3	1.1	2.5
Salad					
All creamy: e.g., French, garlic		2	0.3	1.1	. . .
Creamy with egg or mayonnaise or both: e.g., tartar sauce, Thousand Island		2.5	0.4	1.3	3
Clear: e.g., French, Italian		3	0.5	1.7	. . .
Sandwich spread		2.5	0.3	1.5	2.6
Meat substitutes					
Meat loaf	1 oz	2.5	0.4	1.4	. . .
Sausage, piece					
Link	23 g	4.3	1	1.6	. . .
Patty	38 g	7.2	1.5	2.6	. . .
Ham, slice	1 oz	2.4	0.4	0.8	. . .
Frankfurter	1 oz	5.5	0.8	2.9	. . .
Textured vegetable protein	1 oz	2	0.3	1.1	. . .
Nuts	1/2 oz				
Peanuts					
Runner		7.6	1.3	2.1	. . .
Virginia		7.1	1.2	1.8	. . .
Spanish		7.4	1.4	2.4	. . .
Unspecified		7.3	1.3	2	. . .

FATTY ACID AND CHOLESTEROL CONTENT OF FOODS *(Continued)*

Food	Amount	Total Fat, g	Fatty Acids, g*		Cholesterol, mg
			Saturated	Polyunsaturated	
Nuts *(Continued)*					
Almonds		8.1	0.6	1.5	...
Brazil nuts		10.2	2.6	3.8	...
Cashews		6.8	1.4	1.1	...
Chestnuts		0.4	trace	0.2	...
Filberts		9.7	0.7	1	...
Macadamia nuts		11.3	1.5	0.2	...
Pecans		10.6	0.9	2.7	...
Pistachios		8.1	1.1	1.1	...
Walnuts					
English		9.6	1	6.1	...
Black		8.9	0.7	4.9	...
Peanut butter	2 tbsp				
Hydrogenated		14.4	2.9	4.2	...
Unhydrogenated		13.8	2.5	4.1	...
Avocado, 50 g	1/4	8. 2	1.2	0.9	...
Coconut: shredded, sweetened	1 tbsp	5.3	4.7	1	...
Olives	1/2 oz				
Green		3.6	0.5	0.3	...
Black		3.9	0.5	0.3	...
Cereal products					
Bread, all varieties	1 slice	0.8	0.2	0.3	...
Bagel, small	1/2				
Plain		2	0.3	0.9	...
Egg		2	0.3	0.9	28
English muffin	1/2	0.9	0.2	trace	...
Roll	1	0.8	0.2	0.3	...
Bun, frankfurter or hamburger	1/2	1.5	0.6	0.2	...
Cereals					
Dry	3/4 cup	trace	trace	trace	...
Cooked	1/2 cup	trace	trace	trace	...
Pasta	1/2 cup				
Plain		trace	...	...	...
Egg		2	0.2	0.2	31
Wheat germ	1/4 cup	2.5	0.5	1.6	...
Crackers	5				
Low-fat (< 12%)					
Saltines		<1	<0.7	0.2	...
High-fat (> 12%)					
Ritz		3.2	1.3	0.4	3

FATTY ACID AND CHOLESTEROL CONTENT OF FOODS *(Continued)*

Food	Amount	Total Fat, g	Fatty Acids, g*		Cholesterol, mg
			Saturated	Polyunsaturated	
Prepared foods					
Biscuit	1 oz	2	‡	‡	...
Corn bread, small	1 oz	2.8	‡	‡	...
Muffin, small	1 oz	2.1	‡	‡	...
Potatoes, fried	1 oz	5	‡	‡	...
Potato chips	1 oz	11	‡	‡	...
Pancake, 4 in. round	1 oz	2	‡	‡	...
Waffle, 4 1/2 in. sq	1 1/2 oz	5	‡	‡	...

*Polyunsaturated fats include all unsaturated fats with two or more double bonds. Monounsaturated fats (one double bond) are not listed in the table because they do not affect serum lipids and are not used in calculating the ratio of polyunsaturated to saturated fat (P/S ratio).

†Check label for content of saturates, polyunsaturates, and cholesterol.

‡Fatty acid content depends on type of fat used in preparation.

SELECTED BIBLIOGRAPHY

Comprehensive evaluation of fatty acids in foods (series), J. Am. Diet. Assoc.

   I. Dairy products (Posati, L. P., Kinsella, J. E., and Watt, B. K.). 66:482–488, 1975.
  II. Beef products (Anderson, B. A., Kinsella, J. E., and Watt, B. K.). 67:35–41, 1975.
 III. Eggs and egg products (Posati, L. P., Kinsella, J. E., and Watt, B. K.). 67:111–115, 1975.
  IV. Nuts, peanuts, and soups (Fristrom, G. A., Stewart, B. C., Weihrauch, J. L., and Posati, L. P.). 67:351–355, 1975.
   V. Unhydrogenated fats and oils (Brignoli, C. A., Kinsella, J. E., and Weihrauch, J. L.). 68:224–229, 1976.
  VI. Cereal products (Weihrauch, J. L., Kinsella, J. E., and Watt, B. K.). 68:335–340, 1976.
 VII. Pork products (Anderson, B. A.). 69:44–49, 1976.
VIII. Finfish (Exler, J., and Weihrauch, J. L.). 69:243–248, 1976.
  IX. Fowl (Fristrom, G. A., and Weihrauch, J. L.). 69:517–522, 1976.
   X. Lamb and veal (Anderson, B. A., Fristrom, G. A., and Weihrauch, J. L.). 70:53–58, 1977.
  XI. Leguminous seeds (Exler, J., Avena, R. M., and Weihrauch, J. L.). 71:412–415, 1977.
 XII. Shellfish (Exler, J., and Weihrauch, J. L.). 71:518–521, 1977.

Adams, C. F.: Nutritive Value of American Foods in Common Units. Agriculture Handbook No. 456, Washington, D. C., United States Department of Agriculture, 1975.

Feeley, R. M., Criner, P. E., and Watt, B. K.: Cholesterol content of foods. J. Am. Diet. Assoc., 61:134–149, 1972.

Nazir, D. J., Moorecroft, B. J., and Mishkel, M. A.: Fatty acid composition of margarines. Am. J. Clin. Nutr., 29:331–339, 1976.

SODIUM AND POTASSIUM CONTENT OF FOODS*

Food	Amount	Sodium, meq	Potassium, meq
Meat and meat substitutes			
Bacon	1 strip	2	Tr
Beef potpie, commercial	1	38	5
Beef stew, canned	1 cup	43	10
Casserole, commercial	1 cup	39	11
Cheese, cheddar type	1 oz	9	1
Cheese, processed American	1 oz	15	1
Cheese, processed spread	1 oz	21	2
Chili, canned	1 cup	23	6
Chow mein	1/2 cup	12.5	4
Cold cuts	1 oz	16	2
Corned beef	1 oz	23	1
Dried beef	1 oz	56	2
Fish sticks	1 oz	3	2.5
Frankfurter	1	24	3
Ham	1 oz	14	3
Kosher meat	1 oz	4	2
Peanut butter, regular	2 tbsp	8	5
Peanuts, salted	3/4 cup	18	17
Pizza	1/4 of 16 oz	29	3
Salmon, regular, canned	1/4 cup	7	3
Sardines	1 oz	11	4.5
Sausage, link	2	16.5	3
Sausage, patty	1 oz	12.5	2
Soup, canned, undiluted	1/2 cup	37	3
Spaghetti sauce, canned	1/2 cup	18	4
Tuna, regular, canned	1/4 cup	10	2
TV dinner	10–12 oz	47	†
Fats			
Gravy	2 tbsp	10	†
Olives	3	31	0.5
Salad dressing	1 tbsp	8	1
Milk			
Buttermilk	1 cup	14	8
Starches			
Crackers, saltines	5	7	0.5
Crackers, snack	6	10	0.5
Popcorn, salted	1 cup	15	. . .
Potato chips	1 oz	14	10
Potatoes, packaged	1/2 cup	22	10
Pretzels, round, ring	6–15	14	0.5
Pretzels, very thin	60	28	0.5

SODIUM AND POTASSIUM CONTENT OF FOODS* *(Continued)*

Food	Amount	Sodium, meq	Potassium, meq
Vegetables			
Frozen combination vegetables with sauce	1/3 cup	13	5
Sauerkraut	1/2 cup	33	4
Tomato juice, canned	1/2 cup	9	23
Tomato paste	1 tbsp	3	4
Tomato sauce	1/2 cup	36	11
Desserts			
Cake, commercial	1 piece	6	2
Cookies, commercial	1	3	1
Ice cream	1 cup	4	6
Pie, commercial	1/6 of 9-in. pie	20	4
Pudding, commercial	1/2 cup	6	4
Miscellaneous			
Baking powder	1 tsp	14	. . .
Baking soda	1 tsp	59	. . .
Barbecue sauce	1 tbsp	10	1
Bouillon	1 cube	52	Tr
Catsup, mustard	1 tbsp	8	1
Cheese sauce, packaged	1/4 cup	29	Tr
Cocoa mixes	1 tbsp	1.6	2.5
Coconut	2 tbsp	0.1	3
Meat and vegetable sauces, packaged	1/4 cup	13	1
Monosodium glutamate	1 tsp	33	. . .
Pickles, dill	1 large	62	5
Pickles, dill	1 small	19	1.5
Salt	1 tsp	92	Tr
Salt substitutes	1 tsp	. . .	50–65
Soft water	1 liter	5–8	. . .
Soy sauce	1 tsp	16	

*Data for foods not listed in the sodium food exchange list on page 67.
†Data not available.

SELECTED BIBLIOGRAPHY

Adams, C. F.: Nutritive Value of American Foods in Common Units. Agriculture Handbook No. 456. Washington, D. C., United States Department of Agriculture, 1975.
Kraus, B.: The Dictionary of Sodium, Fats, and Cholesterol. New York, Grosset & Dunlap, 1974.
Church, C. F., and Church, H. N. (Editors): Bowes and Church's Food Values of Portions Commonly Used. Twelfth edition. Philadelphia, J. B. Lippincott Company, 1975.

CALCIUM AND PHOSPHORUS CONTENT OF FOODS

Food	Amount	Calcium, mg	Phosphorus, mg
Meat, fish, poultry			
Beef	1 oz	3	56
Pork	1 oz	3	70
Chicken	1 oz	4	74
Liver	1 oz	4	137
Fish, average	1 oz	12	76
Tuna	1/4 cup	2	95
Sardines, canned, with bones	1 oz	86	101
Salmon, canned, with bones	1 oz	74	98
Luncheon meat	1 oz	3	53
Bacon, strip	1–5 g	1	11
Meat substitutes			
Eggs	1	28	90
Dried beans, average, cooked	1/2 cup	44	144
Lentils, cooked	1/2 cup	25	119
Peanuts and peanut butter	1 tbsp	11	60
Milk	1 cup		
Whole milk		290	227
2% milk		297	232
Skim milk		302	247
Buttermilk		285	219
Chocolate milk		280	251
Hot cocoa		298	270
Other dairy products			
Yogurt, plain, low-fat	8 oz	415	326
Cheddar cheese	1 oz	204	145
Swiss cheese	1 oz	272	171
Processed American cheese	1 oz	174	211
Cottage cheese, creamed	1/4 cup	31	69
Half-and-half	2 tbsp	32	28
Vanilla ice cream	1/2 cup	88	67
Sherbet	1/2 cup	51	37
Cereal and grain products			
Bread, white	1 slice	21	24
Bread, whole wheat	1 slice	23	52
Bread products made from white flour			
Biscuit	2-in. diameter	42	61
Doughnut, cake	1 average	13	61
Doughnut, raised	1 average	11	23
Pancake	4-in. diameter	45	63
Sweet roll	1 average	35	57
Waffle	5-in. diameter	85	130
Cereal, refined	1/2 cup cooked; 3/4 cup dry	35	57
Cereal, whole grain	1/2 cup cooked; 3/4 cup dry	14	109

CALCIUM AND PHOSPHORUS CONTENT OF FOODS *(Continued)*

Food	Amount	Calcium, mg	Phosphorus, mg
Cereal and grain products *(Continued)*			
Crackers, saltines	5 2-in. squares	2	15
Crackers, graham	2 2 1/2 in. squares	6	21
Macaroni; spaghetti; noodles	1/2 cup cooked	8	47
Rice	1/2 cup cooked	7	21
Vegetables	100 g; about 1/2 cup cooked		
Artichokes		51	69
Asparagus		21	50
Bean sprouts		17	48
Broccoli		88	62
Brussels sprouts		32	72
Cabbage		44	20
Corn		4	48
Cress		61	48
Greens			
Beet greens		99	25
Collards		152	39
Dandelion greens		140	42
Kale		134	46
Mustard greens		183	50
Spinach		98	30
Swiss chard		73	24
Turnip greens		184	37
Leeks		52	50
Lima beans		47	121
Mushrooms		6	116
Okra		92	41
Parsnips		45	62
Peas		20	66
Potatoes, white		9	65
Rutabagas		59	31
Winter squash		28	48
Other vegetables, average		25	26
Fruit			
Blackberries	5/8 cup	32	19
Orange	1 small	41	20
Raspberries	2/3 cup	30	22
Rhubarb	3/8 cup	78	15
Tangerine	1 large	40	18
Fresh fruit, average	1/2 cup or 1 medium	16	20
Canned fruit, average	1/2 cup	10	12
Fruit juice	1/2 cup	10	13
Fats and oils			
Butter or margarine	1 tsp	1	1
Nondairy cream substitute, nondairy powder	1 tsp	Tr	8
French dressing	1 tbsp	2	2
Gravy	1 tbsp	...	2
Mayonnaise	1 tsp	1	1

CALCIUM AND PHOSPHORUS CONTENT OF FOODS *(Continued)*

Food	Amount	Calcium, mg	Phosphorus, mg
Sweets			
Candy, sugar	1/2 oz	. . .	. . .
Candy, milk chocolate	1/2 oz	26	28
Honey	1 tbsp	4	3
Jelly	1 tbsp	2	2
Sugar, white	1 tbsp	. . .	. . .
Sugar, brown	1 tbsp	9	6
Syrup, maple	1 tbsp	33	3
Desserts			
Assorted cookies	1 2-in.	7	32
Cake, white	2 in. by 3 in. by 2 in.	34	46
Pie, cream	1/8 of 9-in. pie	62	88
Pie, fruit	1/8 of 9-in. pie	23	30
Snack foods			
Popcorn	1 cup	2	39
Potato chips	5	3	15
Beverages			
Beer	8 oz	10	62
Carbonated beverages			
Colas, average	8 oz	7	42
Ginger ale, average	8 oz	3	. . .
Coffee	6 oz	5	5
Tea	6 oz	5	4

SELECTED BIBLIOGRAPHY

Adams, C. F.: Nutritive Value of American Foods in Common Units. Agriculture Handbook No. 456. Washington, D. C., United States Department of Agriculture, 1975.

Church, C. F., and Church, H. N. (Editors): Bowes and Church's Food Values of Portions Commonly Used. Twelfth edition. Philadelphia, J. B. Lippincott Company, 1975.

United States Agriculture Research Service, Consumer Food Economics Institute: Composition of Foods: Dairy and Egg Products; Raw, Processed, Prepared. Agriculture Handbook No. 8-1. Washington, D. C., United States Department of Agriculture, 1976.

NUTRITIVE VALUE OF DESSERTS AND SNACK FOODS

Food	Amount	Protein g	Fat g	Carbohydrate g	Calories
Bread					
Coffee cake	4 1/2-in. diameter	3	5	26	160
Sweet roll	1 average	5	4	30	175
Cake	1 piece				
Chocolate, iced	2 in. by 3 in. by 2 in.	2	5	33	185
Pound cake	3 in. by 3 in. by 1/2 in.	3	9	27	200
White, iced	2 in. by 3 in. by 2 in.	2	5	30	175
Candy	About 1 oz				
Bar candy, chocolate covered	1 oz	3	8	20	165
Butterscotch	6 pieces	. . .	3	24	125
Caramels	3 medium	1	3	22	120
Chocolate					
Creams	2 average	1	4	18	110
Fudge	1 1/4-in. sq	1	3	24	127
Mints	3 small	1	4	23	130
Hard candy	6 squares	. . .	. . .	30	120
Peanut brittle	2 1/2-in. sq	2	4	18	115
Cookies	1				
Assorted	2-in. diameter	1	4	14	95
Brownies	2-in. square	2	10	15	160
Doughnuts	1				
Cake, plain		2	6	16	125
Yeast-leavened, plain		2	8	11	125
Pudding	1/2 cup				
Chocolate		3	5	26	160
Custard		3	4	23	140
Vanilla		4	4	16	115
Pie	1/6 of 9-in. pie				
Chiffon		7	13	45	325
Cream		7	15	60	400
Custard		9	15	35	310
Fruit		4	15	60	390
Soup	1 cup				
Bean		6	2	26	145
Beef		6	4	12	110
Cream		7	12	18	210
Vegetable		4	2	14	90

SELECTED BIBLIOGRAPHY

Adams, C. F.: Nutritive Value of American Foods in Common Units. Agriculture Handbook No. 456. Washington, D. C., United States Department of Agriculture, 1975.

Church, C. F., and Church, H. N. (Editors): Bowes and Church's Food Values of Portions Commonly Used. Twelfth edition. Philadelphia, J. B. Lippincott Company, 1975.

NUTRITIVE VALUE OF ALCOHOLIC AND CARBONATED BEVERAGES

Beverage	Amount	Calories	Carbohydrate, g	Alcohol,* g
Alcoholic beverages				
Beer	8 oz	100	9	9
Brandy	Brandy glass	75	...	11
Gin; rum; vodka; whiskey	1 jigger			
80 proof		70	...	10
90 proof		80	...	11
100 proof		90	...	13
Liqueurs, average	Cordial glass	65	6	7
Wines	3 1/2 oz			
Champagne		75	3	10
Muscatel		160	14	15
Sauterne		85	4	10
Table wine		85	...	10
Vermouth, French		105	1	15
Vermouth, Italian		165	12	18
Carbonated beverages	1 cup			
Carbonated waters (sweetened quinine soda)		75	19	...
Colas		95	24	...
Ginger ale		75	19	...
Root beer		100	25	...
Soda, cream or fruit-flavored		105	26	...

*Alcohol calculated as 7 calories per gram.

CALORIC VALUE OF ALCOHOLIC BEVERAGES

The caloric contribution of an alcoholic beverage can be estimated by multiplying the number of ounces by the proof and then again by the factor 0.08. For beers and wines, calories can be estimated by multiplying ounces by percentage of alcohol and then by the factor 1.6.

SELECTED BIBLIOGRAPHY

Adams, C. F.: Nutritive Value of American Foods in Common Units. Agriculture Handbook No. 456. Washington, D. C., United States Department of Agriculture, 1975.

Church, C. F., and Church, H. N. (Editors): Bowes and Church's Food Values of Portions Commonly Used. Twelfth edition. Philadelphia, J. B. Lippincott Company, 1975.

Gastineau, C. F.: Alcohol and calories. Mayo Clin. Proc., 51:88, 1976.

CAFFEINE CONTENT OF SELECTED BEVERAGES

Beverage	Caffeine, mg/5-oz cup
Coffee, percolated	110
Coffee, drip	146
Instant coffee	66
Decaffeinated coffee	3
Tea, black	28–46
Tea, green	20–35
Instant tea	20–58
Cocoa beverages	13
Some carbonated beverages (usually colas)	32–65*

*Per 12-oz can.

SELECTED BIBLIOGRAPHY

Bunker, M. L., and McWilliams, M.: Caffeine content of common beverages. J. Am. Diet. Assoc., 74:28–32, 1979.

Graham, D. M.: Caffeine—its identity, dietary sources, intake and biological effects. Nutr. Rev., 36:97–102, 1978.

DRUG–NUTRIENT INTERACTIONS

Drugs may affect utilization of nutrients and, conversely, nutrients may affect drug absorption and bioavailability. The risk of drug-induced nutritional deficiencies is greatest among persons whose diets are marginal.

It is beyond the scope of this manual to list the many potential drug-nutrient interrelations. The following sources are recommended for information on specific drugs.

Grant, A.: Nutritional Assessment: Guidelines for Dietitians. Seattle, Washington, 1977, pp. El-E37.

Hartshorn, E. A.: Food and drug interactions. J. Am. Diet. Assoc., 70:15–19, 1977.

Hathcock, J. N., and Coon, J., eds.: Nutrition and Drug Interrelations (Nutrition Foundation Monograph). New York, Academic Press, 1978, 927 pp.

March, D. C.: Handbook: Interactions of Selected Drugs With Nutritional Status in Man. Chicago, American Dietetic Association, October 1976, 119 pp.

Roe, D. A.: Drug-Induced Nutritional Deficiencies. Westport, Connecticut, Avi Publishing Company, 1976, 272 pp.

DIETARY GUIDELINES FOR AMERICANS*

U.S. DEPARTMENT OF AGRICULTURE AND U.S. DEPARTMENT OF HEALTH, EDUCATION AND WELFARE

1. **Eat a Variety of Foods**

   To assure an adequate diet: eat a variety of foods daily, including selections of fruits; vegetables; whole grain and enriched breads, cereals, and grain products; milk, cheese, and yogurt; meats, poultry, fish, and eggs; and legumes (dry peas and beans). To assure an adequate diet for your baby: breastfeed unless there are special problems, delay other foods until the baby is 3 to 6 months old, and do not add salt or sugar to the baby's food.

2. **Maintain Ideal Weight**

   To improve eating habits: eat slowly, prepare smaller portions, and avoid "seconds." To lose weight: increase physical activity, eat less fat and fatty foods, eat less sugar and sweets, and avoid too much alcohol.

3. **Avoid Too Much Fat, Saturated Fat, and Cholesterol**

   To avoid too much fat, saturated fat, and cholesterol: choose lean meat, fish, poultry, and dry beans and peas as your protein sources; moderate your use of eggs and organ meats (such as liver); limit your intake of butter, cream, hydrogenated margarines, shortenings, coconut oil, and foods made from such products; trim excess fat off meats; broil, bake, or boil rather than fry; and read labels carefully to determine both amounts and types of fat contained in foods.

4. **Eat Foods With Adequate Starch and Fiber**

   To eat more complex carbohydrates daily: substitute starches for fats and sugars and select foods that are good sources of fiber and starch, such as whole grain breads and cereals, fruits and vegetables, beans, peas, and nuts.

5. **Avoid Too Much Sugar**

   To avoid excessive sugars: use less of all sugars, including white sugar, brown sugar, raw sugar, honey, and syrups; eat less of foods containing these sugars, such as candy, soft drinks, ice cream, cakes, and cookies; select fresh fruits or fruits canned without sugar or with light syrup rather than heavy syrup; read food labels for clues on sugar content — if the name "sucrose," "glucose," "maltose," "dextrose," "lactose," "fructose," or "syrup" appears first, there is a large amount of sugar; and remember, how often you eat sugar is as important as how much sugar you eat.

6. **Avoid Too Much Sodium**

   To avoid too much sodium: learn to enjoy the unsalted flavors of foods; cook with only small amounts of added salt; add little or no salt to food at the table; limit your intake of salty foods, such as potato chips, pretzels, salted nuts and popcorn, condiments (soy sauce, steak sauce, garlic salt), cheese, pickled foods, and cured meats; and read food labels carefully to determine the amounts of sodium in processed foods and snack items.

7. **If You Drink Alcohol, Do So in Moderation**

   Remember, if you drink alcohol, do so in moderation.

---

*Modified from: U.S. Department of Agriculture, U. S. Department of Health, Education and Welfare: Nutrition and Your Health, Dietary Guidelines for Americans. Washington, D.C., Government Printing Office, February 1980.

GENERAL DIETARY RECOMMENDATIONS*

AMERICAN HEART ASSOCIATION

1. Adjust caloric intake to achieve and maintain ideal body weight. Avoidance of obesity or participation in a supervised weight reduction program for persons above their ideal body weight is strongly recommended. The food allowance should be eaten in as many small meals as possible; large meals are not recommended.

2. Reduce total fat calories by substantially reducing dietary saturated fatty acids. Reduction from the usual 40 to 45% of total calories from fat to no more than 35% is desirable. Of that amount, less than 10% of the total calories should come from saturated fatty acids and up to 10% from polyunsaturated fatty acids; the remainder of fat is derived from monounsaturated sources. Fat calories should be distributed throughout the day; a massive high saturated fat meal is inappropriate at any time.

3. Substantially reduce dietary cholesterol. It is recommended that the average daily intake of cholesterol approximate 300 mg.

4. Modestly increase carbohydrates if reducing fat intake leads to a deficit in calories from dietary carbohydrate. Use of complex natural carbohydrates is preferable to excessive use of refined sugar.

5. Avoid excessive use of salt.

---

*Data from Committee on Nutrition: Diet and Coronary Disease. New York, American Heart Association, pamphlet EM-379, 1973.

DIETARY GOALS FOR THE UNITED STATES*

SELECT COMMITTEE ON NUTRITION AND HUMAN NEEDS, UNITED STATES SENATE

1. To avoid excess weight, consume only as much energy (calories) as is expended; if overweight, decrease energy intake and increase energy expenditure.

2. Increase the consumption of complex carbohydrates and "naturally occurring" sugars from about 28% of energy intake to about 48% of energy intake.

3. Reduce the consumption of refined and processed sugars by about 45% to account for about 10% of total energy intake.

4. Reduce overall fat consumption from approximately 40% to about 30% of energy intake.

5. Reduce saturated fat consumption to account for about 10% of total energy intake; balance that with polyunsaturated and monounsaturated fats, which should account for about 10% of energy intake each.

6. Reduce cholesterol consumption to about 300 mg per day.

7. Limit the intake of sodium by reducing the intake of salt to about 5 g per day. (This recommendation was later clarified. The 5 g of salt or sodium chloride is that in addition to the salt naturally occurring in foods.)

The goals suggest the following changes in food selection and preparation.

1. Increase consumption of fruits and vegetables and whole grains.

2. Decrease consumption of refined and other processed sugars and foods high in such sugars.

3. Decrease consumption of foods high in total fat, and partially replace saturated fats, whether obtained from animal or vegetable sources, with polyunsaturated fats.

4. Decrease consumption of animal fat, and choose meats, poultry, and fish that will reduce saturated fat intake.

5. Except for young children, substitute low-fat and nonfat milk for whole milk and low-fat dairy products for high-fat dairy products.

6. Decrease consumption of butterfat, eggs, and other high-cholesterol sources. Some consideration should be given to easing the cholesterol goal for premenopausal women, young children, and the elderly in order to obtain the nutritional benefits of eggs in the diet.

7. Decrease consumption of salt and foods high in salt content.

---

*Modified from Select Committee on Nutrition and Human Needs, United States Senate: Dietary Goals for the United States. Second edition. Washington, D. C., Government Printing Office, Dec. 1977.

COMPARISON OF CURRENT AND RECOMMENDED DIETS*

	Current Diet†	American Heart Association‡	Senate Select Committee§
Protein, %	12	12	12
Fat, %	42	35	30
Saturated fats	16	10	10
Monosaturated fats	19	15	10
Polyunsaturated fats	7	10	10
Carbohydrate, %	46	53	58
Complex carbohydrates	22	‖	⎫
"Naturally occurring" sugars	6	. . .	⎬ 48
Refined and processed sugars	18	‖	⎭ 10

*Dietary Guidelines for Americans—U.S. Department of Agriculture and U.S. Department of Health, Education and Welfare (see page 299) does not recommend a specific composition.

†Estimate of composition of current diet is based on United States Department of Agriculture data. From Select Committee on Nutrition and Human Needs, United States Senate: Dietary Goals for the United States. Second edition. Washington, D. C., Government Printing Office, Dec. 1977.

‡See page 300.

§See page 301.

‖Complex carbohydrates preferable to excessive use of refined sugar.

ADDITIONAL INFORMATION FOR GLUTEN–CONTROLLED DIETS

ADDITIONAL INFORMATION

The following sources provide brand-name product lists, recipes, or newsletters.

American Celiac Society, 45 Gifford Avenue, Jersey City, NJ 07304. (Newsletter)

Hartsook, E. I.: Gluten Content of Products and Gluten-Free Diet Instruction (Wheat, Rye, Oat and Barley Free). Write to: Elaine Hartsook, RC-14, University Hospital, Seattle, WA 98195. (Brand-name product list)

Midwestern Celiac Sprue Association, P.O. Box 3554, Des Moines, IA 50322. (Newsletter)

Shaker, M. M.: Low Gluten Diet With Tested Recipes. Ann Arbor, Michigan, University of Michigan. Write to: Dr. Arthur B. French, Clinical Research Unit, W 4644 University Hospital, Ann Arbor, MI 48104. (Special product list, recipes)

Sheedy, C. B., and Keifetz, N.: Cooking for Your Celiac Child. Dial Press, Inc., 705 Third Avenue, New York, NY 10017. (Recipes)

Southeastern Branch, Minnesota Chapter National Cystic Fibrosis Research Foundation, 720 Southwest 25th Street, Rochester, MN 55901. (Recipes)

Wood, M. N.: Delicious and Easy Rice Flour Recipes. Charles C Thomas, Publisher, 301–327 East Lawrence Avenue, Springfield, IL 62717. (Recipes)

Wood, M. N.: Gourmet Food on a Wheat-Free Diet. Charles C Thomas, Publisher, 301–327 East Lawrence Avenue, Springfield, IL 62717. (Recipes)

SUBSTITUTIONS FOR WHEAT FLOUR

Special cookbooks may be helpful. Many other recipes can be modified by the following substitutions.

1 cup of wheat flour may be replaced by
  1 cup of wheat starch
  1 cup of corn flour
  1 scant cup of fine cornmeal
  3/4 cup of coarse cornmeal
  5/8 cup (10 tbsp) of potato flour
  7/8 cup (14 tbsp) of rice flour
  1 cup of soy flour plus 1/4 cup of potato flour
  1/2 cup of soy flour plus 1/2 cup of potato flour
1 tablespoon of wheat flour may be replaced by (for thickening)
  1/2 tbsp of cornstarch, potato flour, rice starch, or arrowroot starch
  2 tbsp of quick-cooking tapioca

SPECIAL PRODUCTS

The following sources provide special flours and other products that can be used on a gluten-controlled diet.

General Mills, Inc.
400 Second Avenue South
Minneapolis, MN 55440

Jolly Joan Products
Ener-G Foods, Inc.
1526 Utah Avenue South
Seattle, WA 98134

Chicago Dietetic Supply, Inc.
P.O. Box 529
La Grange, IL 60525

Vita-Wheat Baked Products, Inc.
1839 Hilton Road
Ferndale, MI 48220

CONVERSION OF MILLIGRAMS TO MILLIEQUIVALENTS

To convert milligrams (mg) to milliequivalents (meq):

$$\frac{\text{Milligrams}}{\text{Atomic weight}} \times \text{Valence} = \text{Milliequivalents}$$

Mineral Element	Chemical Symbol	Atomic Weight	Valence
Chlorine	Cl	35.4	1
Potassium	K	39	1
Sodium	Na	23	1
Calcium	Ca	40	2
Magnesium	Mg	24.3	2
Sulfur	S	32	
Sulfate	SO_4	96	2

To convert specific weight of sodium to sodium chloride:

Milligrams of sodium $\times$ 2.54 = Milligrams of sodium chloride

To convert specific weight of sodium chloride to sodium:

Milligrams of sodium chloride $\times$ 0.393 = Milligrams of sodium

Sodium *Milligrams*	Sodium *Milliequivalents*	Sodium Chloride *Grams*
500	21.8	1.3
1,000	43.5	2.5
1,500	75.3	3.8
2,000	87.0	5.0

APPROXIMATE CONVERSIONS TO METRIC MEASURES*

When You Know	Multiply By	To Find
Length		
Inches	2.5	Centimeters
Feet	30	Centimeters
Yards	0.9	Meters
Miles	1.6	Kilometers
Area		
Square inches	6.5	Square centimeters
Square feet	9.09	Square meters
Square yards	0.8	Square meters
Square miles	2.6	Square kilometers
Acres	0.4	Hectares
Mass (weight)		
Ounces	28	Grams
Pounds	0.45	Kilograms
Short tons (2,000 lb)	0.9	Tonnes
Volume		
Teaspoons	5	Milliliters
Tablespoons	15	Milliliters
Fluid ounces	30	Milliliters
Cups	0.24	Liters
Pints	0.47	Liters
Quarts	0.95	Liters
Gallons	3.8	Liters
Cubic feet	0.03	Cubic meters
Cubic yards	0.76	Cubic meters
Temperature (exact)		
Fahrenheit temperature	5/9 (after subtracting 32)	Celsius temperature

*From United States Department of Commerce, National Bureau of Standards: Metric Conversion Card (NBS Special Publication 365). Washington, D. C., Government Printing Office, 1972.

APPROXIMATE CONVERSIONS FROM METRIC MEASURES*

When You Know	Multiply By	To Find
Length		
Millimeters	0.04	Inches
Centimeters	0.4	Inches
Meters	3.3	Feet
Meters	1.1	Yards
Kilometers	0.6	Miles
Area		
Square centimeters	0.16	Square inches
Square meters	1.2	Square yards
Square kilometers	0.4	Square miles
Hectares (10,000 m^2)	2.5	Acres
Mass (weight)		
Grams	0.035	Ounces
Kilograms	2.2	Pounds
Tonnes (1,000 kg)	1.1	Short tons
Volume		
Milliliters	0.03	Fluid ounces
Liters	2.1	Pints
Liters	1.06	Quarts
Liters	0.26	Gallons
Cubic meters	35	Cubic feet
Cubic meters	1.3	Cubic yards
Temperature (exact)		
Celsius temperature	9/5 (then add 32)	Fahrenheit temperature

*From United States Department of Commerce, National Bureau of Standards: Metric Conversion Card (NBS Special Publication 365). Washington, D. C., Government Printing Office, 1972.

COMMON MEDICAL ABBREVIATIONS

AAA	abdominal aortic aneurysm
ABG	arterial blood gases
ADL	activities of daily living
ALL	acute lymphoblastic leukemia
AML	acute myelocytic leukemia
AODM	adult-onset diabetes mellitus
AP	angina pectoris
ARF	acute renal failure
ASA	aspirin (acetylsalicylic acid)
ASHD	arteriosclerotic heart disease
ASO	arteriosclerosis obliterans
AVM	arteriovenous malformation
BMR	basal metabolic rate
BPH	benign prostatic hypertrophy
Bx	biopsy
Ca	cancer
CAD	coronary artery disease
CAH	chronic active hepatitis
CALD	chronic active liver disease
CBC	complete blood count
CBD	common bile duct
CC	chief complaint
CCK	cholecystokinin
CCU	coronary care unit
CDE	common duct exploration
CHD	coronary heart disease
CHF	congestive heart failure
CNS	central nervous system
C/O	complains of
COPD	chronic obstructive pulmonary disease
CRF	chronic renal failure
CSF	cerebrospinal fluid
CT	collagenous or connective tissue (disease)
	computed tomography
CVA	cerebrovascular accident
CVP	central venous pressure
D & C	dilation and curettage
D/C	discontinue
DIC	disseminated intravascular coagulation
DIP	distal interphalangeal (joint)

COMMON MEDICAL ABBREVIATIONS *(Continued)*

DJD	degenerative joint disease
DKA	diabetic ketoacidosis
DM	diabetes mellitus
DOA	dead on arrival
DOE	dyspnea on exertion
DU	duodenal ulcer
Dx	diagnosis
ECG or EKG	electrocardiogram
ECT	electric convulsive therapy
EEG	electroencephalogram
EENT	eye, ear, nose, and throat
ESR	erythrocyte sedimentation rate
FBS	fasting blood sugar
FFA	free fatty acids
FTT	failure to thrive
FUO	fever of unknown origin
Fx	fracture
GB	gallbladder
GE	gastroenteritis
	gastroenterology
GI	gastrointestinal
GTT	glucose tolerance test
GU	genitourinary
GYN	gynecology
HA	headache
Hb or Hgb	hemoglobin
HBP	high blood pressure
HPI	history of present illness
HPT	hyperparathyroidism
HTN	hypertension
Hx	history
ICU	intensive care unit
IDA	iron deficiency anemia
IHD	ischemic heart disease
IHSS	idiopathic hypertrophic subaortic stenosis
IM	intramuscular
IMP	impression
IPJ	interphalangeal joint
IPPB	intermittent positive pressure breathing
IV	intravenous

COMMON MEDICAL ABBREVIATIONS *(Continued)*

IVC	inferior vena cava
J	joule
KUB	kidney, ureter, and bladder
LBP	low back pain
LFT	liver function tests
LLQ	left lower quadrant
LMD	local medical doctor
LUQ	left upper quadrant
MCT	medium-chain triglycerides
MI	mitral insufficiency
	myocardial infarction
MOM	milk of magnesia
MS	mitral stenosis
	multiple sclerosis
NAD	no apparent distress
N & V	nausea and vomiting
NG	nasogastric
NPN	nonprotein nitrogen
NPO	nothing by mouth (non per os)
NTS	nontropical sprue
OBS	organic brain syndrome
OHD	organic heart disease
OR	operating room
OT	occupational therapy
PA	pernicious anemia
	pulmonary atresia
PAME	preanesthesia medical examination
PAN	periarteritis nodosa
PAT	paroxysmal atrial tachycardia
PBI	protein-bound iodine
PCM	protein-calorie malnutrition
PND	paroxysmal nocturnal dyspnea
PPT	partial prothrombin time
PS	pulmonary stenosis
Pt	patient
PT	physical therapy
	prothrombin time
PTA	prior to admission
PU	peptic ulcer
PVC	premature ventricular contraction

COMMON MEDICAL ABBREVIATIONS *(Continued)*

PVD	peripheral vascular disease
RES	reticuloendothelial system
RHD	rheumatic heart disease
RLQ	right lower quadrant
R/O	rule out
RöRx	radiation therapy
ROS	review of systems
RUQ	right upper quadrant
SAH	subarachnoid hemorrhage
SBE	subacute bacterial endocarditis
SBO	small bowel obstruction
SLE	systemic lupus erythematosus
SOB	shortness of breath
S/P	status postop
STSG	split-thickness skin graft
SVCO	superior vena cava obstruction
Sx	symptoms
T & A	tonsillectomy and adenoidectomy
TCE	transitional cell epithelioma
TEF	tracheoesophageal fistula
TG	triglycerides
THA	total hip arthroplasty
THC	transhepatic cholangiogram
TI	tricuspid insufficiency
TIA	transient ischemic attacks
TKA	total knee arthroplasty
TLA	translumbar aortogram
TPN	total parenteral nutrition
TUR	transurethral resection
U/A	urine analysis
UGI	upper gastrointestinal
URI	upper respiratory infection
UTI	urinary tract infection
V & P	vagotomy and pyloroplasty
VH	vaginal hysterectomy
VS	vital signs
WDHA	watery diarrhea, hypokalemia, achlorhydria (pancreatic cholera)
WNL	within normal limits
ZE	Zollinger-Ellison (syndrome)

MEDICAL TERMINOLOGY: ABBREVIATIONS, PREFIXES, SUFFIXES

COMMON ABBREVIATIONS

Abbreviation	Derivation	Meaning
$\overline{aa}$	ana	of each
ac	ante cibum	before meals
ad lib	ad libitum	as needed or desired
alt dieb	alternis diebus	every other day
alt hor	alternis horis	every other hour
alt noc	alternis noctibus	every other night
bid	bis in die	twice a day
c	cum	with
contin	continuetur	let it be continued
dil	dilutus	dilute
div	divide	divide
fl	fluidus	fluid
h	hora	hour
hd	hora decubitus	at bedtime
hs	hora somni	at sleeping time
m et n	mane et nocte	morning and night
nb	nota bene	note well
od	omni die	daily
om	omni mane	every morning
on	omni nocte	every night
part vic	partibus vicibus	in divided doses
pc	post cibum	after food
prn	pro re nata	as required
pulv	pulvis	powder
qd	quaque die	every day
qh	quaque hora	every hour
q2h	quaque secunda hora	every 2 hours
q3h	quaque tertia hora	every 3 hours
qid	quater in die	four times a day
qs	quantum sufficit	as much as is sufficient
R_X	recipe	take
S or sig	signa	give the following directions
s	sine	without
sos	si opus sit	if necessary
ss	semis	one half
stat	statim	at once
tid	ter in die	three times a day

MEDICAL TERMINOLOGY: ABBREVIATIONS, PREFIXES, SUFFIXES *(Continued)*

COMMON PREFIXES

Prefix	Meaning
a- or an-	without
cardi-	heart
chol-	bile
col-	colon
cyst-	bladder
enter-	intestine
gastr-	stomach
hepat-	liver
hydr-	water
hyper-	too much
hypo-	too little
myel-	marrow
nephr-	kidney
neur-	nerve
oste-	bone
poly-	many
proct-	anus, rectum
pseud-	false
pulm-	lung
pyel-	pelvis

MEDICAL TERMINOLOGY: ABBREVIATIONS, PREFIXES, SUFFIXES *(Continued)*

COMMON SUFFIXES

Suffix	Meaning
-algia	pain
-clysis	drenching
-cyte	cell
-ectomy	excision
-emia	presence in blood (usually implies excess)
-genic or -genesis	formation
-gnosis	knowledge
-itis	inflammation
-lytic or -lysis	destruction
-malacia	softening
-opia	vision
-pathy	disease of
-phagia	eating
-phobia	fear of
-pnea	breath
-privia or -penia	poverty of: without
-ptosis	fallen
-sclerosis	hardening
-scopy	inspection
-stenosis	narrowing
-stomy	mouth (new opening)
-tomy	cutting operation
-trophy	nutrition or growth
-uria	urine

INDEX

315

Drug-nutrient interactions, 298
Dumping syndrome, postgastrectomy,
    dietary management of, 157–158
Dysbetalipoproteinemia, 53, 55, 57

Electrolytes, recommended daily dietary
    allowances, 271
Energy intake, recommended, mean
    heights and weights and, 270
Enfamil, 228
Enfamil Premature Formula, 228
Enfamil with Iron, 228
Ensure, composition of, 242
Ensure Osmolite, composition of, 242
Ensure Plus, composition of, 242
Epilepsy, in children, ketogenic diet for,
    196–209
Esophageal reflux, dietary management
    of, 155–156
Evaporated milk, 228
Exercise, adjustment of diabetic diet for,
    29, 195

Fast foods, nutritional and exchange
    values for, 191–194
Fat, body, and skinfolds, 279
    calories from, in diabetic diet, 28
    defects in lymphatic transport of, fat
        control for, 146
Fat control, 145–150
    food exchanges in, 148
    in cardiac medical patient, 253, 254
    in cystic fibrosis, 209
Fat exchanges, for protein control, 96
    in diabetic diet, 38, 45
    in ketogenic diet, 206
    in sodium control, 69
Fatty acid content of foods, 284–289
Feeding, oral, formulas for, 237–245
    tube, formulas for, 237–245
Fetal alcohol syndrome, 176
Fiber, in diabetic diet, 29
Fiber content of foods, 140–141
Flexical, composition of, 242
Flour, crude fiber content of, 141
Fluid, in urolithiasis, 118
Fluid control, in hemodialysis, 84
    in hepatic coma, 87
Folic acid, in pregnancy, 173, 174
Foods, related, 211–212
Food allergies, 211–212
Food exchanges, in diabetic diet, 33,
    36–45
    in ketogenic diet, 204–208
    in potassium control, 90–93
    in protein control, 90–107
    in sodium control, 65, 67–79, 90–93
    in weight reduction diet, 51
Food nomogram, 282
Food sensitivity elimination diet,
    159–160
Formulas, for tube feeding and oral
        feeding, 237–245
    composition of, 242–245
    infant, 181, 228–233
        caloric distribution of, 182

Fructose, in diabetic diet, 46
Fruit, crude fiber content of, 140
Fruit exchanges, in diabetic diet, 44, 45
    in ketogenic diet, 207–208
    in protein control, 103–104
    in sodium control, 75
Full liquid diet, 10–11
    with frequent feedings, 158

Galactose control, 132–134
Galactosemia, diet for, 132–134
Gastric retention, dietary management
    of, 158
Geriatric nutrition, 20
Glucose tolerance test, diet in preparation
    for, 263
Gluten control, 151–154, 303
Gluten-sensitive enteropathy, gluten
    control for, 151–154
Goat's milk, 230
"Growth-onset" diabetes, 27
Growth percentiles, from birth to 18
    years, 214–221

Heart failure, congestive, sodium control
    in, 62–63
Height, average weight in relation to, 278
Hemodialysis, dietary management in,
    83–84
Hepatic coma, dietary management of,
    86–87
Hepatitis, cholangiolitic, copper control
    in, 126–129
Hepatolenticular degeneration, copper
    control in, 126–129
Hexavitamin, 272
5-HIAA testing, diet in preparation for,
    264
High-fiber diet, 138–142
Hospital diet, general, 7
    with consistency modifications, 8–15
Human milk, 181, 228
    caloric distribution of, 182
Hycal, composition of, 247
Hypercholesterolemia, 53, 54, 57
    with endogenous hypertriglyceridemia,
        53, 55, 57
Hyperchylomicronemia, 53, 54, 57
    fat control for, 146
Hyperlipidemia, diabetic diet in, 31
    mixed, 53, 56, 57
    types I-V, dietary management of,
        52–61
        alcohol in, 61
        foods to allow and foods to avoid,
            58–60
        simple carbohydrates in, 61
Hyperlipoproteinemia(s), 52, 53
    type I, fat control for, 146
    types of, 53–56
Hypertension, sodium control in, 62, 63
Hypertriglyceridemia, 53, 56–57
Hypoglycemia, dietary management of,
    169–170
Hypokalemia, dietary management of,
    108–111